FREE Study Skills Videos/DVD Offer

Dear Customer,

Thank you for your purchase from Mometrix! We consider it an honor and a privilege that you have purchased our product and we want to ensure your satisfaction.

As part of our ongoing effort to meet the needs of test takers, we have developed a set of Study Skills Videos that we would like to give you for <u>FREE</u>. These videos cover our *best practices* for getting ready for your exam, from how to use our study materials to how to best prepare for the day of the test.

All that we ask is that you email us with feedback that would describe your experience so far with our product. Good, bad, or indifferent, we want to know what you think!

To get your FREE Study Skills Videos, you can use the **QR code** below, or send us an **email** at studyvideos@mometrix.com with *FREE VIDEOS* in the subject line and the following information in the body of the email:

- The name of the product you purchased.
- Your product rating on a scale of 1-5, with 5 being the highest rating.
- Your feedback. It can be long, short, or anything in between. We just want to know your impressions and experience so far with our product. (Good feedback might include how our study material met your needs and ways we might be able to make it even better. You could highlight features that you found helpful or features that you think we should add.)

If you have any questions or concerns, please don't hesitate to contact me directly.

Thanks again!

Sincerely,

Jay Willis
Vice President
jay.willis@mometrix.com
1-800-673-8175

SCAN HERE

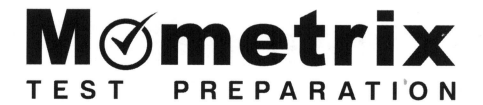

Pediatric Nurse Exam

SECRETS

Study Guide
Your Key to Exam Success

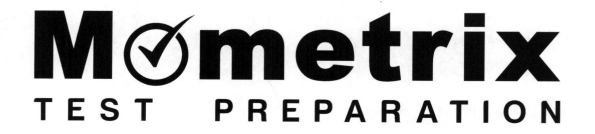

Written and edited by the Mometrix Nursing Certification Test Team

Printed in the United States of America

This paper meets the requirements of ANSI/NISO Z39.48-1992 (Permanence of Paper).

Mometrix offers volume discount pricing to institutions. For more information or a price quote, please contact our sales department at sales@mometrix.com or 888-248-1219.

Mometrix Media LLC is not affiliated with or endorsed by any official testing organization. All organizational and test names are trademarks of their respective owners.

Paperback
ISBN 13: 978-1-61072-498-2
ISBN 10: 1-61072-498-4

Ebook
ISBN 13: 978-1-62120-636-1
ISBN 10: 1-62120-636-X

DEAR FUTURE EXAM SUCCESS STORY

First of all, **THANK YOU** for purchasing Mometrix study materials!

Second, congratulations! You are one of the few determined test-takers who are committed to doing whatever it takes to excel on your exam. **You have come to the right place.** We developed these study materials with one goal in mind: to deliver you the information you need in a format that's concise and easy to use.

In addition to optimizing your guide for the content of the test, we've outlined our recommended steps for breaking down the preparation process into small, attainable goals so you can make sure you stay on track.

We've also analyzed the entire test-taking process, identifying the most common pitfalls and showing how you can overcome them and be ready for any curveball the test throws you.

Standardized testing is one of the biggest obstacles on your road to success, which only increases the importance of doing well in the high-pressure, high-stakes environment of test day. Your results on this test could have a significant impact on your future, and this guide provides the information and practical advice to help you achieve your full potential on test day.

Your success is our success

We would love to hear from you! If you would like to share the story of your exam success or if you have any questions or comments in regard to our products, please contact us at **800-673-8175** or **support@mometrix.com**.

Thanks again for your business and we wish you continued success!

Sincerely,
The Mometrix Test Preparation Team

Need more help? Check out our flashcards at:
http://mometrixflashcards.com/PediatricNurse

TABLE OF CONTENTS

Introduction

Thank you for purchasing this resource! You have made the choice to prepare yourself for a test that could have a huge impact on your future, and this guide is designed to help you be fully ready for test day. Obviously, it's important to have a solid understanding of the test material, but you also need to be prepared for the unique environment and stressors of the test, so that you can perform to the best of your abilities.

For this purpose, the first section that appears in this guide is the **Secret Keys**. We've devoted countless hours to meticulously researching what works and what doesn't, and we've boiled down our findings to the five most impactful steps you can take to improve your performance on the test. We start at the beginning with study planning and move through the preparation process, all the way to the testing strategies that will help you get the most out of what you know when you're finally sitting in front of the test.

We recommend that you start preparing for your test as far in advance as possible. However, if you've bought this guide as a last-minute study resource and only have a few days before your test, we recommend that you skip over the first two Secret Keys since they address a long-term study plan.

If you struggle with **test anxiety**, we strongly encourage you to check out our recommendations for how you can overcome it. Test anxiety is a formidable foe, but it can be beaten, and we want to make sure you have the tools you need to defeat it.

1

Secret Key #1 – Plan Big, Study Small

There's a lot riding on your performance. If you want to ace this test, you're going to need to keep your skills sharp and the material fresh in your mind. You need a plan that lets you review everything you need to know while still fitting in your schedule. We'll break this strategy down into three categories.

Information Organization

Start with the information you already have: the official test outline. From this, you can make a complete list of all the concepts you need to cover before the test. Organize these concepts into groups that can be studied together, and create a list of any related vocabulary you need to learn so you can brush up on any difficult terms. You'll want to keep this vocabulary list handy once you actually start studying since you may need to add to it along the way.

Time Management

Once you have your set of study concepts, decide how to spread them out over the time you have left before the test. Break your study plan into small, clear goals so you have a manageable task for each day and know exactly what you're doing. Then just focus on one small step at a time. When you manage your time this way, you don't need to spend hours at a time studying. Studying a small block of content for a short period each day helps you retain information better and avoid stressing over how much you have left to do. You can relax knowing that you have a plan to cover everything in time. In order for this strategy to be effective though, you have to start studying early and stick to your schedule. Avoid the exhaustion and futility that comes from last-minute cramming!

Study Environment

The environment you study in has a big impact on your learning. Studying in a coffee shop, while probably more enjoyable, is not likely to be as fruitful as studying in a quiet room. It's important to keep distractions to a minimum. You're only planning to study for a short block of time, so make the most of it. Don't pause to check your phone or get up to find a snack. It's also important to **avoid multitasking**. Research has consistently shown that multitasking will make your studying dramatically less effective. Your study area should also be comfortable and well-lit so you don't have the distraction of straining your eyes or sitting on an uncomfortable chair.

 The time of day you study is also important. You want to be rested and alert. Don't wait until just before bedtime. Study when you'll be most likely to comprehend and remember. Even better, if you know what time of day your test will be, set that time aside for study. That way your brain will be used to working on that subject at that specific time and you'll have a better chance of recalling information.

Finally, it can be helpful to team up with others who are studying for the same test. Your actual studying should be done in as isolated an environment as possible, but the work of organizing the information and setting up the study plan can be divided up. In between study sessions, you can discuss with your teammates the concepts that you're all studying and quiz each other on the details. Just be sure that your teammates are as serious about the test as you are. If you find that your study time is being replaced with social time, you might need to find a new team.

Secret Key #2 – Make Your Studying Count

You're devoting a lot of time and effort to preparing for this test, so you want to be absolutely certain it will pay off. This means doing more than just reading the content and hoping you can remember it on test day. It's important to make every minute of study count. There are two main areas you can focus on to make your studying count.

Retention

It doesn't matter how much time you study if you can't remember the material. You need to make sure you are retaining the concepts. To check your retention of the information you're learning, try recalling it at later times with minimal prompting. Try carrying around flashcards and glance at one or two from time to time or ask a friend who's also studying for the test to quiz you.

To enhance your retention, look for ways to put the information into practice so that you can apply it rather than simply recalling it. If you're using the information in practical ways, it will be much easier to remember. Similarly, it helps to solidify a concept in your mind if you're not only reading it to yourself but also explaining it to someone else. Ask a friend to let you teach them about a concept you're a little shaky on (or speak aloud to an imaginary audience if necessary). As you try to summarize, define, give examples, and answer your friend's questions, you'll understand the concepts better and they will stay with you longer. Finally, step back for a big picture view and ask yourself how each piece of information fits with the whole subject. When you link the different concepts together and see them working together as a whole, it's easier to remember the individual components.

Finally, practice showing your work on any multi-step problems, even if you're just studying. Writing out each step you take to solve a problem will help solidify the process in your mind, and you'll be more likely to remember it during the test.

Modality

Modality simply refers to the means or method by which you study. Choosing a study modality that fits your own individual learning style is crucial. No two people learn best in exactly the same way, so it's important to know your strengths and use them to your advantage.

For example, if you learn best by visualization, focus on visualizing a concept in your mind and draw an image or a diagram. Try color-coding your notes, illustrating them, or creating symbols that will trigger your mind to recall a learned concept. If you learn best by hearing or discussing information, find a study partner who learns the same way or read aloud to yourself. Think about how to put the information in your own words. Imagine that you are giving a lecture on the topic and record yourself so you can listen to it later.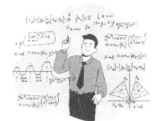

For any learning style, flashcards can be helpful. Organize the information so you can take advantage of spare moments to review. Underline key words or phrases. Use different colors for different categories. Mnemonic devices (such as creating a short list in which every item starts with the same letter) can also help with retention. Find what works best for you and use it to store the information in your mind most effectively and easily.

Secret Key #3 – Practice the Right Way

Your success on test day depends not only on how many hours you put into preparing, but also on whether you prepared the right way. It's good to check along the way to see if your studying is paying off. One of the most effective ways to do this is by taking practice tests to evaluate your progress. Practice tests are useful because they show exactly where you need to improve. Every time you take a practice test, pay special attention to these three groups of questions:

- The questions you got wrong
- The questions you had to guess on, even if you guessed right
- The questions you found difficult or slow to work through

This will show you exactly what your weak areas are, and where you need to devote more study time. Ask yourself why each of these questions gave you trouble. Was it because you didn't understand the material? Was it because you didn't remember the vocabulary? Do you need more repetitions on this type of question to build speed and confidence? Dig into those questions and figure out how you can strengthen your weak areas as you go back to review the material.

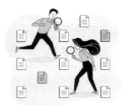 Additionally, many practice tests have a section explaining the answer choices. It can be tempting to read the explanation and think that you now have a good understanding of the concept. However, an explanation likely only covers part of the question's broader context. Even if the explanation makes perfect sense, **go back and investigate** every concept related to the question until you're positive you have a thorough understanding.

As you go along, keep in mind that the practice test is just that: practice. Memorizing these questions and answers will not be very helpful on the actual test because it is unlikely to have any of the same exact questions. If you only know the right answers to the sample questions, you won't be prepared for the real thing. **Study the concepts** until you understand them fully, and then you'll be able to answer any question that shows up on the test.

It's important to wait on the practice tests until you're ready. If you take a test on your first day of study, you may be overwhelmed by the amount of material covered and how much you need to learn. Work up to it gradually.

On test day, you'll need to be prepared for answering questions, managing your time, and using the test-taking strategies you've learned. It's a lot to balance, like a mental marathon that will have a big impact on your future. Like training for a marathon, you'll need to start slowly and work your way up. When test day arrives, you'll be ready.

Start with the strategies you've read in the first two Secret Keys—plan your course and study in the way that works best for you. If you have time, consider using multiple study resources to get different approaches to the same concepts. It can be helpful to see difficult concepts from more than one angle. Then find a good source for practice tests. Many times, the test website will suggest potential study resources or provide sample tests.

Practice Test Strategy

If you're able to find at least three practice tests, we recommend this strategy:

UNTIMED AND OPEN-BOOK PRACTICE

Take the first test with no time constraints and with your notes and study guide handy. Take your time and focus on applying the strategies you've learned.

TIMED AND OPEN-BOOK PRACTICE

Take the second practice test open-book as well, but set a timer and practice pacing yourself to finish in time.

TIMED AND CLOSED-BOOK PRACTICE

Take any other practice tests as if it were test day. Set a timer and put away your study materials. Sit at a table or desk in a quiet room, imagine yourself at the testing center, and answer questions as quickly and accurately as possible.

Keep repeating timed and closed-book tests on a regular basis until you run out of practice tests or it's time for the actual test. Your mind will be ready for the schedule and stress of test day, and you'll be able to focus on recalling the material you've learned.

Secret Key #4 – Pace Yourself

Once you're fully prepared for the material on the test, your biggest challenge on test day will be managing your time. Just knowing that the clock is ticking can make you panic even if you have plenty of time left. Work on pacing yourself so you can build confidence against the time constraints of the exam. Pacing is a difficult skill to master, especially in a high-pressure environment, so **practice is vital**.

Set time expectations for your pace based on how much time is available. For example, if a section has 60 questions and the time limit is 30 minutes, you know you have to average 30 seconds or less per question in order to answer them all. Although 30 seconds is the hard limit, set 25 seconds per question as your goal, so you reserve extra time to spend on harder questions. When you budget extra time for the harder questions, you no longer have any reason to stress when those questions take longer to answer.

Don't let this time expectation distract you from working through the test at a calm, steady pace, but keep it in mind so you don't spend too much time on any one question. Recognize that taking extra time on one question you don't understand may keep you from answering two that you do understand later in the test. If your time limit for a question is up and you're still not sure of the answer, mark it and move on, and come back to it later if the time and the test format allow. If the testing format doesn't allow you to return to earlier questions, just make an educated guess; then put it out of your mind and move on.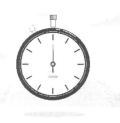

On the easier questions, be careful not to rush. It may seem wise to hurry through them so you have more time for the challenging ones, but it's not worth missing one if you know the concept and just didn't take the time to read the question fully. Work efficiently but make sure you understand the question and have looked at all of the answer choices, since more than one may seem right at first.

Even if you're paying attention to the time, you may find yourself a little behind at some point. You should speed up to get back on track, but do so wisely. Don't panic; just take a few seconds less on each question until you're caught up. Don't guess without thinking, but do look through the answer choices and eliminate any you know are wrong. If you can get down to two choices, it is often worthwhile to guess from those. Once you've chosen an answer, move on and don't dwell on any that you skipped or had to hurry through. If a question was taking too long, chances are it was one of the harder ones, so you weren't as likely to get it right anyway.

On the other hand, if you find yourself getting ahead of schedule, it may be beneficial to slow down a little. The more quickly you work, the more likely you are to make a careless mistake that will affect your score. You've budgeted time for each question, so don't be afraid to spend that time. Practice an efficient but careful pace to get the most out of the time you have.

Secret Key #5 – Have a Plan for Guessing

When you're taking the test, you may find yourself stuck on a question. Some of the answer choices seem better than others, but you don't see the one answer choice that is obviously correct. What do you do?

The scenario described above is very common, yet most test takers have not effectively prepared for it. Developing and practicing a plan for guessing may be one of the single most effective uses of your time as you get ready for the exam.

In developing your plan for guessing, there are three questions to address:

- When should you start the guessing process?
- How should you narrow down the choices?
- Which answer should you choose?

When to Start the Guessing Process

Unless your plan for guessing is to select C every time (which, despite its merits, is not what we recommend), you need to leave yourself enough time to apply your answer elimination strategies. Since you have a limited amount of time for each question, that means that if you're going to give yourself the best shot at guessing correctly, you have to decide quickly whether or not you will guess.

Of course, the best-case scenario is that you don't have to guess at all, so first, see if you can answer the question based on your knowledge of the subject and basic reasoning skills. Focus on the key words in the question and try to jog your memory of related topics. Give yourself a chance to bring the knowledge to mind, but once you realize that you don't have (or you can't access) the knowledge you need to answer the question, it's time to start the guessing process.

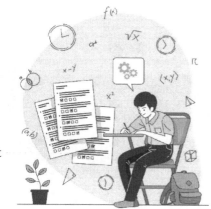

It's almost always better to start the guessing process too early than too late. It only takes a few seconds to remember something and answer the question from knowledge. Carefully eliminating wrong answer choices takes longer. Plus, going through the process of eliminating answer choices can actually help jog your memory.

Summary: Start the guessing process as soon as you decide that you can't answer the question based on your knowledge.

How to Narrow Down the Choices

The next chapter in this book (**Test-Taking Strategies**) includes a wide range of strategies for how to approach questions and how to look for answer choices to eliminate. You will definitely want to read those carefully, practice them, and figure out which ones work best for you. Here though, we're going to address a mindset rather than a particular strategy.

Your odds of guessing an answer correctly depend on how many options you are choosing from.

Number of options left	5	4	3	2	1
Odds of guessing correctly	20%	25%	33%	50%	100%

You can see from this chart just how valuable it is to be able to eliminate incorrect answers and make an educated guess, but there are two things that many test takers do that cause them to miss out on the benefits of guessing:

- Accidentally eliminating the correct answer
- Selecting an answer based on an impression

We'll look at the first one here, and the second one in the next section.

To avoid accidentally eliminating the correct answer, we recommend a thought exercise called **the $5 challenge**. In this challenge, you only eliminate an answer choice from contention if you are willing to bet $5 on it being wrong. Why $5? Five dollars is a small but not insignificant amount of money. It's an amount you could afford to lose but wouldn't want to throw away. And while losing $5 once might not hurt too much, doing it twenty times will set you back $100. In the same way, each small decision you make—eliminating a choice here, guessing on a question there—won't by itself impact your score very much, but when you put them all together, they can make a big difference. By holding each answer choice elimination decision to a higher standard, you can reduce the risk of accidentally eliminating the correct answer.

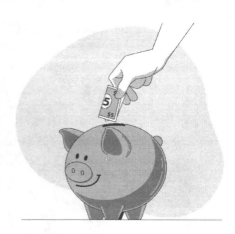

The $5 challenge can also be applied in a positive sense: If you are willing to bet $5 that an answer choice *is* correct, go ahead and mark it as correct.

Summary: Only eliminate an answer choice if you are willing to bet $5 that it is wrong.

8

Which Answer to Choose

You're taking the test. You've run into a hard question and decided you'll have to guess. You've eliminated all the answer choices you're willing to bet $5 on. Now you have to pick an answer. Why do we even need to talk about this? Why can't you just pick whichever one you feel like when the time comes?

The answer to these questions is that if you don't come into the test with a plan, you'll rely on your impression to select an answer choice, and if you do that, you risk falling into a trap. The test writers know that everyone who takes their test will be guessing on some of the questions, so they intentionally write wrong answer choices to seem plausible. You still have to pick an answer though, and if the wrong answer choices are designed to look right, how can you ever be sure that you're not falling for their trap? The best solution we've found to this dilemma is to take the decision out of your hands entirely. Here is the process we recommend:

Once you've eliminated any choices that you are confident (willing to bet $5) are wrong, select the first remaining choice as your answer.

Whether you choose to select the first remaining choice, the second, or the last, the important thing is that you use some preselected standard. Using this approach guarantees that you will not be enticed into selecting an answer choice that looks right, because you are not basing your decision on how the answer choices look.

A. This is wrong.
B. Also wrong.
C. Maybe?
D. Maybe?

This is not meant to make you question your knowledge. Instead, it is to help you recognize the difference between your knowledge and your impressions. There's a huge difference between thinking an answer is right because of what you know, and thinking an answer is right because it looks or sounds like it should be right.

Summary: To ensure that your selection is appropriately random, make a predetermined selection from among all answer choices you have not eliminated.

9

Test-Taking Strategies

This section contains a list of test-taking strategies that you may find helpful as you work through the test. By taking what you know and applying logical thought, you can maximize your chances of answering any question correctly!

It is very important to realize that every question is different and every person is different: no single strategy will work on every question, and no single strategy will work for every person. That's why we've included all of them here, so you can try them out and determine which ones work best for different types of questions and which ones work best for you.

Question Strategies

☑ READ CAREFULLY

Read the question and the answer choices carefully. Don't miss the question because you misread the terms. You have plenty of time to read each question thoroughly and make sure you understand what is being asked. Yet a happy medium must be attained, so don't waste too much time. You must read carefully and efficiently.

☑ CONTEXTUAL CLUES

Look for contextual clues. If the question includes a word you are not familiar with, look at the immediate context for some indication of what the word might mean. Contextual clues can often give you all the information you need to decipher the meaning of an unfamiliar word. Even if you can't determine the meaning, you may be able to narrow down the possibilities enough to make a solid guess at the answer to the question.

☑ PREFIXES

If you're having trouble with a word in the question or answer choices, try dissecting it. Take advantage of every clue that the word might include. Prefixes can be a huge help. Usually, they allow you to determine a basic meaning. *Pre-* means before, *post-* means after, *pro-* is positive, *de-* is negative. From prefixes, you can get an idea of the general meaning of the word and try to put it into context.

☑ HEDGE WORDS

Watch out for critical hedge words, such as *likely, may, can, sometimes, often, almost, mostly, usually, generally, rarely,* and *sometimes*. Question writers insert these hedge phrases to cover every possibility. Often an answer choice will be wrong simply because it leaves no room for exception. Be on guard for answer choices that have definitive words such as *exactly* and *always*.

☑ SWITCHBACK WORDS

Stay alert for *switchbacks*. These are the words and phrases frequently used to alert you to shifts in thought. The most common switchback words are *but, although,* and *however*. Others include *nevertheless, on the other hand, even though, while, in spite of, despite,* and *regardless of*. Switchback words are important to catch because they can change the direction of the question or an answer choice.

☑ FACE VALUE

When in doubt, use common sense. Accept the situation in the problem at face value. Don't read too much into it. These problems will not require you to make wild assumptions. If you have to go beyond creativity and warp time or space in order to have an answer choice fit the question, then you should move on and consider the other answer choices. These are normal problems rooted in reality. The applicable relationship or explanation may not be readily apparent, but it is there for you to figure out. Use your common sense to interpret anything that isn't clear.

Answer Choice Strategies

⊘ Answer Selection

The most thorough way to pick an answer choice is to identify and eliminate wrong answers until only one is left, then confirm it is the correct answer. Sometimes an answer choice may immediately seem right, but be careful. The test writers will usually put more than one reasonable answer choice on each question, so take a second to read all of them and make sure that the other choices are not equally obvious. As long as you have time left, it is better to read every answer choice than to pick the first one that looks right without checking the others.

⊘ Answer Choice Families

An answer choice family consists of two (in rare cases, three) answer choices that are very similar in construction and cannot all be true at the same time. If you see two answer choices that are direct opposites or parallels, one of them is usually the correct answer. For instance, if one answer choice says that quantity x increases and another either says that quantity x decreases (opposite) or says that quantity y increases (parallel), then those answer choices would fall into the same family. An answer choice that doesn't match the construction of the answer choice family is more likely to be incorrect. Most questions will not have answer choice families, but when they do appear, you should be prepared to recognize them.

⊘ Eliminate Answers

Eliminate answer choices as soon as you realize they are wrong, but make sure you consider all possibilities. If you are eliminating answer choices and realize that the last one you are left with is also wrong, don't panic. Start over and consider each choice again. There may be something you missed the first time that you will realize on the second pass.

⊘ Avoid Fact Traps

Don't be distracted by an answer choice that is factually true but doesn't answer the question. You are looking for the choice that answers the question. Stay focused on what the question is asking for so you don't accidentally pick an answer that is true but incorrect. Always go back to the question and make sure the answer choice you've selected actually answers the question and is not merely a true statement.

⊘ Extreme Statements

In general, you should avoid answers that put forth extreme actions as standard practice or proclaim controversial ideas as established fact. An answer choice that states the "process should be used in certain situations, if…" is much more likely to be correct than one that states the "process should be discontinued completely." The first is a calm rational statement and doesn't even make a definitive, uncompromising stance, using a hedge word *if* to provide wiggle room, whereas the second choice is far more extreme.

⊘ Benchmark

As you read through the answer choices and you come across one that seems to answer the question well, mentally select that answer choice. This is not your final answer, but it's the one that will help you evaluate the other answer choices. The one that you selected is your benchmark or standard for judging each of the other answer choices. Every other answer choice must be compared to your benchmark. That choice is correct until proven otherwise by another answer choice beating it. If you find a better answer, then that one becomes your new benchmark. Once you've decided that no other choice answers the question as well as your benchmark, you have your final answer.

⊘ Predict the Answer

Before you even start looking at the answer choices, it is often best to try to predict the answer. When you come up with the answer on your own, it is easier to avoid distractions and traps because you will know exactly what to look for. The right answer choice is unlikely to be word-for-word what you came up with, but it should be a close match. Even if you are confident that you have the right answer, you should still take the time to read each option before moving on.

General Strategies

⊘ Tough Questions

If you are stumped on a problem or it appears too hard or too difficult, don't waste time. Move on! Remember though, if you can quickly check for obviously incorrect answer choices, your chances of guessing correctly are greatly improved. Before you completely give up, at least try to knock out a couple of possible answers. Eliminate what you can and then guess at the remaining answer choices before moving on.

⊘ Check Your Work

Since you will probably not know every term listed and the answer to every question, it is important that you get credit for the ones that you do know. Don't miss any questions through careless mistakes. If at all possible, try to take a second to look back over your answer selection and make sure you've selected the correct answer choice and haven't made a costly careless mistake (such as marking an answer choice that you didn't mean to mark). This quick double check should more than pay for itself in caught mistakes for the time it costs.

⊘ Pace Yourself

It's easy to be overwhelmed when you're looking at a page full of questions; your mind is confused and full of random thoughts, and the clock is ticking down faster than you would like. Calm down and maintain the pace that you have set for yourself. Especially as you get down to the last few minutes of the test, don't let the small numbers on the clock make you panic. As long as you are on track by monitoring your pace, you are guaranteed to have time for each question.

⊘ Don't Rush

It is very easy to make errors when you are in a hurry. Maintaining a fast pace in answering questions is pointless if it makes you miss questions that you would have gotten right otherwise. Test writers like to include distracting information and wrong answers that seem right. Taking a little extra time to avoid careless mistakes can make all the difference in your test score. Find a pace that allows you to be confident in the answers that you select.

⊘ Keep Moving

Panicking will not help you pass the test, so do your best to stay calm and keep moving. Taking deep breaths and going through the answer elimination steps you practiced can help to break through a stress barrier and keep your pace.

Final Notes

The combination of a solid foundation of content knowledge and the confidence that comes from practicing your plan for applying that knowledge is the key to maximizing your performance on test day. As your foundation of content knowledge is built up and strengthened, you'll find that the strategies included in this chapter become more and more effective in helping you quickly sift through the distractions and traps of the test to isolate the correct answer.

Now that you're preparing to move forward into the test content chapters of this book, be sure to keep your goal in mind. As you read, think about how you will be able to apply this information on the test. If you've already seen sample questions for the test and you have an idea of the question format and style, try to come up with questions of your own that you can answer based on what you're reading. This will give you valuable practice applying your knowledge in the same ways you can expect to on test day.

Good luck and good studying!

14

Health Promotion

Health Promotion Activities

HEALTH PROMOTION

Nurses promote health when they assist individuals to change behavior in ways that help them to attain and maintain the highest level of wellbeing possible. Health promotion is a very popular way to control healthcare costs and reduce illness and early death. Health is increasingly the topic of newscasts and literature. The public is demanding more information pertinent to the maintenance of health and to the ways in which the average person can act independently to do so. Health promotion is centered on ideal personal habits, lifestyles, and environmental control that decrease the risk for disease. The US Public Health Service periodically identifies national health goals and most recently published a program called *Healthy People 2030*, with measurable goals to increase the general quality and years of life for all and to increase the health status of all groups to an equal level of wellness. Health promotion programs in the community are now offered by workplaces, clinics, schools, and churches, not just by hospitals as in the past.

HEALTHY PEOPLE 2030

The 5 **main goals** of *Healthy People 2030* are

- Attaining healthy, thriving lives free of preventable disease, disability, injury, and premature death
- Eliminating health disparities, achieving health equality, and increasing health literacy
- Creating environments conducive to health-promotion
- Improving health in all life stages
- Collaborating with leadership and key stakeholders in policy design that improves the health and well-being of all

Healthy People 2030 has 62 topic areas with 355 total objectives divided across five sections:

- Health Conditions
- Health Behaviors
- Populations
- Settings and Systems
- Social Determinants of Health

MAIN COMPONENTS OF HEALTH PROMOTION

Health promotion efforts are concentrated in four areas:

- Individuals must be educated to realize that their **lifestyle and choices** have a large impact on their health. They must then be motivated to choose to modify their personal risk factors and take the responsibility to do so.
- The emphasis on **good nutrition** as the biggest factor that impacts health and the length of life must be brought into general awareness. This is occurring via the media through numerous books and articles educating people about the essential nutrients needed to maintain health.
- **Stress** is a constant in a production-driven society. Individuals must learn ways to manage and decrease stress to achieve and maintain health and to decrease the effects of stress upon chronic illness, risk of infections, and trauma.
- **Physical fitness** helps cardiovascular status, relieves stress, controls weight, delays aging, promotes strength and endurance, and improves appearance and performance. Individuals must have programs that increase activity gradually to prevent injury and are designed to meet individual needs.

15

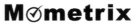

HEALTH SELF-MANAGEMENT

Health self-management includes health maintenance, disease prevention, and health promotion. Health maintenance is defined as strategies that help maintain and/or improve health over time. Health maintenance is dependent on three factors, which include health perception, motivation for behavioral change, and compliance to set goals. Disease prevention is an effort to limit the development or progression of lifestyle-related illness. **Disease prevention** can be categorized into primary, secondary, and tertiary prevention.

- **Primary prevention** measures are employed prior to disease onset and are used in health populations.
- **Secondary prevention** measures are used to screen, detect, and treat disease in earlier stages to prevent further progression or development of other complications.
- **Tertiary prevention** measures are used to prevent the onset of other complications or comorbid conditions.

Health promotion strategies include risk reduction strategies applied to the general population.

INFLUENCES ON DECISION TO MODIFY BEHAVIOR TO ACHIEVE AND MAINTAIN HEALTH

Many factors have an influence on people's efforts to change behavior in a way that improves and maintains their health status. These factors include age, ethnicity, gender, lifestyle, level of education, self-esteem, motivation, and self-image. The patient's support network and the availability of health promotion programs and healthcare systems also have an influence on healthcare behaviors. Some people may be prevented from accessing health promotion programs because of lack of medical insurance. Financial status and employment are important as well. The presence of addictions and diseases, the length of illness, and the severity of disabilities are all factors to be considered. The value placed on health, the threat of potential losses, and the perceived benefits of behavior modification are important motivating factors.

STRATEGIES TO ENCOURAGE SMOKING CESSATION

The **health impact associated with smoking** varies among smokers and can be affected by the number of cigarettes used daily, exposure to smoking-associated stimuli, and educational level. The presence of stress and depression, psychosocial problems, lack of coping mechanisms, low income, and long-term habitual behavior are problematic for the quitter. Nurses can promote smoking cessation by taking every opportunity to bring up the subject, educating about the dangers of smoking and benefits of quitting, and providing **resources** to help patients quit. Strategies include:

- Educating about the personal effects of smoking upon that individual
- Encouraging patients to set a quit date
- Referring to programs and smoking cessation information
- Educating about the use of nicotine replacements including nicotine gum, lozenges, inhalers, transdermal patches, and nasal sprays
- Educating about the use of medications such as Zyban, Catapres, and Chantix
- Providing support via phone calls or office visits
- Discovering the reason for relapses
- Praising and rewarding any success in the quitting process

HEALTHY NUTRITION PRINCIPLES

Healthy nutrition principles include the following:

- Eating a range of different kinds of foods, and eating increased amounts fruits, vegetables, whole grains, poultry, and fish.
- Diets should consist of 55-60% **carbohydrates**, less than 30% **fat**, and the rest should be **protein** (0.8-1.0 g/kg).
- Restrict **saturated fat** to <10%. Restrict **cholesterol** to 300 mg/day.

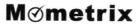

- Utilize moderate amounts of sugar, salt, and sodium.
- Take a **multivitamin** including folic acid if the patient is female and able to have children. Get 200-800 IU/day of vitamin D in order to absorb calcium.
- **Calcium** intake should be: 1,300 mg/day for women age 13-18 or those who are pregnant/nursing; 1,000 mg/day for women age 19-50 years; 1,500 mg/day for age 51 years and older.
- Patients who are pregnant or having chemotherapy should not try to lose weight.
- **Weight loss** may improve diabetes, joint pain, inflammation, cardiovascular disease, hypothyroidism, or renal disease.

WELLNESS EVALUATION

A wellness evaluation is a complete assessment and report of the general health profile of the child, compiling all available pertinent information. A **health profile** should include the following:

- Basic measurements, such as height, weight, and head circumference, and the percentile ranking for age.
- Vital signs, including pulse, respiration, and blood pressure. Body temperature should be included as well.
- Nutrition profile that outlines the child's normal diet and any dietary modifications or adverse reactions, such as allergies or intolerances.
- Mobility/activity level that explains the infant's mobility in accordance to expected development for age. For older children, the type of activities and physical exercise the child engages in and their frequency should be noted.
- Results of any screening tests and, if elective rather than standard, the reason for the test.
- Health promotion/disease prevention activities, including duration, results, and compliance with prescribed interventions.

INFANTS
WELL BABY CHECKUPS DURING THE FIRST YEAR OF LIFE

Most pediatricians will want to check the breastfed baby's weight at one week of age, and the bottle-fed baby's weight at 2 weeks. If the PKU, thyroid, hematocrit and hemoglobin tests were not done after birth, they should be completed at the first visit. Well baby checkups are usually scheduled at 2, 4, 6, 9, and 12 months. A home health assessment and physical exam will be done, along with weight, height, and head circumference. Development, expectations, and concerns are discussed and immunizations will be given according the latest recommendations. If lead testing is warranted, it will be done at 9 or 12 months.

DENTAL HEALTH OF INFANTS

As teeth erupt, the parents can clean them by gently rubbing with a clean wet cloth. Supplemental fluoride is prescribed beginning at 6 months if the parent's water does not contain fluoride or if the baby is breastfed only. Parents should be warned of the dental problems (bottle-mouth caries) that may occur when babies are given a bottle to sleep with or breast feedings are prolonged to pacify the baby. Discuss with parents the symptoms of teething (slight fever, fussiness, drooling) and ways to make the baby more comfortable and facilitate teething (allow baby to chew on a rubber teething ring, rub a clean finger on the baby's gums, and give acetaminophen). Dental visits, by recommendation of the American Academy of Pediatrics, should begin at 6 months.

VISION AND HEARING HEALTH OF INFANTS

Vision will be assessed by having the baby track an object or familiar face. Lack of the following would indicate visual problems: blink reflex, doll's eye reflex (the head is moved to one side and the eyes will not follow right away—disappears as infant grows), tracking by one month, following own hands and feet by 4 months, reaching for toys at 5 months, or good hand-eye coordination at 7 months. Lack of the following would indicate hearing problems: startle or blink reflex at loud noise, responding in some way to loud noises when asleep,

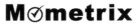

turning head toward sound at 6 months, making babbling sounds at 7 months, or general response to human voice or sound.

TODDLERS AND PRESCHOOLERS

WELL CHILD CHECK UP FOR TODDLERS

Well child visits are scheduled at 15, 18, 24, and 36 months, encompassing a physical exam, home health assessment and immunizations, as appropriate. DTP (DTaP), Hib, polio, and hepatitis B boosters are given by 18 months of age. Other vaccines are given if not begun earlier. The MMR and varicella vaccines are started. Blood pressure, height, weight, head circumference (until anterior fontanel closes), vision, and hearing are checked. Hemoglobin will be tested to detect iron-deficiency anemia and lead levels may be tested in those who live in a high-risk area or show signs of lead poisoning (poor growth or neurological irritability).

COMMON ISSUES FACED BY PARENTS OF TODDLERS AND DISCIPLINE TECHNIQUES TO USE

Toddlers have learned the word "no" and will use it often. Asking open-ended questions, giving choices and ignoring the behavior are ways to handle this frustrating negativism. Toddlers also enjoy rituals (same bedtime routine, same cup, spoon, or bowl) and this helps them to maintain some control over their environment. When routines are altered, the toddler may show signs of regression. Allowing for routines within reason and ignoring regression while giving praise for accomplishments will help the child get through this stage. Sibling rivalry can occur with the birth of a new baby. Setting limits, introducing the concept of a new baby gradually, spending time with both children together, and encouraging the toddler to help with small tasks (get a diaper for mommy) will help with the transition. Temper tantrums begin around 2 years of age and are best ignored, making sure the child does not harm himself. Time-outs can be used before behavior escalates; this may prevent the temper tantrum.

DENTAL HEALTH OF TODDLERS AND PRESCHOOLERS

Toddlers should have regular dental visits. The parents should be brushing their teeth with a small, soft toothbrush, using either water or a very small amount of toothpaste (fluoridated toothpaste, if swallowed, can be harmful). Flossing should be done by the parent to remove food below the gum line and to establish good dental hygiene habits early.

Preschoolers can begin to help with brushing and flossing, although the parents need to supervise and assist them to make sure that all teeth are clean. A pea-sized squeeze of toothpaste should be used to prevent harmful effects of swallowed fluoride. Dental visits every 6 months should be established. Cavities can be prevented with good brushing and flossing habits, limiting foods with lots of sugar, chewing sugar-free gum, and brushing after eating foods with lots of sugar. Teeth-grinding at night is fairly common during these years. If it seems to last longer than it takes the child to fall asleep, a dentist should be consulted. A mouthpiece worn during the night may be needed.

WELL CHILD VISIT AND ANTICIPATORY GUIDANCE FOR PRESCHOOLERS

Checkups are scheduled every year from **age 3 to 6** and include a physical exam, height, weight, vision, hearing, and blood pressure checks. If all immunizations are up-to-date, boosters for DTaP (diphtheria, tetanus, and pertussis), polio, and MMR (measles, mumps, rubella) vaccines will be given. Before entering school, a tuberculin test is required. Lead testing is indicated if the child is at risk (older homes may have lead paint or lead water pipes), as well as hyperlipidemia testing if indicated.

Toilet training is usually completed by age 5. Discipline can be achieved by time-outs, consistency, firm limits, and short explanations of why certain behaviors are wrong. Continue with consistent routines, allowing imaginative play, and limiting TV watching. Read to the child daily. Teach proper hand washing and allow children to do simple chores around the house. Talk to the parents about what to expect when the child begins school.

SCHOOL AGE CHILDREN

WELL CHILD VISITS AND ANTICIPATORY GUIDANCE FOR SCHOOL AGE CHILDREN

Checkups should be scheduled at least every 2 years starting at **age 6 until age 10** and every year thereafter. Included in these visits should be a physical exam, dietary intake, height, weight, hearing, vision, blood pressure, and heart and respiratory rates. The child and family should be questioned about any alcohol, drug, or tobacco use. Assess the home and family dynamics, any extracurricular activities, changes in thought processes (depression), academics, and sexuality problems. High risk children are screened for TB (tuberculosis), and all are screened for scoliosis. The tetanus booster is given at age 11 or 12, along with any missed boosters from the preschool years. The parents should be preparing the child for puberty changes, discussing sex education, as well as talking about drugs, alcohol, and tobacco. TV viewing and computer usage should be limited and monitored for content. Encourage exercise at least one hour a day.

DENTAL HEALTH OF SCHOOL AGE CHILDREN

It is during these years that the baby teeth are lost and replaced by the permanent teeth. Continue with proper brushing (twice a day with fluoride toothpaste) and flossing, assisting as needed until the child is proficient, along with regular dental visits. Make sure the child's toothbrush is small, soft and replaced every 2-3 months. Braces may be needed when the teeth are too crowded or out of alignment. Any permanent tooth that is knocked out should be rinsed in water, placed back into the socket and held in place so that it can be saved. As an alternative, the tooth can be placed in a cup of milk or held in the child's mouth, under the tongue. A dentist should be consulted immediately.

DISCIPLINE AND STRESSORS OF SCHOOL AGE CHILDREN

Set clear limits; taking away privileges is often a successful discipline method for school age children. Use lots of praise for good behaviors. The parent should role model appropriate behaviors and social skills. Show the child that she is a unique person, with much to contribute to the family, and take her thoughts seriously. Explain the whys of rules and consequences. A common misbehavior of this age is dishonesty, which, while distressing to the parents, is a common phase for children to go through.

School age children are exposed to more stress today than ever before. The nurse needs to assess for stressors and whether the child is able to cope or if there is a need for assistance in coping.

SEXUALITY OF SCHOOL AGE CHILDREN

Children of this age are exposed to a great deal of sexual material on TV, in music, in newspapers, and elsewhere. It is common for them to experiment with their own bodies. If parents do not dwell on these behaviors, answer questions honestly, and make themselves available for discussions, the school age child will develop a healthy attitude toward his own sexuality. If the parents do not talk openly with their children, the children will seek answers from their peers, who are not always reliable sources.

ADOLESCENTS

HEALTH CHECKUP AND DENTAL HEALTH FOR ADOLESCENTS

Providing privacy for the adolescent during doctor visits is helpful in gaining a full assessment. A physical exam, including assessing puberty changes, height, weight, vital signs, and growth trajectory, should be done yearly. Consider meningococcal, pneumococcal, influenza, and varicella vaccines for this age. A booster dose of tetanus and diphtheria vaccine is needed 10 years after the pre-kindergarten dose. Hepatitis B vaccines should be started if not given earlier, and hepatitis A vaccines are considered for those at high-risk. The teen should be screened for scoliosis and goiter.

Dental visits should occur every 6 months. Proper brushing and flossing are important, especially when orthodontic devices are in place. Gingivitis is common, usually due to improper cleaning of braces, sugary foods, and hormones. The teen should be encouraged to take special care with their dental hygiene. Trauma to

19

the mouth and teeth is common in sports activities. If the tooth is knocked out, it should be rinsed and placed back in the socket and the teen should be seen by a dentist immediately.

ADOLESCENT ISSUES TO DISCUSS DURING ROUTINE CHECKUPS

Discuss the nutrition requirements of the adolescent and how they are being met. Athletes, teens with eating disorders, and females with heavy menstrual cycles will need additional counseling and possibly supplements to meet their nutritional needs. Ask how much sleep the teen is getting, explain that teens need more sleep than children who are school aged, encourage them to get plenty of rest, and address any sleep problems they might be having. Ask about any risk-taking behaviors (alcohol, drugs, cigarette smoking) and educate as to the consequences of these. Talk about accident prevention, automobile safety, appropriate equipment for sports, and gun safety. Discuss issues of violence and how to prevent date rape. Discuss sexuality and address any issues or concerns such as birth control and STIs. Assess for abnormalities in menstruation. Talk about masturbation and, in males, nocturnal emissions. Assist the teen in addressing any acne concerns.

IMMUNIZATION VS. VACCINATION

Immunization refers to the body's buildup of defenses (antibodies) against specific diseases. It has an important role in preventing the spread of infection. Immunization prevents the individual from contracting a disease or lessens the severity of the disease, and can also prevent the complications (encephalitis, hearing loss, paralysis) associated with the infectious diseases. **Vaccination** is one method of creating immunity through the introduction of a small amount of the virus's or bacteria's antigen to the body, which then stimulates the body's creation of antibodies against that disease. Vaccination prevents the spread of infection to infants who are too young to have developed immunity and to those who are immunocompromised (cancer patients, transplantation recipients). Herd immunity results from a majority of the population being immune to a disease, therefore minimizing transmission. It is defined in terms of the percentage of the population that must be immunized in order to prevent outbreaks. This percentage may range from 80-85% for some disorders, but those that are highly contagious, such as measles, may require a herd immunity of 93-95%. Herd immunity can be obtained via widespread vaccination or widespread infection, though it is not recommended that individuals avoid immunization and rely on herd immunity for protection, as rates of immunization vary from one community to another.

TYPES OF VACCINES

There are a number of different types of vaccines:

- **Conjugated forms**: An organism is altered and then joined (conjugated) with another substance, such as a protein, to potentiate immune response (such as conjugated Hib).
- **Killed virus vaccines**: The virus has been killed but can still cause an immune response (such as inactivated poliovirus).
- **Live virus vaccines**: The virus is live but in a weakened (attenuated) form so that it doesn't cause the disease but confers immunity (such as measles vaccine).
- **Recombinant forms**: The organism is genetically altered and, for example, may use proteins rather than the whole cell to stimulate immunity (such as Hepatitis B and acellular pertussis vaccine).
- **Toxoid**: A toxin (antigen) that has been weakened by the use of heat or chemicals so it is too weak to cause disease but stimulates antibodies.

Some vaccines are given shortly after birth; others begin at 2 months, 12 months, or 2 years and some later in childhood.

DTAP AND TDAP VACCINES

Diphtheria and pertussis (whooping cough) are highly contagious bacterial diseases of the upper respiratory tract. Cases of diphtheria are now rare in the United States, although they still occur in some developing countries. There have, however, been recent outbreaks of pertussis in the United States. Tetanus is a bacterial infection contracted through cuts, wounds, and scratches. The **diphtheria, tetanus, and pertussis (DTaP)**

vaccine is recommended for all children. DTaP is a newer and safer version of the older DTP vaccine, which is no longer used in the United States. **Tdap** is the DTaP booster shot meant to continue immunity to these diseases through adulthood, given every 10 years starting at age 11.

DTaP requires 5 doses:

- 2 months
- 4 months
- 6 months
- 5-18 months
- 4-6 years (or at 11-12 years if booster missed between 4-6)

According to recent ACIP recommendations, DTaP may now also be administered to children ages 7-9 as part of a catch-up series, but children will then require their routine Tdap dose at age 11-12. If DTaP is administered to children ages 10-18 it can be counted as their adolescent Tdap booster. Adverse reactions can occur, but they are usually mild soreness, fever, and/or nausea. About 1 in 100 children will have high fever (>105 °F) and may develop seizures. Severe allergic responses can occur.

HPV Vaccine

Human papillomavirus (HPV) comprises >100 viruses. About 40 are sexually transmitted and invade mucosal tissue, causing genital warts, which are low risk for cancer, or changes in the mucosa, which can lead to cervical cancer. Most HPVs cause little or no symptoms, but they are very common, especially in those 15-25. Over 99% of cervical cancers are caused by HPV and 70% are related to HPVs 16 and 18. The HPV vaccine, Gardasil, protects against HPVs 6 and 11 (which cause genital warts), along with 16 and 18, which can cause cancer. Protection is only conveyed if the female has not yet been infected with these strains. The vaccine is currently recommended for females under 26 but studies have determined that those not adequately covered over the age of 26 and up to 45 can benefit. A series of 3 injections is required over a 6-month period:

- Initial dose 11-12 years (but may be given as young as 9 or ≥18)
- 2 months after first dose
- 6 months after first dose

PPV

Pneumococcal polysaccharide-23 vaccine (PPV) (Pneumovax and Pnu-Immune) is a vaccine that has been available since 1977 to protect against 23 types of pneumococcal bacteria. It is given to adults ≥65 and children ≥2 years in high-risk groups that include:

- Children with chronic heart, lung, sickle cell disease, diabetes, cirrhosis, alcoholism, and leaks of cerebrospinal fluid
- Children with lowered immunity from Hodgkin's disease, lymphoma, leukemia, kidney failure, multiple myeloma, nephrotic syndrome, HIV/AIDS, damaged or missing spleen, and organ transplant

Children ≤2 may not respond to this vaccine and should take PCV-7. Administration is as follows:

- One dose is usually all that is required although a second dose may be advised for children with some conditions, such as cancer or organ/bone marrow transplantations.
- If needed, a second dose is given 3 years after the first for children ≤10 and 5 years after the first for those ≥10.

Hepatitis A Vaccine

Hepatitis A is a contagious virus that causes liver disease and can cause serious morbidity and death. It is spread through the feces of a person who is infected and often causes contamination of food and water. The

Hep A vaccine is now recommended for all children at one year of age. It is not licensed for use in younger infants. Two doses are needed:

- 12 months (12-23 months)
- 18 months (or 6 months after previous dose)

Older children and teenagers may receive the two-injection series if they are considered at risk, depending upon lifestyle, such as young males having sex with other males or those using illegal drugs. It is also recommended if outbreaks occur. Adverse reactions are mild and include soreness, headache, anorexia, and malaise although severe allergic reactions can occur as with all vaccines.

HEPATITIS B VACCINE

Hepatitis B is transmitted through blood and body fluids, including during birth; therefore, it is now recommended for all newborns as well as all those <18 and those in high-risk groups >18. Hepatitis B can cause serious liver disease leading to liver cancer. Three injections of **monovalent HepB** are required to confer immunity:

- Birth (within 12 hours)
- At 1-2 months
- ≥24 weeks

Note: If combination vaccines are given after the birth dose, then a dose at 4 months can be given.

If the mother is Hepatitis B positive, the child should be given both the monovalent HepB vaccination as well as HepB immune globulin within 12 hours of birth. Adolescents (11-15) who have not been vaccinated require 2 doses, 4-6 months apart. Adverse reactions include local irritation and fever. Severe allergic reactions can occur to those allergic to baker's yeast.

ROTAVIRUS VACCINE

Rotavirus is a cause of significant morbidity and mortality in children, especially in developing countries. Most children, without vaccination, will suffer from severe diarrhea caused by rotavirus within the first 5 years of life. The new **rotavirus vaccine** is advised for all infants but should not be initiated after 12 weeks or administered after 32 weeks, so there is a narrow window of opportunity. Three doses are required:

- 2 months (between 6 and 12 weeks)
- 4 months
- 6 months

An earlier vaccine was withdrawn from the market because it was associated with an increase in intussusception, a disorder in which part of the intestine telescopes inside another. Rates of intussusception in those receiving the current (RotaTeq) vaccine have been investigated and incidence of intussusception was within the range of normal occurrences with no evidence linking the occurrences to the vaccine.

INACTIVATED POLIOVIRUS VACCINE

Poliomyelitis is a serious viral infection that can cause paralysis and death. Prior to introduction of a vaccine in 1955, there were >20,000 cases of polio in the United States each year. There have been no cases of polio caused by the poliovirus for >20 years in the United States, but it still occurs in some third world countries, so continuing vaccinations is very important. Oral polio vaccine (OPV) is no longer recommended in the United States because it carries a very slight risk of causing the disease (1:2.4 million). Children require 4 doses of injectable polio vaccine (IPV):

- 2 months
- 4 months

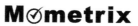

- 6-18 months
- 4-6 years (booster dose)

IPV is contraindicated for those who have had a severe reaction to neomycin, streptomycin, or polymyxin B. Rare allergic reactions can occur, but there are almost no serious problems caused by this vaccine.

VARICELLA VACCINE

Varicella (chickenpox) is a common infectious childhood disease caused by the varicella zoster virus, resulting in fever, rash, and itching, and it can also cause skin infections, pneumonia, and neurological damage. After infection, the virus retreats to the nerves by the spinal cord and can reactivate years later, causing herpes zoster (shingles), a significant cause of morbidity in adults. Infection with varicella conveys immunity, but because of associated problems, it is recommended that all children receive varicella vaccine. Two doses are needed:

- 12-15 months
- 4-6 years (or at least 3 months after first dose)

Children ≥13 years and adults who have never had chickenpox or previously received the vaccine should receive 2 doses at least 28 days apart. Children should not receive the vaccine if they have had a serious allergic reaction to gelatin or neomycin. Most reactions are mild and include soreness, fever, and rash. About 1:1000 may experience febrile seizures. Pneumonia is a very rare reaction.

MMR VACCINE

Measles is a viral disease characterized by fever and rash but can cause pneumonia, seizures, severe neurological damage, and death. Mumps is a viral disease that causes fever and swollen glands but can cause deafness, meningitis, and swelling of the testicles. Rubella, also known as German measles) is also a viral disease that can cause rash, fever, and arthritis, but the biggest danger is that it can cause a woman who is pregnant to miscarry or deliver a child with serious birth defects. The **measles, mumps, and rubella (MMR) vaccine** is given in 2 doses:

- 12-15 months
- 4-6 years

Children can get the injections at any age if they have missed them, but there must be at least 28 days between injections. Children with severe allergic reactions to gelatin or neomycin should not get the injection. Severe adverse reactions are rare, but fever and mild rash are common. Teenagers may have pain and stiffness in joints. Occasional seizures (1:3000) and thrombocytopenia (1:30,000) occur.

PCV-7

Heptavalent pneumococcal conjugate vaccine (PCV-7) (Prevnar) was released for use in the United States in 2001 for treatment of children under 2 years old. It provides immunity to 7 serotypes of *Streptococcus pneumoniae* to protect against invasive pneumococcal disease, such as pneumonia, otitis media, bacteremia, and meningitis. Because children are most at risk ≤1, vaccinations begin early:

Administration is in 4 doses:

- 6-8 weeks
- 4 months
- 6 months
- 12-18 months

Although less effective for older children, PCV-7 has been approved for children between 2 and 5 years of age who are at high risk because of the following conditions:

- Chronic diseases: sickle cell disease, heart disease, lung disease, liver disease
- Damaged or missing spleen
- Immunosuppressive disorders: diabetes, cancer
- Drug therapy: chemotherapy, steroids

PCV-7 may also be considered for all children ≤ 5, especially those ≤3 and in group day care and in some ethnic groups (Native American, Alaska Natives, and African Americans).

MENINGOCOCCAL VACCINE

Meningitis is severe bacterial meningitis that can result in severe neurological compromise or death. A number of different serotypes of *meningococci* can cause meningitis and current vaccines protect against 4 types although not against subtype B, which causes about 65% of meningitis cases in children. However, the vaccines provide 85-100% protection against sub-types A, C, Y, and W-135. There are 2 types of vaccine:

- **Meningococcal polysaccharide vaccine (MPSV4)** is made from the outer capsule of the bacteria and is used for children 2-10.
  - One dose is given at 2 years, although those at high risk may receive 2 doses, 3 months apart.
  - Under special circumstances, children 3-24 months may receive 2 doses, 3 months apart.
- **Meningococcal conjugate vaccine (MCV4)** is used for children ≥11 (who have not received MPSV4). One dose is required:
  - Ages 11-12, all children should receive the vaccine.
  - If not previously vaccinated, high school and college freshmen should be vaccinated.
- Side effects are usually only local tenderness.

HIB VACCINE

Haemophilus influenzae **type b (Hib) vaccine** (HibTITER and PedvaxHIB) protects against infection with *Haemophilus influenzae,* which can cause serious respiratory infections, pneumonia, meningitis, bacteremia, and pericarditis in children ≤5 years old. *Administration* is as follows:

- 2 months
- 4 months
- 6 months (may be required, depending upon the brand of vaccine)
- 12-15 months (this booster dose must be given at least 2 months after the earlier doses for those who start at a later age than 2 months)

Children over age 6 usually do not require Hib, but it is recommended for older children and adults. Here are some conditions that place them at risk:

- Sickle cell disease
- HIV/AIDS
- Bone marrow transplant
- Chemotherapy for cancer
- Damaged or missing spleen

Some chemotherapy drugs, corticosteroids, and other immunosuppressive drugs may interact with the vaccine.

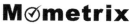

INFANT IMMUNIZATION SCHEDULE SUMMARY

The recommended schedule for immunizations for the infant is summarized below:

- All newborns receive **ophthalmic drops or ointment**, to prevent blindness from possible gonorrhea infection, and an injection of vitamin K to prevent hemorrhagic disease.
- Before discharge, newborns are tested for **phenylketonuria** and **hypothyroidism**, and will possibly have their **hematocrit** and **hemoglobin** checked.
- **Hepatitis B vaccine** is given at birth, 1-2 months, and 6-18 months.
- **Diphtheria/tetanus/pertussis vaccine** is administered at 2 months, 4 months, 6 months, and 15-18 months.
- **Hib (Haemophilus influenza type b) vaccine** is given at 2 months, 4 months, and 12 months or later.
- **Poliovirus vaccine** is given at 2 months, 4 months, and 6-18 months.
- **MMR vaccine** is given at 12-18 months.
- **Varicella (chickenpox) vaccine** can be given at 12 months.

REQUIRED IMMUNIZATION HISTORY FOR CHILDREN UP TO 6 YEARS OF AGE

According to the Centers for Disease Control and Prevention, by 6 years of age, children in the United States should receive a three-part series of hepatitis B, three doses of rotavirus prevention; four injections protecting against diphtheria, tetanus, and pertussis; four doses of *Haemophilus influenzae* type b; four doses of pneumococcal vaccine; four doses of polio vaccine; two injections that protect against measles, mumps, and rubella; two varicella vaccinations; one hepatitis A vaccination; and a yearly influenza prevention injection.

VACCINATION OF CHILDREN WITH UNCERTAIN IMMUNIZATION HISTORIES

Children who have uncertain immunization histories may need vaccinations to meet guidelines. The number of vaccinations needed depends on the child's history. For children who are not up-to-date on immunizations, the necessary injections must be determined. These vaccinations can then be given on a schedule so that the child can catch up. For children with no immunization history or uncertain status, such as refugees or internationally adopted children, restarting the immunization series may be necessary to ensure adequate coverage with all vaccines, particularly measles, mumps, and rubella; varicella; hepatitis B; *Haemophilus influenzae* type b; and polio.

POSSIBLE SIDE EFFECTS

Immunization reactions can be minimized and the child made more comfortable by giving acetaminophen prior to the immunizations. Common reactions to immunizations include irritability, decrease in appetite, fever less than 102 °F, and swelling, redness and tenderness at injection site. These may last for the first 1-2 days and can be treated with acetaminophen every 4-6 hours for the first day. If more severe reactions occur, such as fever greater than 102 °F, severe prolonged irritability, or high-pitched crying, or the symptoms last more than 2 days, the parents should call the healthcare provider immediately.

IMPORTANT CONSIDERATIONS WHEN GIVING IMMUNIZATIONS

Every time a child comes into contact with the healthcare system, his **immunization status** should be assessed. Children are required, by all states, to be immunized before entering a licensed school or day care. Specific requirements will vary from state to state. Vaccines must be handled and stored according the manufacturers guidelines. Immunizations must be documented according to specific guidelines and parents must sign a consent form every time a vaccine is administered. Common illnesses such as colds, ear infections and diarrhea will not usually preclude giving vaccines. The MMR and varicella vaccines should not be given during pregnancy. There are two situations in which immunizations are contraindicated: a previous severe allergic reaction to a vaccine or one of its components and encephalopathy occurring within 7 days of giving a DTP or DTaP vaccine.

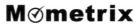

THE ANTI-VACCINATION MOVEMENT

While **opposition to vaccination** is not a new concept, it is a movement that has gained momentum with the power of information sharing via social media. Opposers to vaccination, often referred to as "Anti-Vaxxers," believe that vaccinations can cause complications such as autism and SIDS, especially when administered in infancy and early childhood, and believe that these risks far outweigh the benefits. There are also those who oppose such medical interventions due to religious beliefs.

While the therapeutic effects of vaccinations have been supported by evidence for both individuals and communities, it is important that healthcare professionals be equipped to respectfully inform and care for those that oppose vaccinations. Individuals should be educated regarding the evidence supporting vaccinations and the vaccinations required by law. The CDC offers a wealth of resources for healthcare workers and for individuals regarding vaccinations. The most notable resource is the CDC's Vaccine Information Statement, a living document that outlines the benefits and risks of vaccines, that healthcare workers can use to inform individuals and parents. If, despite efforts to educate, the individual or caregiver still refuses vaccination, there are ICD codes that providers are required to use to document this refusal (for example, ICD-10-CM: Z28.82: Immunization not carried out because of caregiver refusal). The healthcare worker must also document that preventive medical counseling was provided.

VACCINATIONS PROGRAMS

Vaccination programs seek to promote health by preventing large-scale outbreaks of preventable disease. Public health has the responsibility of weighing the benefits and risks of a vaccine before recommending widespread vaccination for any given disease. Vaccines consist of an **antigen** in solution designed to stimulate the immune system of an individual to produce **antibodies** against the antigen to prevent disease from future exposure. The antigen may be alive or dead. The CDC periodically updates recommendations for all ages and has information concerning each vaccine's composition, contraindications, dosage, administration, and storage. Vaccines are recommended for adults who travel, have occupational risks of exposure, have chronic disease, or are immunocompromised. Some individuals may not receive certain vaccines due to allergies or the presence of certain diseases. Vaccines that are currently recommended for adults include tetanus, diphtheria, pneumococcal, Hepatitis A and B, measles, mumps, rubella, varicella, influenza, and meningococcal.

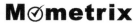

Anticipatory Guidance

LEADING CAUSES OF DEATH BY AGE GROUP

BIRTH TO 10-YEAR AGE GROUP

For the **birth to 10-year** age group, the US Preventive Services Task Force has assembled a list of the **five leading causes of death**. The number one cause of death in this age group is actually a group of conditions that arise in the time period surrounding birth (the "**perinatal period**"). There are a number of conditions that arise surrounding birth that are fatal, including placental problems (premature separation, abruption), umbilical cord problems (cord prolapse, nuchal cord, single umbilical artery), infections (chorioamnionitis, congenital pneumonia), trauma during the birthing process (nerve damage, intracranial hemorrhage), and hemolytic disease of the newborn. The second leading cause of death is attributed to **congenital defects**, including tetralogy of Fallot, transposition of the great arteries, spina bifida, and anencephaly. Other leading causes of death include **sudden infant death syndrome (SIDS)**, **motor vehicle injuries**, and **other unintentional injuries**.

INJURY PREVENTION COUNSELING

Injury prevention counseling is a strong recommendation for the **birth to 10-year** age group, owing to the fact that motor vehicle accidents and other unintentional accidents are leading causes of death for this population. Children and their parents should be advised to use car safety seats until the age of 5 (this is subject to state law, however, as some states require the use of booster seats until a certain height or age is reached). After the age of 5, standard safety belts should always be used. When biking, skating, or skateboarding, a helmet should always be worn; these activities should not take place in the street. Parents should be advised to become CPR certified. They should also be advised to keep drugs, poisons, guns, other weapons, and matches out of the reach of children; to install smoke detectors and plan an escape route in the event of fire; and to make sure that stairs, windows, and pools are safe for children.

11- TO 24-YEAR AGE GROUP

The list of the top five leading causes of death in the **11-24** age population differs significantly from the leading causes of death in the birth to 10-year age population. Leading the list for ages 11-24 are deaths caused by either **motor vehicle accidents or other unintentional accidents**. Second on the list is **homicide**, followed by **suicide**. The fourth leading cause of death in the 11-24 age population is **cancer**. The most common fatal cancers in this age group include leukemia (acute lymphocytic leukemia and acute myeloid leukemia), brain tumors (medulloblastoma, astrocytoma, and brainstem glioma), rhabdomyosarcoma, neuroblastoma, Wilms tumor, Ewing sarcoma, and Hodgkin's lymphoma. The fifth leading cause of death in this age population is due to **general heart diseases**, which may include cardiomyopathies and faulty valves.

YOUTH RISK BEHAVIOR SURVEILLANCE SYSTEM

The **Youth Risk Behavior Surveillance System** (YRBSS) is a program conducted through the CDC that monitors eight different categories of health-risk behaviors of adolescents:

- Unintentional injuries and violence
- Tobacco use
- Alcohol and other drug use
- Sexual behaviors
- Dietary behaviors
- Physical activity
- Obesity, overweight, and weight control
- Other health topics

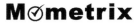

The YRBSS gathers data from participating states and local surveys (such as large cities) from grades 9-12 and then compiles the information, assessing for trends. Current results reflect data collected in 2021 and released in 2023. Responses are either weighted (≥60% participation) or unweighted (relates only to those completing survey). Weighted results can be generalized to the teenage population at large in the area of the survey. The data obtained in the YRBSS is used to determine progress in national health objectives for health promotion.

YRBSS 2021 Results

Tobacco Use

The CDC conducts the Youth Risk Behavior Surveillance System to determine health-risk behaviors that contribute to significant morbidity in adolescents. **Tobacco,** often thought of as an adult issue, is a cause of concern for children and teenagers. Tobacco use is one of the leading preventable causes of death in the United States, but 2021 results showed that about 6.3% of children (down from 9.5% in 2019) have tried smoking before high school, often beginning by age 12, putting themselves at risk for heart and lung disease as adults. Almost 18% of children have tried smoking in total according to 2021 results, which is a downward trend. A newer trend is the use of electronic vapor products, with 36% of children reporting having tried this product at some point, and 18% reporting current use. Those most at risk are males in low-income families with parents who smoke. Male adolescents may smoke to be rebellious, but females often smoke to lose weight. Other factors include the desire to be part of a group, lack of supervision, and accessibility of tobacco. Intervention includes identifying those smoking, providing information about the dangers of smoking, beginning with children at about 9 years old, and providing programs to help teenagers quit smoking.

Drug Use

Drug use continues to be a serious problem for children and teenagers, with some starting as young as 9 or 10, using a wide variety of drugs, including marijuana, crack, prescription drugs, cocaine, inhalants (such as glue and lighter fluid), hallucinogens, and steroids. Marijuana is the most reported drug in the high school data, with about 28% of children reporting having used marijuana in their lifetime. Approximately 13% of children reported having used illicit drugs (e.g., cocaine, heroin, inhalants, methamphetamines, ecstasy, or hallucinogens) at least once in their lifetime. Risk factors for drug use include aggressive behavior, poor social skills, and poor academic progress coupled with lack of parental supervision, poverty, and availability of drugs. Small children who use drugs are often reacting to circumstances within the family, while teenagers are more likely to use drugs in response to peer pressure from outside the family. Studies have shown that early intervention to teach children better self-control and coping skills is often more effective than trying to change behavior patterns that are established, so family-based programs often show positive results. Teenagers may need help with basic academic skills and social skills to improve communication. Methods of resisting drugs must be provided and reinforced. Drug recovery programs can be helpful but are often too expensive or not available for those who need them.

Alcohol Use

Alcohol use is a significant problem in adolescence and even in younger children. It is the most-commonly abused substance. Of high schoolers who responded to the survey question in 2021, about 23% reported having had at least one drink within the past 30 days (down from 30% in 2019). While alcohol can impair development of almost all body systems in a growing child, it is of particular concern for the effects on the neurological system and liver. Additionally, because it interferes with impulse control, adolescents who drink are often involved in violence, abuse, and at-risk sexual behavior. Drinking should be suspected if a child has memory problems, changes in behavior, poor academic progress, emotional lability, and physical changes, such as slurring of speech, general lethargy, or lack of coordination. Intervention includes teaching children from around age 9 about the dangers of drinking, identifying those who are drinking, identifying underlying problems, and providing programs to help teenagers stop drinking, such as counseling or Alcoholics Anonymous.

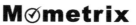

HIGH-RISK SEXUAL BEHAVIOR

High-risk sexual behavior in teenagers is often coupled with other health-risk behaviors, such as drinking and drug use. In 2021, about 30% of high school students reported having previously had sex (a significant decline from the 38.4% reported in 2019), with around 3% becoming sexually active before the age of 13. Risk factors include poverty, single-family homes, lack of supervision, and siblings or peers who are sexually active. Those who have sex before age 15 are especially vulnerable, often having multiple partners and unprotected sex, leading to sexually transmitted infections (STIs) and pregnancy. They are often emotionally vulnerable and unable to deal effectively with relationships. Intervention should begin early with age-appropriate honest sex education. Abstinence education, while the ideal, has not been successful in changing the sexual behavior of teenagers, with studies showing that many of those signing pledges to remain virgins are already sexually active. Teenagers who are sexually active should be advised regarding the use of condoms, birth control, and protection from STIs in a non-judgmental manner.

PREVENTION OF STIs

The **CDC** has developed five strategies to prevent and control the spread of STIs:

- **Educate** those at risk about how to make changes in sexual practices to prevent infection.
- **Identify** symptomatic and asymptomatic infected persons who might not seek diagnosis or treatment.
- **Diagnose** and treat those who are infected.
- **Prevent infection** of sex partners through evaluation, treatment, and counseling.
- Provide pre-exposure **vaccination** for those at risk.

Practitioners are advised to inquire of patients' **sexual histories** and to assess risk. The 5-P approach to questioning is advocated. Practitioners should ask about:

- **Partners**: Gender and number
- **Pregnancy prevention**: Birth control
- **Protection**: Methods used
- **Practices**: Type of sexual practices (oral, anal, vaginal) and use of condoms
- **Past history of STIs**: High-risk behavior (promiscuity, prostitution) and disease risk (human immunodeficiency virus [HIV]/ hepatitis)

The CDC recommends a number of specific preventive methods as part of the clinical guidelines for prevention of sexually transmitted infections:

- **Abstinence or reduction** in number of sex partners.
- Pre-exposure **vaccination**: All those evaluated for STIs should receive hepatitis B vaccination, and men who have sex with men (MSM) and illicit drug users should receive hepatitis A vaccination.
- **Male latex (or polyurethane) condoms** should be used for all sexual encounters with only water-based lubricants used with latex.
- **Female condoms** may be used if a male condom cannot be used properly.
- Condoms and diaphragms should not be used with spermicides containing **nonoxynol-9 (N-9)**, and N-9 should not be used as a lubricant for anal sex.
- **Non-barrier contraceptive measures** provide no protection from STIs and must not be relied on to prevent disease.

MEASURES TO PREVENT INJURY/ILLNESS OF TODDLERS

HOME AND AUTO SAFETY

Toddlers are curious and very mobile, so accidents can occur easily in and outside the home. **Auto safety** includes using the appropriate size child-safety seat in the back seat, and buckling the child up every time they are in a moving vehicle. Toddlers need to be supervised closely when playing outside, to prevent them from running into the street in front of moving vehicles. Parents can begin to teach them how to stop, look, and listen before crossing a street.

The home environment needs to be child-proofed, moving all poisonous substances well away from the toddler's reach (keeping in mind that toddlers will learn to climb). Poisons should be stored in a locked or inaccessible location to the child. Medication should be stored up high and children should not be told that medication is candy when they are taking it.

WATER, TOY, AND GUN SAFETY, AND BURNS

The following are some measures the parents can take to prevent injury and illness of their toddler, focusing on burns and water, toy, and gun safety:

- Never leave a toddler alone in or near water, as they can drown in as little as one inch of water. Toddlers are still unstable and prone to falling, possibly into a puddle or bucket.
- When appropriate, life jackets should be worn by toddlers (in a boat or near a lake, pond, or pool).
- Toddlers should wear helmets when riding tricycles.
- Make sure any toys given to toddlers are appropriate for their age and safe. Balloons, small toys, and plastic bags are potential choking hazards.
- A big concern today is guns kept in the home. Toddlers don't know the difference between a toy gun and a real gun, so all guns kept in the home must be properly secured.
- Teach the toddler the meaning of "hot," while using safety plugs on appliances, keep matches and lighters up high, turn pot handles toward the back of the stove, and don't use tablecloths in the home (toddlers can pull on these and topple hot food/liquids on themselves).

MEASURES TO PREVENT INJURY/ILLNESS OF PRESCHOOLERS

HOME AND AUTO SAFETY

Preschoolers are aware of potential dangers and can be taught safety rules. Poisonous substances, including medicines, need to have safety caps and be locked up. Watch for unsafe areas at playgrounds. Enforce the wearing of safety equipment when playing sports. Use the appropriate safety seat (booster) in the back seat until the child weighs 80 lb. After 80 lb, use a seat belt in the back seat. Do not leave a child alone in a car or home. Use close supervision when playing outside and near streets. Have the child wear a bike helmet when riding and teach him the rules for safe riding. Parents should have the poison control number saved to their phones or written down somewhere it can be quickly accessed.

AUTO, SPORTS, AND WATER SAFETY

School age children are especially prone to accidents, due to their mobility and participation in sports and other physical activities. The following rules should be taught to children and enforced by the parents/caregivers:

- Children should always wear a seatbelt, and sit in the backseat, in a moving vehicle.
- When riding anything with wheels, the child should always wear a helmet and elbow and knee pads.
- The child must obey traffic signals when walking on or across streets.
- The school-aged child should participate in swim lessons and be taught to swim with a buddy, wear a life jacket when in a boat, and not dive into shallow water.

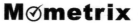

MEASURES TO PREVENT INJURY/ILLNESS OF SCHOOL AGE CHILDREN

The following are some measures parents can take to prevent injury/illness of their school age child, focusing on drug, fire, stranger, and gun safety:

- Keep medicine locked and teach children the dangers of taking any medicine without adult supervision.
- Begin teaching the child about illegal drug use and smoking.
- Use sunscreen when playing outside.
- Establish an escape route for each member of the family in case of fire and practice the route monthly.
- Don't allow the child to use the stove without adult supervision.
- Teach the child to stay away from guns. Parents should keep guns unloaded and in a locked location with ammunition stored in a separate location.
- Teach the child to not talk to strangers or approach strange vehicles.
- Make sure the child knows their phone number, their address, and how to call 911.
- Find a neighbor's house that can serve as a safe place for the child if needed.

MEASURES TO PREVENT INJURY/ILLNESS OF ADOLESCENTS

Adolescents think they are invincible, which can contribute to risk-taking behaviors.

- Motor vehicle accidents claim many teenagers' lives every year. Teens should take driver's education courses, wear seat belts at all times, obey traffic laws, and refrain from drinking and driving.
- If an adolescent legally uses firearms, they need to be taught safety rules and how to use and store firearms.
- Adolescents should be taught the risks of using drugs, alcohol, and nicotine.
- Sports teams should focus on safety, proper equipment, and appropriate conditioning.
- Adolescents should know proper swimming and water safety and use sunscreen when outside.
- Sexual activity is a high-risk behavior that should be addressed on a family level. If appropriate, the adolescent should be taught sexual responsibility.

APPROPRIATE SUNSCREEN USE

While children need some exposure to the sun, sunscreen protects against harmful ultraviolet rays that can cause burns, sun damage, premature aging, and skin cancer. Sunscreen should be generously applied before children go out in the sun, covering the parts of the body that are exposed, including the face, lips, tops of the ears, and back of the neck. It should be reapplied at least every 2 hours, and if children are going to be around water, the sunscreen should be waterproof. The sun protection factor (SPF) should be a minimum of 30 for children older than 6 months, as recommended by the American Academy of Dermatology. The American Academy of Pediatrics recommends that children under the age of 6 months be kept out of direct sunlight. If they must be in direct sunlight, children should be covered by clothing and hats. A small amount of SPF 15 sunscreen is allowed on children under the age of 6 months, but only to small areas such as their face and the backs of their hands.

GUIDELINES FOR USING INSECT REPELLANT

Insect repellant may be used on children to prevent insect bites, but it should be used with caution. Many insect repellants contain N,N-diethyl-meta-toluamide (DEET), which has been shown to be safe for limited use with children over 2 months of age. Repellants used on children should have less than a 30% concentration of DEET and should only be applied once a day. It should be sprayed on a caregiver's hand and then put on the child, rather than spraying the child directly. This decreases the likelihood of the child ingesting the repellant. Insect repellant can also be applied to clothing to provide some protection without applying it directly to the skin.

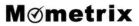

ENVIRONMENTAL ASSESSMENT
ENVIRONMENTAL HEALTH HISTORY

The environmental health history is important to determine potential hazards in the child's surroundings that may contribute to poor health or injuries. Examples of potential exposures that should be considered when taking a pediatric environmental health history include air pollution, including industrial exposure, cigarette smoke, carbon monoxide from furnaces or machinery; lead exposure through paint or plumbing in older homes; allergen exposure, such as pet dander, pollen, or mold; exposure to ultraviolet radiation during outdoor activities; water quality; and nutrition.

ENVIRONMENTAL INFLUENCES ON THE PEDIATRIC PATIENT'S HEALTH

Safety in the home environment is a big influence on the health of the child. Accidental injuries in and around the home can include burns from scalding liquids or cooking appliances, drownings in pools or bathtubs, falls from climbing or from bicycles, and motor vehicle accidents or pedestrian-car accidents. Children who spend a great deal of time watching TV or playing video games are at risk for obesity and health issues that accompany obesity. Some children may try to be like characters they see on TV shows or other media, which can lead to aggressive behavior and risk-taking.

CONSIDERATION OF ENVIRONMENTAL FACTORS PRIOR TO A CHILD'S RETURN HOME

Environmental factors should be assessed within the **actual environment** if at all possible. If not, careful questioning and drawing of diagrams and approximate floor plans with the patient (or the patient's parent)— or asking for a drawing—can be useful, especially when showing the patient needed modifications. Family members may also assist with the assessment, providing useful information. Some patients or their parents, may be reluctant to admit that the home is cluttered or that they are unable to maintain the home environment in a sanitary condition. Brochures and handouts about home safety and assistive devices should be provided to the patient and caretaker as well as contact names and numbers for equipment needed in the home. A checklist should be compiled of all necessary changes or additions, with specific details, such as "Install 18-inch grab bar across from toilet." In some cases, a social worker or occupational therapist should visit the home.

GENERAL ELEMENTS OF ENVIRONMENTAL SAFETY

Some elements of an environmental assessment are not specific to rooms in the house but are **general needs** that must be met in order for individuals, especially the disabled child and their caregivers, to remain safe:

- **Environmental hazards** such as piles of papers or junk on the floors, loose carpet or rugs, and cluttered pathways can cause falls and must be cleared, organized, or repaired.
- **Lighting** should be adequate enough for reading in all rooms and stairways.
- **Heat and air conditioning** must be adequate. The young and the elderly are especially susceptible to heat and cold injury.
- **Sanitation** should ensure that health hazards do not exist, such as from rotting food or infestations of cockroaches or rodents.
- **Animals** should be cared for adequately with access to food, water, toileting, and routine veterinary care.
- **Smoke/chemicals** in the environment may pose a hazard, such as exposure to cigarette smoke or cleaning materials.

DANGEROUS WEAPONS AND TOYS

Parents should be advised that any guns kept in the home must be secured, with the guns unloaded and with the ammunition separately secured in a different location. All children, from an early age, should be taught to never pick up a gun or point it at anyone, even in play, and to immediately tell a trusted adult if they see anyone with a gun or know of anyone, such as a peer, who is carrying a gun or intends to harm someone with a gun.

Children should be protected from **dangerous toys**, which can include toys with small parts that may cause choking, especially for infants and toddlers. Toys that shoot projectiles, have cords or strings attached, or have sharp edges may pose a risk as well. Some products, such as some types of slime, have been found to contain toxins, so parents should regularly check with the US Consumer Product Safety Commission for alerts and should always read and adhere to warning labels. Smart toys and electronic devices that connect to the internet may provide identifying information about the child to unauthorized individuals.

RECOMMENDATIONS FOR PARENTS AND CHILDREN REGARDING SOCIAL SITUATIONS

Recommendations for social situations include:

- **Strangers**: Parents should stress the importance of going places and playing outside with a friend or an adult and not being alone. Children should know to run and yell if a stranger asks them to carry something, help get something out of a car, or to help look for or see a puppy or kitten. Parents should stress that children should never get into a car with a stranger or an acquaintance who says that the child's parent has sent the person unless this person uses a password. Children should know to yell what is happening ("This woman is taking me!") and should know their full name, address, and phone number as soon as they are old enough to learn them.
- **Violence**: Parents should limit children's exposure to violent media content (TV, movies, video games) and use blocking tools when appropriate. Parents should encourage children to talk about their feeling if they've experienced or observed violence and to reassure them. If violence is common, children should play only in safe areas and learn safety rules, such as dropping to the ground if they hear gunshots.
- **Bullying**: Parents should recognize the signs that a child is being bullied (depression, withdrawal, dislike of school, change in affect, lack of friends, change of sleep patterns, bruises) and teach children the impact that bullying has on others. Advise parents to teach children to tell an adult if they are being bullied and to respond assertively, act unimpressed, make a joke out of mean comments, and get involved in activities, such as clubs, where they feel safe. If children are cyberbullied, they should block the senders, change passwords, and report it to an adult.
- **Automobile safety/distracted driving**: Children should be seated and secured properly for their age and size and should be taught to avoid yelling, throwing things, and scuffling while in the car as this may distract the driver. Teenage drivers should be taught safe driving (including never driving while drinking), should have clear consequences for unsafe driving (such as a loss of driving privileges), and should have an app on their phones that prevents texting while driving and provides their location to their parents.

RECOMMENDATIONS FOR SPORTS AND RECREATION

Recommendations regarding sports and recreation include:

- **Concussion risks**: Greatest risks are from sports activities (football, hockey, soccer, lacrosse) and accidents (fall, car/bicycle). Parents should ensure that any sports team a child participates in has adequate safety rules (limits to tackling, for example) and that coaches carefully monitor the children. Children should always wear appropriate safety gear, such as helmets, when engaged in sports activities and should never continue playing if exhibiting any signs of head injury (headache, dizziness, confusion).
- **Helmet use**: Helmets (the appropriate type) should be worn for sports activities that may involve falls or blows to the head (hockey, football, skateboarding, baseball, bicycling). Helmets should fit snugly so that they don't move if they are rotated, turned, or tilted, and the helmet should be pressed down at the crown to check for fitting of the jaw pads and chin straps. Football helmets may be air/fluid filled or padded.

VEHICLE SAFETY

BOAT SAFETY

According to the US Coast Guard's recommendations for **boat safety**, infants who are not of the appropriate weight and size to wear approved personal flotation devices (PFDs) should not be taken on recreational boats (rowboats, motorboats, kayaks, sailboats). All other children should wear life jackets that are properly fitted and secured. PFDs do not include swimming aids intended for play, such as water wings or pool noodles. If an infant is on a boat, a caregiver wearing a life jacket should hold the infant at all times and should not place the child in a car seat (which will not float). Infants and young children are more likely to develop hypothermia, so they should be wrapped with a dry blanket or towel if cold and shivering. Children by about age 3 should be taught safety rules, such as keeping hands and feet inside the boat and walking instead of running. All children should take swimming lessons. Older children should take a boat safety course if possible. Adolescents should be cautioned to never engage in drinking or recreational drug use while boating.

CAR SEATS

All infants, regardless of age, must be placed properly in an **infant car seat** during transit. Holding an infant while the car is in motion is not safe. Car seats should be new or in very good condition and fastened according to manufacturer's guidelines to ensure safety:

- Place the car seat in the back seat and away from any side airbags.
- Always securely buckle the child into the seat.
- Face the infant seat toward the rear of the car.
- Recline the seat so that the infant's head does not fall forward.
- Place padding around (not under) the infant if the infant slouches to one side.
- Place blankets OVER the straps and buckles, not under.

The infant/toddler should be placed in the rear-facing seat to the maximum weight and height allowed by the seat (some accommodate up to 65 pounds). Once transitioned to front-facing seats, children should be placed in belt-positioning booster seats until the vehicle's seat/shoulder belts fit properly (usually until 4' 9" and 8-12 years old). Until age 13, children should sit secured in the back seat and not the front.

TOXIC EXPOSURES

CARBON MONOXIDE POISONING

Carbon monoxide (CO) poisoning occurs with inhalation of fossil fuel exhausts from engines, emission of gas or coal heaters, indoor use of charcoal, and smoke and fumes. The CO binds with hemoglobin, preventing oxygen carriage and impairing oxygen delivery to tissue.

Diagnosis includes history, on-site oximetry reports, neurological examination, and CO neuropsychological screening battery (CONSB) done with patient breathing room air, CBC, electrolytes, ABGs, ECG, chest radiograph (for dyspnea); *pulse oximetry is not accurate in these patients.*

Symptoms:

- Cardiac: chest pain, palpitations, decreased capillary refill, hypotension, and cardiac arrest
- CNS: malaise, nausea, vomiting, lethargy, stroke, coma, and seizure
- Secondary injuries: Rhabdomyolysis, AKI, non-cardiogenic pulmonary edema, multiple organ failure (MOF), DIC, and encephalopathy

Treatment includes:

- Immediate support of airway, breathing, and circulation
- Non-barometric oxygen (100%) by non-breathing mask with reservoir or ETT if necessary

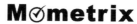

- Mild: Continue oxygen for 4 hours with reassessment
- Severe: hyperbaric oxygen therapy (usually 3 treatments) to improve oxygen delivery

CYANIDE POISONING

Cyanide poisoning, from hydrogen cyanide (HCN) or cyanide salts, can result from sodium nitroprusside infusions, inhalation of burning plastics, intentional or accidental ingestion or dermal exposure, occupation exposure, ingestion of some plant products, and the manufacture of PCP. Inhalation of HCN causes immediate symptoms, and the ingestion of cyanide salts causes symptoms within minutes.

Diagnosis is by history, clinical examination, normal PaO_2 and metabolic acidosis.

Symptoms: Increase in severity and alter with the amount of exposure: tachycardia, hypertension, leading to bradycardia, hypotension, and cardiac arrest. Pink or cherry-colored skin because of oxygen remaining in the blood. Other symptoms include headaches, lethargy, seizures, coma, dyspnea, tachypnea, and respiratory arrest.

Treatment includes:

- Supportive care as indicated
- Removal of contaminated clothes
- Gastric decontamination
- Copious irrigation for topical exposure
- Antidotes:
  - Amyl nitrate ampule cracked and inhaled 30 seconds
  - Sodium nitrite (3%) 10 mL IV
  - Sodium thiosulfate (25%) 50 mL IV

CAUSTIC INGESTIONS

Caustic ingestions of acids (pH <7) such as sulfuric, acetic, hydrochloric, and hydrofluoric found in many cleaning agents and alkalis (pH >7) such as sodium hydroxide, potassium hydroxide, sodium tripolyphosphate (in detergents) and sodium hypochlorite (bleach) can result in severe injury and death. Acids cause coagulation necrosis in the esophagus and stomach and may result in metabolic acidosis, hemolysis, and renal failure if systemically absorbed. Alkali injuries cause liquefaction necrosis, resulting in deeper ulcerations, often of the esophagus, but may involve perforation and abdominal necrosis with multi-organ damage.

Diagnosis is by detailed history, airway examination (oral intubation if possible), arterial blood gas, electrolytes, CBC, hepatic and coagulation tests, radiograph, and CT for perforations.

Symptoms may vary but can include pain, dyspnea, oral burns, dysphonia, and vomiting.

Treatment includes:

- Supportive and symptomatic therapy
- NO ipecac, charcoal, neutralization, or dilution
- NG tube for acids only to aspirate residual
- Endoscopy in first few hours to evaluate injury/perforations
- Sodium bicarbonate for pH <7.10
- Prednisolone (alkali injuries)

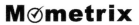

ALLERGIC REACTIONS

Exposure to certain toxins, medications, illegal substances, and allergens can cause life threatening effects in some patients. The physiologic response of the patient is dependent on the agent and the degree of exposure. Tissue hypoperfusion and lactic acidosis often occur as a result of the exposure. This can lead to metabolic acidosis, shock, organ failure, and death.

Signs and symptoms: In allergic type reactions, urticaria, pruritus, chest, back or abdominal pain, facial flushing, shortness of breath, wheezing and stridor may occur. Beta- and alpha-adrenergic responses may occur with exposure to amphetamines, cocaine, ephedrine, and pseudoephedrine. This response is manifested by diaphoresis, hypertension, tachycardia, and mydriasis. Diarrhea, nausea, and vomiting can occur with exposure to certain toxins.

Diagnosis: Physical assessment and testing to discover the toxin, drug, or allergen the patient was exposed to. Labs—blood gases, BMP, complete blood count, toxicology screen, urinalysis, and allergy testing.

Treatment: Priority is to eliminate exposure to the drug/toxin/allergen. Antidotes (if available) may be administered in the case of toxin exposure. Activated charcoal may be administered in the case of medication/drug overdose. For allergic reactions, antihistamines and corticosteroids may be administered. Severe allergic reactions may need to be treated with epinephrine. Dialysis may be indicated in some patients. Sodium bicarbonate may be administered for the treatment of metabolic acidosis caused by many toxic reactions.

ACETAMINOPHEN TOXICITY

Acetaminophen toxicity from accidental or intentional overdose has high rates of morbidity and mortality unless promptly treated. **Diagnosis** is by history and acetaminophen level, which should be completed within 8 hours of ingestion if possible. Toxicity occurs with dosage >140 mg/kg in one dose or >7.5g in 24 hours.

Symptoms occur in stages:

1. (Initial) Minor gastrointestinal upset
2. (Days 2-3) Hepatotoxicity with RUQ pain and increased AST, ALT, and bilirubin
3. (Days 3-4) Hepatic failure with metabolic acidosis, coagulopathy, renal failure, encephalopathy, nausea, vomiting, and possible death
4. (Days 5-12) Recovery period for survivors

Treatment includes:

- GI decontamination with activated charcoal (orally or NG) <24 hours
- Toxicity is plotted on the Rumack-Matthew nomogram with serum levels >150 requiring antidote. The antidote is most effective ≤8 hours of ingestion but decreases hepatotoxicity even >24 hours.
- Antidote: 72-hour N-acetylcysteine (NAC) protocol includes 140 mg/kg initially and 70 mg/kg every 4 hours for 17 more doses (orally or IV)
- Supportive therapy: Continuous dialysis, fluids, blood pressure medications

AMPHETAMINE AND COCAINE TOXICITY

Amphetamine toxicity may be caused by IV, inhalation, or insufflation of various substances that include methamphetamine (MDA or "ecstasy"), methylphenidate (Ritalin), methylenedioxymethamphetamine (MDMA), and ephedrine and phenylpropanolamine. Cocaine may be ingested orally, IV or by insufflation while crack cocaine may be smoked. Amphetamines and cocaine are CNS stimulants that can cause multi-system abnormalities.

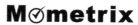

Symptoms may include chest pain, dysrhythmias, myocardial ischemia, MI, seizures, intracranial infarctions, hypertension, dystonia, repetitive movements, unilateral blindness, lethargy, rhabdomyolysis with acute kidney failure, perforated nasal septum (cocaine), and paranoid psychosis (amphetamines). Crack cocaine may cause pulmonary hemorrhage, asthma, pulmonary edema, barotrauma, and pneumothorax. Swallowing packs of cocaine can cause intestinal ischemia, colitis, necrosis, and perforation. **Diagnosis** includes clinical findings, CBC, chemistry panel, toxicology screening, ECG, and radiography.

Treatment includes:

- Gastric emptying (<1 hour). Charcoal administration
- IV access. Supplemental oxygen
- Sedation for seizures: Lorazepam 2 mg, diazepam 5 mg IV titrated in repeated doses
- Agitation: Haloperidol
- Hypertension: Nitroprusside/nicardipine, phentolamine IV
- Cocaine quinidine-like effects: Sodium bicarbonate

SALICYLATE TOXICITY

Salicylate toxicity may be acute or chronic and is caused by ingestion of OTC drugs containing salicylates, such as ASA, Pepto-Bismol, and products used in hot inhalers.

Diagnosis is by ferric chloride or Ames Phenistix tests. Symptoms vary according to age and amount of ingestion. Co-ingestion of sedatives may alter symptoms.

Symptoms include:

- <150 mg/kg: Nausea and vomiting
- 150-300 mg/kg: Vomiting, hyperpnea, diaphoresis, tinnitus, and alterations in acid-base balance
- >300 mg/kg (usually intentional overdose): Nausea, vomiting, diaphoresis, tinnitus, hyperventilation, respiratory alkalosis, and metabolic acidosis
- Chronic toxicity results in hyperventilation, tremor, and papilledema, alterations in mental status, pulmonary edema, seizures, and coma

Treatment includes:

- Gastric decontamination with lavage (≤1 hour) and charcoal
- Volume replacement (D5W)
- Sodium bicarbonate 1-2 mEq/kg
- Monitoring of salicylate concentration, acid-base, and electrolytes every hour
- Whole-bowel irrigation (sustained release tablets)

BENZODIAZEPINE TOXICITY

Benzodiazepine toxicity may result from accidental or intentional overdose with such drugs as Xanax, Librium, Valium, Ativan, Serax, Versed, and Restoril. Mortality is usually the result of co-ingestion of other drugs.

Diagnosis is based on history and clinical exam, as benzodiazepine level does not correlate well with toxicity.

Symptoms: Non-specific neurological changes: Lethargy, dizziness, alterations in consciousness, and ataxia. Respiratory depression and hypotension are rare complications. Coma and severe central nervous depression are usually caused by co-ingestions.

Treatment includes:

- Gastric emptying (<1 hour)
- Charcoal
- Concentrated dextrose, thiamine, and naloxone if co-ingestions suspected, especially with altered mental status
- Monitoring for CNS/respiratory depression
- Supportive care
- Flumazenil (antagonist) 0.2 mg each minute to total 3 mg may be used in some cases but not routinely advised because of complications related to benzodiazepine dependency or co-ingestion of cyclic antidepressants. Flumazenil is contraindicated in patients with increased ICP.

ETHANOL OVERDOSE

Ethanol overdose affects the central nervous system as well as other organs in the body. Alcohol is an inhibitory neurotransmitter that depresses the central nervous system. In most states, the legal intoxication blood alcohol level is defined as 100 mg/dL. Blood alcohol levels of **500 mg/dL or greater** are associated with a high mortality rate. The central nervous system depressant effect is further enhanced when alcohol is mixed with other agents.

Ethanol is absorbed through the mucosa of the mouth, stomach, and intestines, with concentrations peaking about 30-60 minutes after ingestion. If people are easily aroused, they can usually safely sleep off the effects of ingesting too much alcohol, but if the person is semi-conscious or unconscious, emergency medical treatment should be initiated.

Symptoms include:

- Altered mental status with slurred speech and stupor
- Nausea and vomiting
- Hypotension
- Bradycardia with arrhythmias
- Respiratory depression and hypoxia
- Cold, clammy skin or flushed skin (from vasodilation)
- Acute pancreatitis with abdominal pain
- Lack of consciousness
- Circulatory collapse

Treatment includes:

- Careful monitoring of arterial blood gases and oxygen saturation
- Ensure patent airway with intubation and ventilation if necessary
- Intravenous fluids
- Dextrose to correct hypoglycemia if indicated
- Maintain body temperature (warming blanket)
- Dialysis may be necessary in severe cases

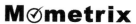

GASTRIC EMPTYING FOR TOXIC SUBSTANCE INGESTION

Gastric emptying for toxic substance ingestion should be done ≤60 minutes of ingestion for large life-threatening amounts of poison. The patient requires IV access, oximetry, and cardiac monitoring. Sedation (1-2 mg IV midazolam) or rapid sequence induction and endotracheal intubation may be necessary. Patients should be positioned in left lateral decubitus position with head down at 20° to prevent passage of stomach contents into duodenum, although intubated patients may be lavaged in the supine position. With a bite block in place, an orogastric Y-tube (36-40 Fr. for adults) should be inserted after estimating length. Placement should be confirmed with injection of 50 mL of air confirmed under auscultation and aspiration of gastric contents, as well as abdominal x-ray (pH may not be reliable depending on substance ingested). Irrigation is done by gravity instillation of about 200-300 mL warmed (45 °C) tap water or NS. The instillation side is clamped and drainage side opened. This is repeated until fluid returns clear. A slurry of charcoal is then instilled, and the tube is clamped and removed when procedures completed.

TOXIC EXPOSURES IN CHILDREN

Children may be exposed to a wide range of **toxic exposures**. Contaminants can include toxins (produced by organisms) and toxicants (natural or synthetic chemicals). Contaminants are often produced by industry but may also be disseminated through acts of terrorism. Some types of exposure, such as from radiation, may have long-term effects not evident after initial exposure. Children tend to be more vulnerable to toxic exposures than adults. Risk factors for toxic exposures include:

- Parental employment with toxic substances
- Home built before 1978 or with recent renovations
- Lack of adequate safety alarms for radon, carbon monoxide, and smoke
- Pica

Environmental toxic exposures can include pesticides, outdoor pollution (smoke, emissions), and indoor pollution (mold, lead, wood smoke, cigarette smoke). Children may develop toxic reactions from breastfeeding, skin contact, inhalation, or ingestion of contaminated food and fluids. Symptoms vary depending on the agent, but usually occur within 2 hours.

LEAD TOXICITY

Normal values for lead are as follows:

- Whole blood: Less than 10 mcg/dL
- Urine: Less than 80 mcg/dL

Children at risk for **lead toxicity** may have lead levels checked through a blood test. Normal values for lead levels among children are less than 10 mcg/dL. Children at risk of lead toxicity include those who live in older homes that may have lead-based paint or plumbing; lead can also be found in soil, batteries, items made from pewter, and in the paint of some toys. Children can develop lead toxicity if they ingest any materials, dust, or water that has been exposed to lead. Lead toxicity causes complications associated with memory and learning, decreased attention span, and chronic problems with nerves, muscles, and kidneys.

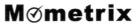

LEAD POISONING

Lead poisoning occurs with serum levels >10µg/dL although some children may experience cognitive impairment at lower levels. Lead poisoning is especially dangerous for developing children ages <7 because it interferes with normal cell function, especially in the nervous system, blood cells, and kidneys. **Treatment** involves removing the source of lead and providing chelation therapy for levels >25 µg/dL. Agents used for chelation include calcium disodium ethylenediamine tetraacetate (CaNa2 EDTA), dimercaprol (BAL), d-penicillamine, or succimer (DMSA), usually for 5-7 days and then repeated. Classification of lead exposure/poisoning is as follows:

Class	Serum Level	Signs and Symptoms
Class I	<9 µg/dL	Usually asymptomatic or slight neurological deficits
Class II A	10-14 µg/dL	Anemia; mild cognitive, growth, and fine motor impairment
Class II B	15-19 µg/dL	Same as Class II A
Class III	20-44 µg/dL	Anemia, fatigue, difficulty concentrating, headache, motor impairment, tremors, paresis, paralysis, abdominal pain, nausea, vomiting, constipation, weight loss
Class IV	45-69 µg/dL	Anorexia, vomiting, severe intermittent abdominal cramping, hyperirritability, increased lethargy, blue-black lead line on gums
Class V	>70 µg/dL	Encephalopathy, ataxia, seizures, coma, death

ANIMAL BITES

Animal bites, including human, are frequent causes of traumatic injury. There is not a single preferred topical therapy for traumatic wounds because they vary so widely in the type and degree of injury.

General treatment includes:

- **Cleanse** wound by flushing with 10 to 35 cc syringe with 18-gauge Angiocath to remove debris and bacteria using normal saline or diluted Betadine solution.
- Hand, puncture, and infected wounds or those more than 12 hours old may be closed by **secondary intention**.
- **Moisture-retentive dressings** are used as indicated by the size and extent of the wound left open. Dry dressings may be applied to injuries with closure by primary intention.
- **Topical antibiotics** may be indicated, although systemic antibiotics are commonly prescribed for animal bites.
- **Tetanus toxoid** or **immune globulin** is routinely administered.

SPIDER BITES

Spider bites are frequently a misdiagnosis of a *Staphylococcus aureus* or MRSA infection, so unless the spider was observed, the wound should be cultured and antibiotics started. If the wound responds to the antibiotic, then it probably was not a spider bite. There are two main types of venomous spider bites:

- Those producing **neurological symptoms** (black widow).
- Those producing **local necrosis** (brown recluse, yellow sac, and hobo spiders).

General treatment includes:

- Cleanse wound, apply cool compress, and elevate body part if possible.

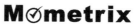

Treatment for black widow bites:

- Narcotic analgesics.
- Nitroprusside to relieve hypertension.
- Calcium gluconate 10% solution IV for abdominal cramps.
- Antivenin *Latrodectus mactans* for those with severe reaction.

Treatment for necrotic/ulcerated bites (e.g., brown recluse):

- There is no consensus on the best treatment, as ulceration caused by the venom may be extensive and **surgical repair** with grafts may be needed.
- Necrotic ulcers should be treated **moisture-retentive dressings** as indicated, and monitored for complications.
- **Hyperbaric oxygen therapy** (HBOT) has been used in some cases.

SNAKE BITES

About 45,000 snake bites occur in the United States each year, with about 8,000 from poisonous snakes. In the United States, about 25 species of snakes are venomous. There are two types of snakes that can cause serious injury, classified according to the type of fangs and venom.

CORAL SNAKES

Coral snakes have short fixed permanent fangs in the upper jaw and venom that is primarily neurotoxic, but may also have hemotoxic and cardiotoxic properties:

- Wounds show no fang marks but there may be scratches or semi-circular markings from the teeth.
- There may be little local reaction, but neurological symptoms may range from mild to acute respiratory and cardiovascular failure.

Treatment includes the following:

- Cleanse the wound thoroughly of dirt and debris and either leave it open to air or cover it with a dry dressing.
- Administer antivenin immediately even without symptoms, which may be delayed.
- Administer tetanus toxoid or immune globulin.
- Antibiotics are not usually indicated.

PIT VIPERS

A second type of snake that can cause serious injury is the pit viper. Pit vipers (**rattlesnakes, copperheads, and cottonmouths)** have erectile fangs that fold until they are aroused, and venom is primarily hemotoxic and cytotoxic but may also have neurotoxic properties:

- Wounds usually show one or two fang marks.
- Edema may begin immediately or may be delayed up to six hours.
- Pain may be severe.
- There may be a wide range of symptoms, including hypotension and coagulopathy with defibrination that can lead to excessive blood loss, depending upon the type and amount of venom.
- There may be local infection and necrosis.

Treatment includes the following:

- Cleanse the wound thoroughly and apply dressings as indicated.
- Administer tetanus toxoid or immune globulin.
- Administer analgesics, such as morphine sulphate, as needed.

41

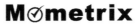

- Avoid NSAIDs and aspirin because of anticoagulation properties.
- Mark edema every 15 minutes.
- Administer antivenin therapy if indicated. Observe for serum sickness if horse serum used.
- Administer prophylactic antibiotics for severe tissue necrosis.
- Administer platelets, plasma, or packed RBCs for coagulopathy.

SHARK BITES

Even small shark bites can crush bones. Hit and run attacks may cause small lacerations or minimal damage, but other types of attacks can result in loss of limbs or large chunks of flesh, with loss of muscle and bone. Internal organs may be exposed and damaged. Extensive soft tissue trauma and damage to arteries and veins may occur, as well as crushing internal injuries. The wounds are often contaminated with sand, algae, fragments of shark teeth, and other materials and pathogens, such as *Mycobacterium marinum* and *Vibrio spp.* Life-threatening injuries need to be addressed first, including control of hemorrhage:

- Administer IV fluids and blood products.
- Administer tetanus toxoid or tetanus immune globulin.
- Wounds must be flushed with copious amounts of normal saline and debris removed.
- Treat for hypothermia if needed.
- X-rays are ordered to identify fractures or debris in wound.
- Fixation of fractures.
- Administer prophylactic antibiotics:
  o Ciprofloxacin
  o Trimethoprim-sulfamethoxazole
  o Doxycycline
- Surgical repair, debridement, and/or skin grafting if indicated.

ALLIGATOR BITES

Alligators are found in ten coastal states in the southeastern United States with the largest population in Florida, where most injuries are reported. Animals between four and eight feet often bite once and release, but larger animals may bite repeatedly, engaging in typical biting and feeding activities, which result in severe injury, amputations, or death. Most wounds involve the limbs, with the hands and arms the most frequently bitten.

Treatment includes:

- Treat for shock and blood loss.
- Apply pressure to wound.
- Retrieve amputated limbs if possible.
- Flush wound(s) with copious amounts of normal saline to reduce contamination.
- Collect wound cultures.
- Administer prophylactic broad-spectrum antibiotics for gram-negative organisms, such as *Aeromonas hydrophila* and *Clostridium.*
- Observe for signs of infection, such as erythema, cellulitis, exudate, and necrosis.
- Administer tetanus toxoid or immune globulin.
- Repair fractures.
- Surgical repair and debridement as indicated, with wounds usually healing by secondary intention or delayed primary closure.

STINGRAY STINGS

Stingrays can induce injury when their tail is thrust forward, driving serrated spines into the victim, resulting in a jagged laceration. The spines of the stingray tail contain a venom that is injected upon impact, causing severe pain. The resulting wounds often become infected.

Symptoms include:

- Intense, excruciating pain with envenomation lasting two to three days.
- Bleeding.
- Systemic symptoms: Dizziness, GI upset, seizures, hypotension.

Treatment includes the following:

- **Rinse** the wound with fresh water or saline and remove visible pieces of spine with forceps or tweezers.
- **Heat immersion**: Deactivate the venom and relieve pain by immersing the wound in hot water for 30 to 90 minutes at 110-115°F (45°C). May repeat up to 2 hours.
- **Radiographs** may be necessary to locate the spine or fragment.
- Administer tetanus toxoid or tetanus immune globulin.
- Inject the wound with a **local anesthetic**, such as lidocaine or bupivacaine, to relieve severe pain.
- Administer **opiates** for pain.
- **Open wounds** are usually allowed to heal without primary closure or with loose primary closure.
- **Prophylactic antibiotics** may be given for five days to prevent infections.

INSECT STINGS AND BITES
BEE STINGS

Bees and wasps sting by puncturing the skin with a hollow stinger and injecting venom. Wasps and bumblebees can sting more than once but honeybees have barbs on their stingers, and the barbs embed the stinger into the skin. **Local reactions** to bee sting include the following:

- Raised white **wheal** with central red spot of about 10 mm appearing within a few minutes and lasting 20 minutes (honeybees).
- **Edema and erythema**, which may last several days (vespid wasps).
- Pain, swelling, and redness confined to sting site.
- Swelling may extend **beyond the sting site** and may, for example, involve swelling of an entire limb.

Some people may develop an anaphylactic reaction, including a **biphasic reaction**, in which the symptoms recede and then return two to three hours later. About 50% of deaths occur within 30 minutes of the sting, and 75% within four hours.

Symptoms of an allergic reaction/anaphylaxis may become increasingly severe with generalized urticaria, edema, hypotension, and respiratory distress.

Treatment of bee stings initially includes the following:

- Wash the site with soap and water.
- Remove stinger using 4 x 4 inch gauze wiped over the area or by scraping a sharp instrument over the area.
- NEVER squeeze the stinger or use tweezers, as this will cause more venom to go into the skin.
- Apply ice to reduce the swelling (10 to 20 minutes on, 10 to 20 minutes off, for 24 hours).
- Antihistamines may be prescribed.
- A paste of baking soda and water or meat tenderizer and water may reduce itching.

- Topical corticosteroids may relieve itching.
- Administer tetanus toxoid or tetanus immune globulin as needed.

Allergic responses/anaphylaxis requires immediate, aggressive medical intervention:

- Administer epinephrine.
- Administer antihistamines.
- Administer corticosteroids.
- Administer IV fluids as needed.
- Provide oxygen and other supportive treatments.

People with extensive local or anaphylactic reactions should be advised to carry an epinephrine autoinjector for emergency use if stung.

SCORPION STINGS

Symptoms

- Note: Children <6 are most at risk of death from severe reactions. Symptoms vary widely depending on individual reaction and amount of venom.
- **Local (most common):** Neurotoxic effects include itching, redness, edema, and ascending hyperesthesia. Tap test: Paresthesia worsens if area tapped.
- **Cytotoxic effects** include development of macule or papule within an hour. Purpuric plaque becomes necrotic and ulcerates and venom spreads through the lymph system.
- **Nonlethal response** includes pain, induration, redness, and wheal.
- **Neurologic**: Severe wide-ranging symptoms include strokes, altered consciousness, muscle rigidity, paralysis, and seizures.
- **Multiple organ:** Can include hypertension, tachycardia, respiratory distress, generalized allergic response, dysphagia, hepatitis, priapism, acute tubular necrosis, DIC, hyperglycemia, lactic acidosis.

Treatment

- Note: Meperidine and morphine may potentiate symptoms.
- Hospital admission for 24 hours unless symptoms very mild.
- Cool compresses, acetaminophen, topical anesthetics for pain.
- Tetanus toxoid or tetanus immune globulin as needed.
- Antivenom (available only for Centruroides).
- Complex supportive care may include intubation and ventilation.

FIRE ANT BITES

Symptoms

- Note: Multiple bites, sometimes hundreds, are common. Deaths are rare but do occur if children have a severe systemic reaction or bites about the head and neck.
- **Local reaction:** A severely itching wheal develops and subsides in 30–60 minutes, followed by a blister within 4 hours. The blister fills with milky dead tissue in 8 to 24 hours with redness at base and severe itching and burning. The blister ruptures and crusts over within 72 hours but redness pain and itching may persist for days.
- **Systemic reaction**: Edema, urticaria, nausea, vomiting, bronchospasm, dyspnea, slurred speech, anaphylaxis.

Treatment

- **Local reaction**: Cold compresses, weak bleach solution (within 15 minutes of bites), or topical anesthetic for pain. Cleanse with soap and water without breaking blisters. NSAIDS for pain. Topical corticosteroids for itching. Antihistamines. Tetanus toxoid or tetanus immune globulin as needed.
- **Systemic reaction**: As for anaphylaxis, depending on degree of symptoms, including epinephrine.

HUMAN BITES

Human "bites" occur when the teeth of one person injure another. This is not uncommon in contact sports. Intentional biting is common among children but usually presents mild injury. Human bites may also be the result of altercations and are referred to as "fist-bites." There are 3 common **types** of fist-bites:

- Closed fist bite resulting in small wound on the metacarpophalangeal joint of the middle finger. Bacteria enter the wound when the person extends the fingers, carrying bacteria to the extensor tendons, which can result in infection.
- Finger bite in which a finger may be partially or completely severed
- Puncture bite, usually on the face, from contact with another person's tooth

Immediate treatment of bites includes applying pressure to stop bleeding and then thoroughly flushing the wound with dilute Betadine, dilute peroxide, or normal saline solution. Protective dressings should be applied. Large wounds or those with skin flaps or signs of more serious tissue injury may require surgical repair.

RISK ANALYSIS AS PART OF DISEASE PREVENTION

Risk analysis is an important part of health promotion and disease prevention because it can help to identify those factors (normed for age and sex) that put a child at risk for current or future disease. Typically, risk analysis uses observations, interviews, and questionnaires to gain information about a child and their family so that interventions and diagnostic testing can be targeted to areas of increased risk. Risk factors may be controllable (diet and exercise) or non-controllable (genetic), but once identified, a plan of care can be formulated. Risk analysis is an important component of cost-containment because early identification and treatment or intervention can reduce future costs of care. **Areas for risk analysis** may include:

- Nutrition
- Exercise
- Cardiovascular
- Diabetes
- Hypertension
- Cancer
- Osteoporosis
- Vision
- Behavior and lifestyle

Results of risk analysis are not diagnostic, but they indicate if the child is at a low, medium, or high risk of developing a disease or health problem.

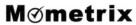

COMPONENTS OF RISK ANALYSIS

Risk analysis can be used to assess individual risks or to assess the risk and effectiveness of different treatments and programs in a broader sense. Risk analysis should be carried out for all new treatments and procedures to determine if the benefits outweigh the risks and if they are cost-effective. Risk analysis should be an ongoing part of the nurse's role. There are three primary **components** to risk analysis:

- **Assessing** requires gaining information by questioning, observing, or analyzing data, which may be derived from active study or review of the research.
- **Intervening** involves taking information from the assessment and making changes in management, treatments, or procedures to reflect the risk analysis with the aim of providing the most beneficial and cost-effective care.
- **Communicating** requires publishing the results or sharing those with the organization, family, child, or the general public, depending on the scope of the risk analysis.

RISK FACTORS FOR NEONATES ASSOCIATED WITH MATERNAL DISEASE

There are a number of **maternal factors** that put the infant at increased risk:

- **Diabetes mellitus**: Both gestational and pre-existing diabetes put the infant at risk of stillbirth, hypoglycemia, and macrosomia (larger size than normal) as well as birth injury. Maternal pre-existing diabetes is also associated with birth defects, including abnormal development of the cardiovascular and gastrointestinal systems, neurological and spinal cord disorders, and urinary tract abnormalities.
- **HIV/Hepatitis B**: Infectious diseases may be transmitted during pregnancy or delivery.

IMPLICATIONS OF FETAL DRUG EXPOSURE

There are many drugs that can profoundly affect the growing fetus. Some are prescribed drugs, such as Accutane, but the greatest numbers are illicit drugs, such as crack, heroin, or cocaine. Increasing numbers of children are born to addicted mothers. While each drug has specific effects, there are many effects that are common with any type of fetal drug exposure:

- Premature weight and low birth weight with infants who are small for gestational age (SGA)
- Failure to thrive often related to poor sucking and dysphagia
- Increased risk of congenital infectious disease (HIV, hepatitis, CMV)
- Increased risk of SIDS
- Withdrawal symptoms typically manifest within 72 hours of birth:
  - Tremors, excitability, seizures
  - Vomiting, diarrhea, diaphoresis
  - Dry, red, irritated skin
- Developmental and cognitive problems that vary with age. Initial problems often subside within the first couple of years, but in a small number of children learning disabilities and behavioral problems persist.

IMPLICATIONS OF FETAL ALCOHOL SYNDROME

Fetal alcohol syndrome (FAS) is a syndrome of birth defects that develop as the result of maternal ingestion of alcohol. Despite campaigns to inform the public, women continue to drink during pregnancy, but no safe amount of alcohol ingestion has been determined. FAS results in:

- **Facial abnormalities**: Hypoplastic (underdeveloped) maxilla, micrognathia (undersized jaw), hypoplastic philtrum (groove beneath the nose), and short palpebral fissures (eye slits between upper and lower lids).

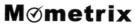

- **Neurological deficits**: May include microcephaly, intellectual disability, motor delay, and hearing deficits. Learning disorders may include problems with visual-spatial and verbal learning, attention disorders, and delayed reaction times.
- **Growth retardation**: Prenatal growth deficit persists with slow growth after birth.
- **Behavioral problems**: Irritability and hyperactivity. Poor judgment in behavior may relate to deficit in executive functions.

Indication of brain damage without the associated physical abnormalities is referred to as alcohol-related neurodevelopmental disorder (ARND).

INFANT WITHDRAWAL FROM FETAL EXPOSURE TO DRUGS

Fetal exposure to drugs, such as opioids, methadone, cocaine, crack, and other recreational drugs causes **withdrawal symptoms** in about 60% of infants. There are many variables, which include the type of drug, the extent of drug use, and the duration of maternal drug use. For example, children may have withdrawal symptoms within 48 hours for cocaine, heroin, and methamphetamine exposure, but there may be delays of up to 2-3 weeks for methadone. Short hospital stays after birth make it imperative that children who are at risk are identified so that they can receive supportive treatment, particularly since they often feed poorly and can quickly become dehydrated and undernourished. Polydrug use makes it difficult to describe a typical profile of **symptoms**, but they usually include:

- Tremors
- Irritability
- Hypertonicity
- High-pitched crying
- Diarrhea
- Dry skin
- Seizures (in severe cases)

Treatment is supportive, but children with opiate exposure may be given decreasing doses of opiates, such as morphine elixir, with close monitoring until the child is weaned off of the medication.

FETAL NICOTINE/CARBON MONOXIDE EXPOSURE

About 25% of women who smoke regularly before becoming pregnant continue to smoke throughout pregnancy, and others are exposed to second-hand smoke, putting the fetus at risk for a number of abnormalities from **exposure to nicotine and carbon monoxide**:

- Fetal growth retardation with damage to neurotransmitters accompanied by nervous system cell death with concomitant damage to peripheral autonomic nervous system
- Vasoconstriction from nicotine and interference with oxygen transport caused by carbon monoxide can lead to fetal hypoxia
- Vasoconstriction leading to increased risk of spontaneous abortion, prematurity, and low birth weight
- Increased risk for perinatal death and SIDS
- Cognitive deficiency and learning disorders, such as auditory processing defects (Children of mothers who smoke have a 50% increase in idiopathic intellectual disability.)
- Increased cancer risk, especially for acute lymphocytic leukemia and lymphoma

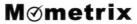

RISK FACTORS FOR INFANTS OR CHILDREN RELATED TO POVERTY

Poverty places children at increased risk of stress disorders and disease, especially if the children are homeless. The following problems are common:

- **Incomplete or no immunizations** because of a lack of health care and regular well-baby or child visits.
- **Frequent infections**, such as respiratory infections or skin infections, because of lack of adequate shelter, living in close quarters, and lack of adequate hygiene.
- **Insufficient sleep**, especially if children are sleeping in cars, on the ground, or in shelters.
- **Nutritional deficiencies** because of poor diet.
- **Dental caries** because of poor nutrition and lack of dental care or lack of toothbrushing supplies.
- **Depression** is common in all ages.
- **Sexual abuse, pregnancies, and sexually transmitted infections** are frequent, especially with homeless teenagers.
- **Injuries** from lack of safety equipment or dangers of the street.

RISK REDUCTION FOR CHILDREN WITH DIABETES

There has been a marked increase in **diabetes mellitus** in children, correlating with increasing obesity and lack of exercise. This is especially true for minority children. Until recent years, Type I (insulin-dependent) diabetes was most common in children and Type II was rare, but now 8-45% of children presenting with diabetes have Type II (insulin deficiency), although it may be difficult to determine the type with initial diagnosis. Most cases are diagnosed during puberty when hormone changes affect insulin, but children with Type II as young as 4 have been identified. Since obesity is a significant risk, health risk reduction efforts are aimed at improving diet and increasing exercise, but intervention aimed at the whole family is often more effective than tailoring diet and exercise just to the needs of the child. The family should work with a nutritionist. Screening with fasting blood sugar is normally done about every 2 years for those at risk or presenting with symptoms.

CARDIOVASCULAR RISK REDUCTION

Some children are at increased risk of developing **cardiovascular disease**, such as coronary artery disease, including those with diabetes mellitus, Kawasaki disease, and familial hypercholesterolemia, which can lead to severe coronary artery disease in less than ten years from onset. Screening children at risk should begin at age 2 and include cholesterol levels to assess for an elevation of low-density lipoprotein (LDL):

- Total cholesterol <170 and LDL <110: Normal level
- Total cholesterol 170-199 and LDL 110-120: Borderline elevation
- Total cholesterol >200 with LDL >130: Elevated

Early dietary intervention to reduce cholesterol and prevent increase in LDLs can significantly reduce morbidity and mortality. Dietary recommendations to reduce LDLs include guidelines provided in the *Therapeutic Lifestyle Changes* diet created by the National Institutes of Health for those at risk or with elevated cholesterol.

- 25-30% of diet should be from fat and <7% from saturated fat
- 10-25 g of soluble fiber per day
- <200 mg dietary cholesterol per day
- ≥2 g of plant sterols or stanols per day (found in vegetables, fruits, and nuts)
- 30 minutes of moderate to vigorous exercise per day

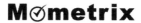

Collaboration and Referral

SKILLS NEEDED FOR COLLABORATION

Nurses must learn the set of skills needed for collaboration in order to move nursing forward. Nurses must take an active role in gathering data for evidence-based practice to support nursing's role in health care, and they must share this information with other nurses and health professionals in order to plan staffing levels and to provide optimal care to patients. Increased and adequate staffing has consistently been shown to reduce adverse outcomes, but there is a well-documented shortage of nurses in the United States, and more than half currently work outside the hospital setting. Increased patient loads not only increase adverse outcomes but also increase job dissatisfaction and burnout. In order to manage the challenges facing nursing, nurses must develop the following skills needed for collaboration:

- Be willing to compromise
- Communicate clearly
- Identify specific challenges and problems
- Focus on the task
- Work with teams

COMMUNICATION SKILLS

Collaboration requires a number of communication skills that differ from those involved in communication between nurse and patient. These skills include:

- **Using an assertive approach**: It's important for the nurse to honestly express opinions and to state them clearly and with confidence, but the nurse must do so in a calm, non-threatening manner.
- **Making casual conversation**: It's easier to communicate with people with whom one has a personal connection. Asking open-ended questions, asking about others' work, or commenting on someone's contributions helps to establish a relationship. The time before meetings, during breaks, and after meetings presents an opportunity for this type of conversation.
- **Being competent in public speaking**: Collaboration requires that a nurse be comfortable speaking and presenting ideas to groups of people. Speaking and presenting ideas competently also helps the nurse to gain credibility. Public speaking is a skill that must be practiced.
- **Communicating in writing**: The written word remains a critical component of communication, and the nurse should be able to communicate clearly and grammatically.

COMMUNICATION AND HAND OFFS

The nurse is usually the primary staff member responsible for **external and internal hand off transitions of care**, and should ensure that communication is thorough and covers all essential information. The best method is to use a standardized format:

- **DRAW**: Diagnosis, recent changes, anticipated changes, and what to watch for.
- **I PASS the BATON**: Introduction, patient, assessment, situation, safety concerns, background, actions, timing, ownership, and next.
- **ANTICipate**: Administrative data, new clinical information, tasks, illness severity, contingency plans.
- **5 Rs**: Record, review, round together, relay to team, and receive feedback.

A reporting **form** or checklist may be utilized to ensure that no aspect is overlooked.

For external transitions, the nurse must ensure that the type of transport team and monitoring is appropriate for patient needs, and provide insight when determining the most appropriate mode of transportation: ground transfer for short distance, helicopter for medium to long distance, and fixed-wing aircraft for long distances.

SBAR TECHNIQUE

The SBAR technique is used to hand-off a patient from one caregiver to another to provide a systematic method so that important information is conveyed:

- **(S) Situation**: Overview of current situation and important issues
- **(B) Background**: Important history and issues leading to current situation
- **(A) Assessment**: Summary of important facts and condition
- **(R) Recommendation**: Actions needed

COLLABORATION BETWEEN NURSE AND PATIENT/FAMILY

One of the most important forms of collaboration is that between the nurse and the patient/family, but this type of collaboration is often overlooked. Nurses and others in the healthcare team must always remember that the point of collaboration is to improve patient care, and this means that the patient and patient's family must remain central to all planning. For example, including family in planning for a patient takes time initially, but sitting down and asking the patient and family, "What do you want?" and using the Synergy model to evaluate patient's (and family's) characteristics can provide valuable information that saves time in the long run and facilitates planning and expenditure of resources. Families, and even young children, often want to participate in care and planning and feel validated and more positive toward the medical system when they are included.

COLLABORATION WITH EXTERNAL AGENCIES

The nurse must initiate and facilitate collaboration with external agencies because many have direct impacts on patient care and needs:

- **Industry** can include other facilities sharing interests in patient care or pharmaceutical companies. It's important for nursing to have a dialog with drug companies about their products and how they are used in specific populations because many medications are prescribed to women, children, or the aged without validating studies for dose or efficacy.
- **Payers** have a vested interest in containing health care costs, so providing information and representing the interests of the patient is important.
- **Community groups** may provide resources for patients and families, both in terms of information and financial or other assistance.
- **Political agencies** are increasingly important as new laws are considered about nurse-patient ratios and infection control in many states.
- **Public health agencies** are partners in health care with other facilities and must be included, especially in issues related to communicable disease.

INTERDISCIPLINARY TEAMS

There are a number of skills that are needed to lead and facilitate coordination of **intra- and inter-disciplinary teams**:

- Communicating openly is essential. All members must be encouraged to participate as valued members of a cooperative team.
- Avoiding interrupting or interpreting the point another is trying to make allows free flow of ideas.
- Avoiding jumping to conclusions, which can effectively shut off communication.
- Active listening requires paying attention and asking questions for clarification rather than to challenge other's ideas.
- Respecting others' opinions and ideas, even when opposed to one's own, is absolutely essential.
- Reacting and responding to facts rather than feelings allows one to avoid angry confrontations and diffuse anger.

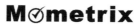

- Clarifying information or opinions stated can help avoid misunderstandings.
- Keeping unsolicited advice out of the conversation shows respect for others and allows them to solicit advice without feeling pressured.

LEADERSHIP STYLES

Leadership styles often influence the perception of leadership values and commitment to collaboration. There are a number of different leadership styles:

- **Charismatic**: Relies on personal charisma to influence people, and may be very persuasive, but this type leader may engage followers and relate to one group rather than the organization at large, limiting effectiveness.
- **Bureaucratic**: Follows organization rules exactly and expects everyone else to do so. This is most effective in handling cash flow or managing work in dangerous work environments. This type of leadership may engender respect but may not be conducive to change.
- **Autocratic**: Makes decisions independently and strictly enforces rules. Team members often feel left out of process and may not be supportive of the decisions that are made. This type of leadership is most effective in crisis situations, but may have difficulty gaining the commitment of staff.
- **Consultative**: Presents a decision and welcomes input and questions, although decisions rarely change. This type of leadership is most effective when gaining the support of staff is critical to the success of proposed changes.
- **Participatory**: Presents a potential decision and then makes final decision based on input from staff or teams. This type of leadership is time-consuming and may result in compromises that are not entirely satisfactory to management or staff, but this process is motivating to staff who feel their expertise is valued.
- **Democratic**: Presents a problem and asks staff or teams to arrive at a solution, although the leader usually makes the final decision. This type of leadership may delay decision-making, but staff and teams are often more committed to the solutions because of their input.
- **Laissez-faire ("free reign")**: Exerts little direct control but allows employees/teams to make decisions with little interference. This may be effective leadership if teams are highly skilled and motivated, but in many cases, this type of leadership is the product of poor management skills and little is accomplished because of this lack of leadership.

TEAM BUILDING

Leading, facilitating, and participating in performance improvement teams requires a thorough understanding of the dynamics of team building:

- **Initial interactions**: This is the time when members begin to define their roles and develop relationships, determining if they are comfortable in the group.
- **Power issues**: The members observe the leader and determine who controls the meeting and how control is exercised, beginning to form alliances.
- **Organizing**: Methods to achieve work are clarified and team members begin to work together, gaining respect for each other's contributions and working toward a common goal.
- **Team identification**: Interactions often become less formal as members develop rapport, and members are more willing to help and support each other to achieve goals.
- **Excellence**: This develops through a combination of good leadership, committed team members, clear goals, high standards, external recognition, spirit of collaboration, and a shared commitment to the process.

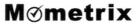

TEAM MEETINGS

Leading and facilitating improvement teams requires utilizing good techniques for meetings. Considerations include:

- **Scheduling**: Both the time and the place must be convenient and conducive to working together, so the leader must review the work schedules of those involved, finding the most convenient time. Venues or meeting rooms should allow for sitting in a circle or around a table to facilitate equal exchange of ideas. Any necessary technology, such as computers or overhead projectors, or other equipment, such as whiteboards, should be available.
- **Preparation**: The leader should prepare a detailed agenda that includes a list of items for discussion.
- **Conduction**: Each item of the agenda should be discussed, soliciting input from all group members. Tasks should be assigned to individual members based on their interest and part in the process in preparation for the next meeting. The leader should summarize input and begin a tentative future agenda.
- **Observation**: The leader should observe the interactions, including verbal and nonverbal communication, and respond to them.

COMMON VISION

Facilitating the creation of a common vision for care within the healthcare system begins with the organization/facility, working collaboratively to create teams and an organization focused on serving the patient/family. A common vision should be the ideal in any organization, but achieving such a goal requires a true collaborative effort:

- Inclusion of all levels of staff across the organization/facility, both those in nursing and non-nursing positions
- Consensus building through discussions, inservice, and team meetings to bring about convergence of diverse viewpoints
- Facilitation that values creativity and provides encouragement during the process
- Vision statement incorporating the common vision that is accessible to all staff
- Recognition that a common vision is an organic concept that may evolve over time and should be reevaluated regularly and changed as needed to reflect the needs of the organization, patients, families, and staff

FACILITATING CHANGE

Performance improvement processes cannot occur without organizational change, and resistance to change is common for many people, so coordinating collaborative processes requires anticipating resistance and taking steps to achieve cooperation. Resistance often relates to concerns about job loss, increased responsibilities, and general denial or lack of understanding and frustration. Leaders can prepare others involved in the process of change by taking these steps:

- Be honest, informative, and tactful, giving people thorough information about anticipated changes and how the changes will affect them, including positives.
- Be patient in allowing people the time they need to contemplate changes and express anger or disagreement.
- Be empathetic in listening carefully to the concerns of others.
- Encourage participation, allowing staff to propose methods of implementing change, so they feel some sense of ownership.
- Establish a climate in which all staff members are encouraged to identify the need for change on an ongoing basis.
- Present further ideas for change to management.

CONFLICT RESOLUTION

Conflict is an almost inevitable product of teamwork, and the leader must assume responsibility for conflict resolution. While conflicts can be disruptive, they can produce positive outcomes by opening dialogue and forcing team members to listen to different perspectives. The team should make a plan for dealing with conflict. The best time for conflict resolution is when differences emerge but before open conflict and hardening of positions occur. The leader must pay close attention to the people and problems involved, listen carefully, and reassure those involved that their points of view are understood. Steps to conflict resolution include:

- Allow both sides to present their side of conflict without bias, maintaining a focus on opinions rather than individuals.
- Encourage cooperation through negotiation and compromise.
- Maintain the focus, providing guidance to keep the discussions on track and avoid arguments.
- Evaluate the need for re-negotiation, formal resolution process, or third-party involvement.
- Utilize humor and empathy to diffuse escalating tensions.
- Summarize the issues, outlining key arguments.
- Avoid forcing resolution if possible.

IDENTIFYING THE NEED FOR PATIENT REFERRAL

Issues to consider when making patient referrals include:

- **Necessity**: The referral may be needed if the patient's needs are outside of the provider's scope or practice or field of expertise and if the provider cannot provide adequate assessment and treatment for the patient's condition.
- **Insurance requirements**: The provider should determine whether the patient's carrier requires preauthorization or other steps to make sure the patient's referral is covered.
- **Selection of specialist/therapist**: The specialist, in many cases, must be selected from a group of physicians who are participating in an insurance plan if the service is to be covered completely or at all by the insurance company. When possible, the patient should be given choice of referrals.
- **Submission**: The referral should be sent along with appropriate records and releases. The provider may need to make personal contact if specialists are selective, have waiting lists, and may not approve a referral.

FIVE RIGHTS OF DELEGATION

Prior to delegating tasks, the nurse should assess the needs of the patients and determine the task that needs to be completed, assure that he/she can remain accountable and can supervise the task appropriately, and evaluate effective completion. The **5 rights of delegation** include:

- **Right task**: The nurse should determine an appropriate task to delegate for a specific patient. This would not include tasks that require assessment or planning.
- **Right circumstance**: The nurse has considered the setting, resources, time factors, safety factors, and all other relevant information to determine the appropriateness of delegation. A task that is usually in one's scope (such as feeding a patient) may require assessment that makes it inappropriate to delegate (feeding a new stroke patient).
- **Right person**: The nurse is in the right position to choose the right person (by virtue of education/skills) to perform a task for the right patient.
- **Right direction**: The nurse provides a clear description of the task, the purpose, any limits, and expected outcomes.
- **Right supervision**: The nurse is able to supervise, intervene as needed, and evaluate performance of the task.

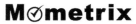

DELEGATION OF TASKS IN TEAMS

On major responsibility of leadership and management in performance improvement teams is using delegation effectively. The purpose of having a team is so that the work is shared, and leaders can cripple themselves by taking on too much of the workload. Additionally, failure to delegate shows an inherent distrust in team members. Delegation includes:

- Assessing the skills and available time of the team members, determining if a task is suitable for an individual
- Assigning tasks, with clear instructions that include explanation of objectives and expectations, including a timeline
- Ensuring that the tasks are completed properly and on time by monitoring progress but not micromanaging
- Reviewing the final results and recording outcomes

Because the leader is ultimately responsible for the delegated work, mentoring, monitoring, and providing feedback and intervention as necessary during this process is a necessary component of leadership. Even when delegated tasks are not completed successfully, they represent an opportunity for learning.

Assessment

Growth and Development

PRINCIPLES OF HUMAN DEVELOPMENT

Principles of human development as they relate to the pediatric population are as follows:

- Development follows a basic sequence. Developmental changes will always occur in a specific order.
- Development follows a specific pathway. Development that progresses from the head downward through the body is termed cephalocaudal. Proximodistal denotes development that progresses from the inside to the outside of the body.
- Each child will progress through the developmental stages at their own pace.
- The different areas of development are dependent on each other.
- As the child develops, the responses of the systems become more specific.
- As the child grows, the skills learned will become more complex.
- From infancy, children have inborn survival tactics.
- While a new skill is being learned, that skill takes precedence over learning other new skills.

HUMAN DEVELOPMENT FROM INFANCY THROUGH ADOLESCENCE

The stages and characteristics of human development through adolescence are outlined below:

- **Infant stage**: From birth to 1 year: rapid growth occurs, bonding and development of trust with family members
- **Toddler stage**: From age 1-3: development of basic motor, sensory and coordination skills, beginning understanding of self, seeks autonomy
- **Preschool stage**: From age 3-6: continue to develop better motor, sensory and coordination skills, learning to dress self and take care of basic hygiene, plays with other children, increased understanding of who they are
- **School age stage**: Age 6-12 years: seek academic success, interests broaden to include activities outside the home, competitive
- **Adolescent stage**: Age 12-19: physical changes related to puberty, begin to question their own and their family's values and beliefs, transitioning between childhood and adulthood

PHYSICAL GROWTH AND DEVELOPMENT DURING INFANCY

The newborn sleeps about 16 hours/day during the **first month** and is growing and developing.

- **Growth**: Infant loses 5–7% of birth weight and then gains 4–7 ounces/week (about 2 lb/month). Head circumference increases 1.5 cm/month and length 1.5 cm.
- **Mobility**: The infant makes fists and flexes arms and legs. Reflexes such as Moro, sucking, grasping, startle, rooting, and asymmetric tonic neck are present.
- **Feeding**: About every 2–3 hours with breastfeeding.
- **Urine/feces**: Urination should occur about 8 times per day. Breastfed babies may have frequent loose stools or may skip 2–3 days. If bottle-fed, stools are usually firmer. Color varies (yellow, tan, green, brown).
- **Sensory**: Follows items in line of vision and often prefers faces and contrasting geometric designs. Vision is somewhat blurry with ability to focus at about 8–15 inches. Color distinction is poor. Babies hear well and respond with startle reflex. Sense of smell is strong.
- **Communication**: Infant signals distress with crying, gagging, and arching body and responds to comfort measures.

During **months 2–4**, the infant continues to sleep much of the time but is often awake for periods in the morning, afternoon, and evening.

- **Growth**: Gains 5–7 oz/wk and 1.5 cm length/month and 1.5 cm head circumference/month. Posterior fontanel closes.
- **Mobility**: Loses grasp reflex and hands start to stay open and grasp. Able to lift head while prone or supine and turn from side to side. Can roll stomach to back by 4 months. Moro reflex fades. Plays with hands. Can be pulled to standing position.
- **Feeding**: Needs about 2 oz/lb per 24 hours, usually feeding every 4 hours.
- **Urine/feces**: Urine is about 5–6 times/day. Stools vary from one each feeding to every 2–3 days, but usually are firmer and more regular.
- **Sensory**: Can focus at about 12 inches and follows objects 180° with eyes.
- **Communication**: Crying differentiates to show hunger, pain, frustration. Infant can smile indiscriminately by 2 months and socially responsive smile by 3 months. Child shows preference for mother and may turn from strangers.

During **4–6 months** the child sleeps about 10–11 hours at night, with 2–3 daytime naps (total 15 hours).

- **Growth**: Doubles weight by 5–6 months, gains 5–7 oz/week.
- **Mobility**: Infant can roll over and roll from back to side by 6 months; can hold head up at 90° and turn head in both directions when sitting or lying. Can sit with support for 10–15 minutes. Grasp improves and may hold bottle and play with feet. By 6 months, the infant can pick up items and move items from one hand to the other. Manipulates and mouths objects and watches objects fall.
- **Feeding**: Still having about 2 feedings at night and every 4 hours during the day, 1.5 oz/lb per 24 hours.
- **Urine/feces**: Urination and defecation are becoming regular.
- **Sensory**: Eyes focus well; the infant follows items/people with eyes.
- **Communication**: Vocalizes more and mimics tones. Squeals and laughs. Yells with anger. Vocalizes to get attention and recognizes family members.

During **6–8 months** the child begins to have more waking hours, sleeping 10–11 hours with 2 naps.

- **Growth**: Growth slows. Gains 3–5 oz/wk and 1 cm in length/month.
- **Mobility**: Can sit alone by 8 months. Can stand supported and bounces on legs. Starting to use pincer grasp. Easily manipulates and moves objects. Most birth reflexes have faded. Bangs objects together and mouths objects freely.
- **Feeding**: Starting to take solid foods (cereal, vegetables, and fruit) 2–3 times daily as well as breastfeeding/bottle-feeding 3–5 times daily. Teething biscuits, graham crackers, and Melba toast may be introduced.
- **Urine/feces**: Stool larger with solid foods. Urinating 5–6 times daily.
- **Sensory**: Watches and listens actively, turning head to sounds and to follow objects.
- **Communication**: Increased babbling and mimicking of sounds, including two syllable sounds and vowels, such as "mama" or "dada" but doesn't use intentionally. Has babbling conversations. May be fearful of strangers.

During **8–10 months,** the child continues to sleep about 10–11 hours at night and usually sleeps through the night, with 2 naps in the daytime.

- **Growth**: Gains 3–5 oz/wk and 1 cm in length/month.
- **Mobility**: Uses pincer grasp well and can pick up small objects. Crawls or creeps readily. Can sit up and by 10 months can pull to standing position by holding onto furniture.

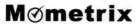

- **Feeding**: Meat introduced. Breastfeeding or bottle-feeding 3–4 times daily with 3 meals. Eggs may be introduced, but must be cooked completely. Will enjoy finger foods, such as meat sticks.
- **Urine/feces**: Fairly regular.
- **Sensory**: Watches and listens freely, attentive.
- **Communication**: Babbles and may be able to say one or two words besides "mama" or "dada." Understands basic vocabulary, such as "no" and "cookie." Babbling follows speech-like rhythm when "talking."

During **10–12 months**, the child continues to sleep 10–11 hours at night with 2 naps in the daytime.

- **Growth**: Gains 3–5 oz/week and 1 cm/month. Head and chest circumference are equal. Birth weight tripled by 12 months.
- **Mobility**: Can make marks on paper with pens or crayons. Fits objects through holes. Can stand alone and walk holding onto furniture. Can sit from standing position.
- **Feeding**: Breastfeeding or bottle-feeding 3–4 times daily and starting with "sippy" cup. Eating solid foods, both prepared baby foods and soft home-cooked foods. Enjoys finger foods and may resist being fed.
- **Urine/feces**: May smear feces. Holding urine for longer periods of time, especially girls.
- **Sensory**: Watches and listens, engaging in activities.
- **Communication**: Understands many words. Uses "mama" and "dada" intentionally and may use a few other words. Plays patty-cake and peek-a-boo games. Enjoys repetition.

Between **1 and 2 years**, the child is growing in size and independence.

- **Growth**: Gains 8 oz/month and 3–5 in/year. Anterior fontanel closes.
- **Mobility**: Begins with first steps and by 2 walks and runs and can go up and down stairs. Scribbles on paper, throws toys, and learns to stack blocks. Begins independent exploration of environment.
- **Diet**: Child eats 3 meals and 2–3 snacks daily. Whole cow's milk can be taken after 1 year, 2–3 cups daily. Some may breastfeed. Child can consume a wide range of foods.
- **Toileting**: Between 18–24 months, some children show an interest in potty training.
- **Communication**: Begins with one word and grows. Learns names for common objects and begins trying to communicate with simple words leading to short sentences around 2 with vocabulary of 30–50 words. May show apprehension with strangers and anger with temper tantrums.

The **2- to 3-year-old** makes significant changes over the course of a year.

- **Growth**: Gains 3–5 lb/year and 3.5–5 in/year
- **Mobility**: Can run steadily, jump on two feet, and climb. Scribbling becomes more intentional and can draw simple shapes. Makes effort to color in the lines. Able to undress at 2 and dress at 3. Can throw a ball overhand. Plays side by side and begins to interact with others.
- **Diet**: Can switch to lowfat milk, 2–3 cups daily along with a regular well-balanced meal of meat, fruits, vegetables, and grains. Parents should limit fruit juice to 2–4 oz/day because of high sugar content. The child should not be receiving bottle feedings.
- **Toileting**: Most children become potty-trained sometime during this year.
- **Communication/cognition**: Begins to talk in short 3-word sentences and to understand rules. Begins to use pronouns (I, me, you) and can talk about feelings. Usually knows at least 5 body parts and colors and can categorize by size (big, little).

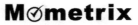

LANGUAGE MILESTONES

While children develop at different rates, there are a number of **language milestones** of developmentally appropriate communication for infants and toddlers.

- **5–6 weeks**: Vocalizations usually small and throaty, sometimes during crying
- **2 months**: Single vowel sounds (ah, oh, oo, eh)
- **3 months**: Gurgling, laughing, and some consonant sounds (n, k, g, b, p)
- **8 months**: Add consonants (t, d, w) and may combine syllables ("mama") although may not attach meaning
- **10 months**: Understand simple words, such as "no" and "mama"
- **12 months**: Say a few words with comprehension, such as "mama," "dada," and can imitate some animal sounds
- **13–15 months**: Have a 4- to 6-word expressive vocabulary but understand many more words and can point to indicate a desire for something, such as a toy
- **16–18 months**: Use 7- to 20-word vocabulary and point to 5 body parts
- **20 months**: Can combine 2 words
- **24 months**: Understand 300 words and uses 2- to 3-word sentences

PHYSICAL GROWTH AND DEVELOPMENT DURING PRESCHOOL YEARS

At ages **3-6**, the child moves from being a toddler to a child.

- **Growth**: Gains 3–5 lb/yr and 1.5–2.5 in/yr. Most growth occurs in long bones as child increases in stature and proportionate head size decreases.
- **Mobility**: Becomes increasingly adept, drawing various shapes, coloring in the lines, using scissors to cut along lines. Can brush teeth. Can tie shoes by 6. Able to climb, run, jump, balance, and ride tricycle or bicycle with training wheels. Interacts with others.
- **Diet**: Eats 3 meals with snack and can manage spoon, fork, and knife independently by age 6.
- **Communication/cognition**: Becomes increasingly verbal and social and commands a large complex vocabulary by 6. Understands concepts of right and wrong, good and bad, and can lie. Learns letters and numbers and by age 6 is beginning to read. May focus on one thing to the exclusion of others.

PHYSICAL GROWTH AND DEVELOPMENT DURING SCHOOL AGE YEARS

During the school years **(ages 6-12)**, children go through many changes.

- **Dental**: Children lose deciduous teeth and begin acquiring permanent teeth.
- **Height and weight**: These should progress slowly and steadily, gaining an average of 2 inches each year, beginning at about 45 inches at 6 and attaining about 59 inches at 12. Weight usually doubles during this time from 46 pounds at 6 to 88 pounds at 12. Boys and girls are similar in size but by 12, some girls will be undergoing pubertal changes and may gain height and weight over boys.
- **Proportions**: The body becomes slimmer and better proportioned with an increase in muscle mass and decrease in fat. In relation to height, head circumference decreases, leg length increases, and waist circumference decreases. Facial characteristics change.
- **Body systems**: Systems mature with respirations and heart rate decreasing. Bladder capacity is usually better in girls than boys. Muscles strengthen and bones begin to ossify. Physical variation increases with age.

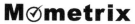

PHYSICAL GROWTH AND DEVELOPMENT PROBLEMS DURING SCHOOL-AGE YEARS

Routine health assessments should be done at ages 6, 8, 10, 11, and 12 to determine if there are developmental delays or problems, which may include:

- **6 years**: Peer problems, depression, cruelty to animals, poor academic progress, speech problems, lack of fine motor skills, and inability to catch a ball or state age.
- **8 years**: No close friends, depression, cruelty to animals, interest in fires, very poor academic progress with inability to do math, read, or write adequately and poor coordination.
- **10 years**: No team sports or extracurriculars and poor choices in peers (gangs), failure to follow rules, cruelty to animals, interest in fires, depression, failure to understand causal relationships, poor academic progress in reading, writing, math, and penmanship, and problems throwing or catching.
- **12 years**: Continuation of problems at 10 years with increasing risk-taking behaviors (drinking, drugs, sex) and continued poor academic progress in reading, following directions, doing homework, and organization.

PHYSICAL GROWTH AND DEVELOPMENT ISSUES FOR EARLY ADOLESCENCE

Early adolescence, ages **11-14,** is a transitional time for children as their hormones and their bodies go through changes. Children mature at varying rates, so there are wide differences. Emotions may be labile, and the child may feel isolated and confused at times, trying to find an identity. Peers take on more influence and the child may challenge the values of the family. Children may have much anxiety about their bodies and sexuality as secondary sexual characteristics develop. Developmental concerns include:

- Delayed maturation
- Short stature (female)
- Spinal curvature (females)
- Poor dental status (caries, malocclusion)
- Chronic illnesses, such as diabetes
- Lack of adequate physical activity
- Poor nutrition, anorexia, obesity
- Concerns about sexual identity
- Negative self-image, depression
- Lack of close friends, fighting or violent episodes, lack of impulse control
- Poor academic progress with truancy and failure to complete assignments

NORMAL GROWTH AND DEVELOPMENT ISSUES FOR MIDDLE ADOLESCENCE

In middle adolescence, ages **15-17,** most body changes have occurred, so there is less concern about this but more concern about the image they are projecting to others. Girls may worry about weight and boys about muscle development. Teenagers are interested in sexuality and many begin sexual experimentation. There is strong identification with peer groups, including codes of dress and behavior, often putting the individual at odds with family. **Developmental concerns** include:

- Spinal curvature (females) and short stature (males)
- Lack of testicular maturation/ persistent gynecomastia
- Acne
- Anorexia, obesity
- Sexual experimentation, multiple partners, and unprotected sex
- Sexual identification concerns
- Depression, poor self-image
- Lack of adequate exercise, poor nutrition, and poor dental health
- Chronic diseases
- Experimentation with drugs and alcohol and problems with authority figures

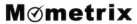

- Lack of peer group identification, gang association
- Poor academic progress, failing classes, truancy, attention deficits and disruptive class behavior, and poor judgment and impulse control

Normal Growth and Development Issues for Late Adolescence

Late adolescence, ages **18-21,** is the time when adolescents begin to take on more adult roles and responsibilities, entering the world of work or going to college. Most have come to terms with their sexuality and have a more mature understanding of people's motivations. Some young people will continue to engage in high-risk behaviors. Many of the problems associated with middle adolescence may continue if unresolved, interfering with the transition to adulthood. Developmental concerns include:

- Failure to take on adult roles, no life goals or future plans
- Low self-esteem, lack of impulse control
- Lack of intimate relationships, sexual identification concerns
- Gang association
- Continued identification with peer group or dependence on parents
- High-risk sexual behavior, multiple partners, and unprotected sex
- Poor academic progress or ability
- Psychosomatic complaints, depression
- Poor nutrition, obesity, anorexia
- Poor dental health
- Chronic disease
- Lack of exercise

Maturity Assessment

A maturity assessment should be part of the examination for children and adolescents to determine their level of sexual, dental, and skeletal maturity. **Skeletal maturity** is usually assessed by measurements of the hand and wrist as well as weight/height for age. Skeletal maturity and chronological age may differ. For example, if the chronological age is 14.3 and the skeletal age is 15.5, this would be expressed as 15.5–14.3 = SA +1.2. Another method is to divide the skeletal age by the chronological age: a score >1.0 equates with advanced skeletal maturity and <1.0 a delay in skeletal maturity.

The most common assessment tool for **sexual maturity** is Tanner's 5 stages of assessment. This tool assesses maturity for both males and females, based on direct observation of breasts and genitals.

- Females: Breast development, onset of menses, and pubic hair distribution
- Males: Penis and testes development and pubic hair distribution

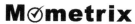

History and Physical Exam

CLIENT-NURSE COMMUNICATION

Client-nurse communication may include:

- **Emails or texts**: Email allows for fast communication and mass mailings at little cost, but emails are often screened and may be ignored if the receiver doesn't know or recognize the sender. Documents can be easily transmitted through email as text or PDF files. Some people prefer to be reminded of appointments by email or text messages. Reminders and alerts can be sent to patients regarding appointments or guidelines. Texts can be used in-house to reduce the number of audible pages in order to provide a quieter environment. Confidential information must be delivered over secure lines so that confidentiality is not compromised.
- **Patient portal**: Allows the patients to access all or parts of their medical records, including lists of medications and laboratory results, and usually contains a messaging function that allows the nurse to send messages to a patient and vice versa. Some patient portals also allow the patient to enter information into the medical record.

TELEPHONE USE FOR TRIAGE

Often the first contact that a parent has with the nurse is by telephone when calling or in person at an appointment. Parents are often not good judges of the seriousness of a condition, so that first contact is critical. The nurse must establish a clear plan for **telephone triage** and protocols that must be followed:

- **Receptionists/nurse aides** should not dispense medical advice. They should be provided a "script" of questions to ask when people call with a complaint, request, or to make an appointment in order to screen those who need the attention, and they should make appointments or refer them to a staff nurse or the nurse practitioner as necessary.
- **Staff nurses and the nurse practitioner** should also have guidelines and protocols, depending upon whether a call constitutes a severe medical emergency (call 911), a non-life-threatening emergency (see immediately), an urgent problem (see within 4 hours), a less urgent problem (see in 1 day), or a recurrent problem (see within 2 weeks).

MEDICAL AND SURGICAL HISTORY

The pediatric nurse is expected to demonstrate competency in assessment, including **medical and surgical history**, as part of identifying and managing health concerns in infants and children. Complete and accurate documentation of findings is an essential element of the plan of care. **History** may be collected in the classic manner that begins with a complaint and includes health history, surgical history, review of systems, nutrition, developmental status, family history, and socioeconomic factors that may affect the health issue. This should include detailed information about medical conditions, treatments, and surgery.

A **problem-oriented history** builds upon the classic history by focusing on developmental health problems, functional problems, and diseases, moving from subjective information (history) to objective (physical/laboratory data):

- Developmental assessment includes motor, speech, cognitive, social, and adaptive behaviors.
- Functional assessment includes issues related to basic health behavior patterns, such as diet, sleeping, coping, sexuality, and elimination.
- Diseases are those diagnoses according to the *International Classification of Diseases,* Clinical Modification (ICD-10-CM, used to classify morbidity data), and interventions are planned based on diagnosis.

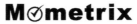

MEDICAL AND SURGICAL HISTORY OF THE ADOLESCENT

While the essential elements of assessment and medical and surgical history for **adolescents** are similar to those for infants and children, there are some differences because often the adolescent is providing, or in some cases withholding, information. Additionally, the risk factors associated with adolescence vary from those of infancy or earlier childhood. Assessment should include lifestyle information, such as whether the teenager has been homeless, engaged in high-risk sexual behavior, violence, tobacco use, or drug use. Documenting nutrition, weight concerns, peer relationships, and coping mechanisms can help to identify health concerns. A complete history should include information about medical conditions, treatment, and surgery. Successful assessment includes:

- Listen and show respect for the adolescent
- Question adolescent/parent cause for concern
- Interview both the adolescent and the parent(s) alone
- Observe nonverbal behavior and interactions among children and parents

DIFFERENCE FROM ADULT HISTORY

Pediatric histories differ from adult histories in both their content and the method of obtaining the history. The content differs because of the patient's age, and parents are the most likely source of information for a pediatric history. Differences between a pediatric history and an adult history include the following: the prenatal history, including significant events during pregnancy and the history of the child's development, including the ages of developmental milestones.

TYPES OF HEALTH HISTORIES

Depending on the status of the child at the exam, the nurse may need to take one or more of three different **types of health histories**.

- The **initial history** is the child's health history from gestation until the present time; it includes the birth history, developmental milestones, and any illnesses. The initial history is often taken at a preliminary visit to a pediatric practitioner when no other history is available.
- The **well interim history** is taken when an initial history is on file. The well interim history outlines any significant health events that have occurred since the last visit.
- The **episodic history** is taken to confirm events that have led up to the current visit. For example, an episodic history for a child with an arm fracture would involve a description of the activities that resulted in the injury.

ENVIRONMENTAL CONSIDERATIONS WHEN COLLECTING HISTORY

Obtaining a pediatric history may be challenging because of the time it takes to gather data while managing the behavior of a child. If siblings are also present, there may be more distractions. An **environment** that is most suitable for taking a pediatric history is one that is conducive to gaining information in the quickest and most accurate way possible, with minimal distractions. Depending on the age of the child, the nurse may take the history in a quiet room that is separate from others, which protects the privacy of the family as well. While minimal distractions may help with collecting information, some locations may offer toys or activities to keep the child busy so the nurse has adequate time to talk with the caregiver without interruption.

METHODS OF GATHERING INFORMATION FOR PEDIATRIC HISTORY

The information from a pediatric history may be **gathered** through several means, depending on the location. Some offices have preprinted forms that allow parents to fill out the information about their child, whether it is before the office visit or on admission. With these forms, parents must "fill in the blanks," but there is also space to describe illnesses and conditions that may be affecting the child. A face-to-face interview is another method of gathering information when no forms are available; this is suitable when the child is seen emergently or when the present illness or injury must be addressed quickly.

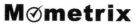

TYPES OF INFORMANTS

The **most common person to give information** about the pediatric patient is the parent. Foster parents, adoptive parents, and legal guardians may also be informants; however, depending on the length of time the adult has known the child, the information may not be as comprehensive as that from a parent who has cared for the child since birth. Older children and teens may provide information about themselves if they are capable of answering questions. In emergent situations or if a parent is not available, the person who has brought the child for care may be the informant. This may be emergency personnel, teachers, neighbors, or friends. In the absence of parents, a child's medical record may also be a source of valuable information.

IN LOCO PARENTIS

In loco parentis is a Latin term used to describe a person standing in place of the parent. Legally, the term means the responsibility of a caregiver for a child whose parent may be unavailable during assessment or treatment. Examples of *in loco parentis* include cases where a child is taken for medical treatment by someone in authority at school, daycare, or another organization, when the parent is unavailable or in cases of guardianship or foster placement. In these situations, the caregiver would provide as much information about the patient's history as possible.

EFFECTS OF FAMILY MEMBERS ON PATIENT HISTORY AND ABILITY TO GAIN INFORMATION

Family members can be great sources of information when taking a patient history, but they may also be distracting or disruptive, prohibiting attempts at gathering information. The nurse should assess the situation before attempting the patient history to minimize distractions as much as possible. Ideas include providing toys and activities that may keep the patient's siblings busy during the interview; offering reading materials, television, or other pursuits during the interview to prevent interruptions; or asking another nurse or professional to monitor or talk with family members while assessing the patient.

IDENTIFYING CAREGIVERS' PERCEPTION OF CHILD'S BASELINE

During times of emergency, a child's caregivers may be stressed, but the nurse must have information regarding the caregivers' perception of the **child's baseline status**, especially with infants and younger children or those who are developmentally delayed. The nurse should ask specific questions rather than very general questions, such as "What behavior or activity is normal for your child?" Questions relate to the child's age, but those for infants and young children should include:

- **Height (length) and weight:** Considered in conjunction with one another to establish appropriate nutritional status and growth/development. These are compared against standardized curves.
- **Diet**: Whether the child is nursing or bottle-fed, including the frequency and duration of nursing or ounces of milk per feeding. Question the number of meals daily and typical diet and eating habits.
- **Mobility**: Varies by age, but includes the ability to grasp, roll, turn, sit up, walk, run, and manipulate items.
- **Elimination**: Includes bowel and urinary output, problems, habits, routine, and continence. If the patient is an infant, include the number of wet diapers daily.
- **Sensory**: Includes age-appropriate indications of hearing and vision.
- **Communication**: Includes age-appropriate communication, such as vocalizing, babbling, saying words, saying sentences, comprehension.

USING DEVELOPMENTALLY APPROPRIATE COMMUNICATION

Children, even toddlers, should always receive an explanation of treatment or other aspects of care, but the explanations should be given with **developmentally appropriate communication**, avoiding technical terms the child may not understand. Short explanations are better for small children as they may become very anxious. If more detailed explanations are needed for the parents, these explanations should be given away from the child.

Avoid	Use
Shot, injection, bee sting, needle stick	Medication under the skin
Incision, cut	Special opening
Pain	Hurt, "owie," or other term used by the child
Take temperature	See how warm you are
Monitor	TV/Computer screen
Stool, feces	Use child's term (poop, doo-doo)
Urine	Use child's term (pee-pee)
Gurney	Rolling bed
X-ray	Special pictures
Catheter	Tube
Anesthetize, deaden	Make sleepy, numb
Treat	Fix, make better

POTENTIAL BARRIERS WHEN TAKING A PEDIATRIC HISTORY

When taking a pediatric health history, several **barriers** can inhibit the nurse's ability to gather information:

- The **environment** may not be conducive to conducting an examination or talking to the family because of noise or an inadequate space.
- **Parents** often are a great source of background information for the pediatric patient, but cultural differences, ethnic practices, and language barriers may all inhibit gathering information. Parents who are under the influence of medication or alcohol, those with psychiatric histories, those who are very young, and those who face financial pressures, illness, or time constraints may have difficulty supplying accurate information.
- **Siblings** or other **family members** who are present in the room may also be a distraction when trying to obtain a history.

CHIEF COMPLAINT TAKEN DURING MEDICAL HISTORY

The **chief complaint** is a description of symptoms that brought the patient in for treatment, such as shortness of breath, nausea, vomiting, abdominal pain, rash, or headache. Determining the chief complaint is part of taking the patient history, as this explains the reasons for seeking medical care. Other parts of the history related to the chief complaint include circumstances that may have led to the current symptoms, factors that make the symptoms better or worse, and a history of illnesses that may exacerbate the current chief complaint.

HISTORY OF PRESENT ILLNESS

The history of the present illness follows a description of the chief complaint. The history of the present illness explains circumstances that drove the patient and family to seek care. Determining the history of the present illness is important for diagnostic purposes and for guiding treatment plans. The nurse can ask questions such as the following:

- How long have you experienced these symptoms?
- What makes the symptoms worse or better?
- Are symptoms worsening?
- What does the family believe to be the cause of the symptoms?

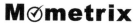

PREGNANCY AND BIRTH HISTORY

The **history of health during pregnancy and delivery** is an important component of the pediatric history. If the information is available, the nurse should record all significant events that occurred during pregnancy, labor, and delivery. Components of this type of history include the following:

- The health of the mother, such as any illnesses associated with pregnancy, bed rest, medication use, or complications
- The infant's gestational age at birth and whether the child was considered pre-term or full-term
- The type of delivery and any complications that occurred during delivery, such as fetal distress, cord compression, or emergent cesarean section
- The infant's health after birth, including Apgar scores, health complications, or time spent in the neonatal intensive care unit

NEONATAL HISTORY

The parents of young infants and children should give an account of any significant events that occurred during the neonatal period, which may impact the child's health and behavior at the visit. The **neonatal history** should include the following:

- Complications associated with delivery, such as cord compression or excessive bleeding
- Assistance needed in delivery, such as vacuum extraction or forceps
- Apgar scores
- The need for oxygen or resuscitation at birth
- Complications in the prenatal period, such as hypoglycemia, transient tachypnea, infection, or jaundice
- Medications
- Periods of apnea
- Time spent in the neonatal intensive care unit, if applicable

PEDIATRIC FEEDING HISTORY

The pediatric feeding history indicates the type of feedings the child has taken from birth until the present visit. The feeding history is important because it determines whether the child has met developmental milestones for feeding, if the child is gaining weight appropriately, and if there are any health issues that may interfere with feedings, such as gastrointestinal issues or allergies. The pediatric nutrition portion of the history includes whether the child was breastfed or bottle-fed. If the child was fed by bottle, the type and amount of formula are noted. Any feeding issues, such as reflux or breast milk jaundice, are also noted. Older infants and toddlers have complete health histories concerning the introduction of solid foods, the timing of these foods, and the variety of foods eaten. Older child histories describe the number of meals and snacks each day, food preferences and dislikes, and any health problems associated with certain foods, such as gluten intolerance or food allergies.

PEDIATRIC BEHAVIORAL HISTORY

The pediatric behavioral history describes social or environmental situations that may affect children's health, both physically and emotionally. Behavioral issues at home may lead to increased risks of injury or may be the result of physical illnesses that affect the children's ability to cope. Components of a behavioral history for the pediatric patient include assessing the children's environment at home, such as the number of siblings; family dynamics (e.g., parents together, divorced, separated); behavioral concerns, such as excessive temper tantrums, breath holding, controlling or manipulative behavior, responses to strangers, relationships with peers, and rapport with teachers and persons of authority. Sleep issues should be assessed to determine how much sleep the children are getting each night, if they still take naps, their bed times and waking times, and the state of their sleeping quarters. Older children and adolescents should be assessed for tobacco, alcohol, or drug use, peer relationships, and sexual development.

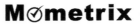

MEDICATION RECONCILIATION DURING COLLECTION OF PATIENT HISTORY

Maintaining an **accurate list of current and previous medications** is an essential component of medication reconciliation. A patient (or parent) who maintains a list of personal medications becomes more involved in the care received and serves alongside the health care team as part of managing this care. The patient may have better health or improved outcomes when medication use is tracked and communicated to the health care team. In addition, maintaining a knowledge base of medications will benefit the patient/family and allow the opportunity for education about side effects and complications associated with certain medications. This also supports long-term compliance with the prescribed medication regimen.

ASSESSING FOR DRUG AND FOOD ALLERGIES WHEN COLLECTING PATIENT HISTORY

Assessing for **drug allergies** is especially important when collecting patient history in order to identify drugs that may cause reactions and to predict what other drugs may also trigger allergic reactions. For example, a patient who is allergic to penicillin may have cross reactivity to other antibiotics as well. The list of drug allergies should be reviewed with every new prescription. Food allergies should also be assessed, as they may provide indications of possible drug allergies. For example:

- Allergic reaction to bananas, kiwi, melons, papaya, raw potatoes, tomato and/or avocado increases the risk of allergy to latex.
- Allergic reaction to eggs or chicken is a contraindication for use of hyaluronic acid intra-articular injections because the substance is derived from chicken.
- The culture media for some vaccines can include eggs and horse serum.
- Allergic reaction to seafood may be associated with allergic reaction to IV iodine contrast.

INTERACTION BETWEEN SOME FOOD/FOOD ELEMENTS AND MEDICATIONS

Grapefruit may interact with many drugs (statins, SSRIs, CCBs, sildenafil, sirolimus, tacrolimus, buspirone, midazolam, cyclosporine), and the interaction may occur up to 3 days after ingestion of grapefruit. Grapefruit inhibits CYP3A4, an isoenzyme of cytochrome P450, which is found in the wall of the intestines and the liver, but the inhibitory action takes place primarily in the intestines, decreasing the intestinal metabolism of various drugs and increasing absorption so that blood levels rise. This may intensify therapeutic effects or result in toxicity.

Vitamin K (phytonadione) may also interact with drugs. It is used to reverse excessive doses of warfarin but may decrease the effects of other drugs as well (anisindione, dicumarol). Some drug interactions decrease the effects of the vitamin K (cholestyramine, colesevelam colestipol, and sevelamer).

Tyramine-containing foods can cause a severe reaction when taken with MAOIs. Neuronal MAO is inhibited, resulting in increased levels of norepinephrine in sympathetic nerve terminals. Because MAO is inhibited in the intestinal walls and liver, dietary tyramine enters the circulatory system intact and promotes release of the epinephrine that has built up, resulting in severe vasoconstriction and stimulation of the heart.

ASSESSING HISTORY FOR GENETIC OR FAMILIAL RISKS

Assessing family history for **genetic or familial risks** is an important part of disease prevention because, in some cases, early identification and intervention may reduce future health risks. Creating a genogram with the family is helpful. A thorough history should be broad and include assessment of the following:

- Early onset disorders, such as cardiovascular disease, hypertension, or Alzheimer's disease
- Progressive neurological or neuromuscular diseases
- Diabetes mellitus
- Mental illness, such as depression, bipolar disorder, and schizophrenia
- Intellectual disability, including Trisomy 21 (Down syndrome)
- Any unusual disabilities or abnormalities, such as birth defects

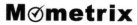

Once risk factors are determined, then the question of screening tests arises. If there is a possibility that the child is a carrier, then screening is usually deferred until the child can give informed consent. Screening is done with parental permission when it is in the best interests of the child, allowing for appropriate care and intervention.

RELATIONSHIP BETWEEN ETHNICITY AND RISK OF GENETIC DISORDERS

Some ethnic groups have increased risk for **genetic disorders** with high carrier rates, ranging from 1:6 to 1:40. The nurse should be aware of these risks and observant for symptoms in the child. A careful maternal and paternal family history may provide information about occurrence of the disease in other family members. Some disorders are covered in routine neonatal screening, but others are not. In some cases, it may be appropriate to recommend testing to ensure that early diagnosis is made so that treatment can be initiated. The following groups are at increased risk for specific genetic disorders:

- Ashkenazi Jews: Canavan disease, Tay-Sachs disease, cystic fibrosis, and familial dysautonomia
- African Americans: Sickle cell disease (carrier rate 1:6 to 1:12), other hemoglobinopathy
- European Caucasians: Cystic fibrosis
- Mediterranean: Beta thalassemia
- South Asian: Beta thalassemia
- Southeast Asian: Alpha and beta thalassemia

USE OF INFORMATION FROM PEDIATRIC HISTORY IN CURRENT PRACTICE

Information from the pediatric history can be a valuable resource for the nurse and offers a **framework for providing treatment**. The pediatric history not only gives clues to the current complaint and offers direction for treatment, but it may also be used to educate parents about better health practices at home. Thus, the history serves as a teaching tool for better parenting. Additionally, a pediatric history may identify patterns of illness that can be genetic, which may indicate further testing for other family members who may be at risk. Finally, the pediatric history supports public health measures for identifying and treating children who are at risk for chronic disease, such as diabetes, asthma, or obesity.

PRIMARY SURVEY

Elements of the primary survey, which can be remembered using the **ABCDE mnemonic**, include the following:

- **Airway**: Check airway for obstruction. Open airway with head tilt chin maneuver (lift chin with one hand and apply pressure to forehead with the other) or if trauma is present, the jaw thrust (stabilize cervical spine and pull mandible forward).
- **Breathing**: Look, listen, and feel for breathing for no more than 10 seconds. If not breathing, institute bag-valve-mask (BVM) ventilation followed by nasotracheal or orotracheal intubation if there is no response to BVM.
- **Circulation**: Provide basic life support (BLS). Check the carotid pulse in children >1 year of age, the brachial pulse in infants, and the umbilical pulse in neonates. Begin CPR: 120 compressions per minute in neonates and 100-120 per minute for infants and children. Defibrillate. If no response, institute Pediatric Advanced Life Support (PALS).
- **Disability**: Evaluate neurological status by checking pupillary response, level of alertness, Glasgow Coma Scale, CT for suspected stroke, blood glucose level and naloxone for suspected narcotic overdose.
- **Exposure/environmental control**: Remove clothes, check body for lesions, rashes, and trauma and maintain thermoregulation.

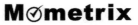

SECONDARY SURVEY

Elements of the secondary survey include the following:

- **History**: Question medical problems, current medications, onset of illness or injury, allergies, time of last meal, and pregnancy status when applicable.
- **Head**: Examine eyes, ears, nose, throat, skull, and skin for lacerations and bruises.
- **Neck**: Note carotid pulses, stiffness, bruit, jugular venous distention and trauma.
- **Chest**: Complete inspection, palpation, percussion, and auscultation. Note hyperresonance, dullness, adventitious sounds, or absent breath sounds.
- **Heart**: Note rhythm, heart sounds, and murmurs.
- **Abdomen**: Complete careful examination with supporting laboratory (blood counts) and imaging assessment (ultrasound, radiograph, CT, MRI) as needed.
- **Rectal, genital, perineal**: Perform examination if indicated.
- **Musculoskeletal**: Inspect and palpate all extremities for fractures, lacerations, dislocations, motor function, sensation, and pulses with supporting imaging as indicated. Multiple trauma patients should have pelvis x-ray.
- **Neurological**: Assess level of consciousness and complete evaluation of pupils and cranial nerves, reflexes, motor function, and sensory level with supporting imaging, such as CT scans. Note evidence of spinal cord injury.

HEIGHT, WEIGHT, HEAD CIRCUMFERENCE, AND CHEST CIRCUMFERENCE

Height and weight are plotted on a standard growth chart. If the child is below the 5th percentile or above the 95th percentile, or falls two standard deviations below his normal curve, further investigation is required.

Normal head growth is 1.0-1.5 cm per month during the first year. A smaller than normal head circumference could be due to prematurity or microcephaly, a congenital abnormality resulting in mental deficits due to a small brain and small skull. A larger than normal head circumference could be due to hydrocephalus, an enlargement of the head due to buildup of CSF in the brain.

The **chest circumference** should be less than the head circumference up to one year of age. After this age, the chest circumference should be larger than the head circumference. A smaller than average chest circumference can be due to prematurity.

NORMAL AND ABNORMAL FINDINGS DURING PHYSICAL EXAMINATION

SKIN

The **color of skin** should be assessed for jaundice or cyanosis, especially apparent in the nose, external ear, lips, hands, and feet. Note any lesions. Birthmarks, freckles, and moles, flat or raised, are normal. **Eczema** is common in children; **erythema toxicum** (erythematous, maculopapular lesions) is also common in newborns, as well as stork bites on the back of the neck and diaper dermatitis. **Mongolian spots** (dark blue areas in the lumbar and sacral areas, buttocks, shoulders, or upper back) are normal in African, Latino, and Asian babies. One abnormal finding is a dimple or a dark patch of hair over the lumbosacral area (spina bifida occulta).

Skin temperature should be the same bilaterally. Very warm skin indicates fever, hyperthyroidism, or exercise. Hypothermia can be due to shock or a circulatory problem.

The skin should be soft and smooth. **Milia** (small white papules on the face) are common in newborns, as is **vernix caseosa** (a cheesy coating present at birth). Decreased skin turgor indicates dehydration. Edema is abnormal.

HEAD

The head should be symmetrical without bumps or depressions. The anterior fontanel may pulsate with the heartbeat. An occiput that is flattened with hair loss is caused by lying in the same position for long periods of time. Head lag after 4 months can be caused by prematurity, hydrocephalus, and developmental delays. Head lag remaining after 6 months can indicate brain damage. The fontanels should be flat and soft. Bulging, tense fontanels result from increased intracranial pressure and sunken fontanels from dehydration. Fontanels that fail to close or are larger than normal can indicate rickets or congenital hypothyroidism. Suture lines should line up, without gapping or overriding. Craniotabes (soft outer layers of the skull bones behind and above the ears that can be depressed) is abnormal, indicating rickets, hydrocephaly, syphilis, or hypervitaminosis. Cephalhematoma and caput succedaneum are abnormal findings resulting from pressure during delivery.

EAR AND NOSE

Hearing tests are usually performed starting at 3-4 years. The top of the ear should be level with or a little above the outer corner of the eye. If it is lower, it can indicate renal abnormalities or Down syndrome. When looking at the tympanic membrane, it should be pearly gray to light pink and transparent with a smooth membrane.

The **nose** should be symmetrical and centered. Congenital abnormalities may be present if the nose is short and small, flat, or large. Flaring can indicate respiratory distress, odor can indicate a foreign object stuck in the nasal canal, and discharge can indicate an infection. The mucous membrane should be pink and moist. The newborn should be assessed for patent nares. An obstruction indicates choanal atresia, a septum between the nose and pharynx.

EYES

Upon physical assessment of the **eyes**, the sclera is normally bluish (newborns), white, or slightly darker in color (dark-skinned children). A yellow sclera indicates jaundice. The iris in newborns is blue or gray (light-skinned children) or brown (dark-skinned). The color may change up until 12 months. Brushfield's spots (small white spots around the edge of the iris) are abnormal and related to Down syndrome. Pupils should be equal size and react equally to light. If one or both pupils don't react to light, it can indicate a CNS abnormality. The newborn should exhibit the optical blink reflex. The red reflex should be assessed; black spots or opacities are abnormal (possible cataract resulting from eye trauma, infection during pregnancy or chromosomal disorders). A cat's eye reflex (yellow or white light) can indicate retinoblastoma, a malignant tumor of the eye. The retina is usually pink in color; red color is abnormal and usually indicates bleeding. The optic disc is examined for color and shape. If the margins are irregular or blurred, it can indicate papilledema or intracranial pressure.

VISION AND EYELIDS

A **vision test**, appropriate for age, should be done every 1-2 years through adolescence. Vision is abnormal if the child sees 20/40 or greater at 3 years of age or 20/30 or greater over 6 years of age (using the Snellen E chart). Congenital cataracts, tumors or retinal trauma can result in nearsightedness. Screening should be done for strabismus (eye muscle weakness), using an appropriate test. The **opening of the eyes** should be symmetrical, the upper lid should cover part of the iris and the lower lid should meet the iris. Asian children may have an epicanthal fold. Hydrocephalus can cause sunset eyes (part of the sclera is seen above the iris). Down syndrome children have a fold of skin covering the inner canthus and lacrimal caruncle. By 3 months, the lacrimal duct should be patent. Tearing and discharge from the eye can result from dacryocystitis (blockage of the lacrimal duct causes infection of the lacrimal sac.

NECK

Observe the **neck** for abnormal appearance, such as shortness, thickening, or swelling. Swelling of the parotid gland indicates mumps. The thyroid glands should be assessed for swelling, tenderness or masses, possibly indicative of hyperthyroidism. Lymph nodes can't normally be felt. Enlarged lymph nodes indicate infection; the site of which depends on which lymph nodes are affected. Bacterial infections of the pharynx are indicated by swelling of the anterior cervical nodes; tinea capitis and otitis media are indicated by swelling of the occipital or posterior cervical nodes. Small, cool nodes that are not fixed are common in children; these "shotty" nodes indicate a prior infection or allergies.

MOUTH AND THROAT

The edges of the **lips** should meet. Cleft lip is present if there is a separation of the lip area. The mucosa of the mouth should be pink, smooth, and moist; a thick white coating can indicate thrush. The number of **teeth** should be noted and compared with normal teething guidelines. If normal teeth are not present and tooth buds are not noted on x-ray, genetic abnormalities may be present. Teeth should be without brown-black spots. These spots indicate cavities. The hard and soft **palates** should be continuous and have a slight arch. A separation of the palate indicates cleft palate. Epstein's pearls (small, white, hard cysts on the gums and hard palate) are abnormal. The **tonsils** are normally enlarged in early childhood, decreasing in size after age 10. The **uvula** should be pink and centered. The **mucosa** of the oropharynx should also be pink and smooth. Excess saliva production can be a sign of a tracheoesophageal fistula.

HEART

Abnormalities should be of primary concern when assessing the **heart**. Dextrocardia, when the apex of the heart points toward the right side of the chest, will affect the landmarks used in examining the heart. The apical pulse should be assessed for any deviation from its normal placement, indicating an enlarged heart or pneumothorax. The apical pulse is visible on the precordium, but no other movements should be seen. If the cardiac area heaves, or lifts, the left ventricle is working too hard and can indicate CHF or shunt defects. Septal defects will produce a thrill, a vibration of the chest similar to a purring cat. Peripheral pulses should be equal and simultaneous. If there is a lag or weakness in some pulses, consider heart defects, such as coarctation of the aorta. Some children have innocent murmurs and sinus arrhythmias, which are normal. Other abnormalities in heart sounds can indicate heart defects or CHF.

RESPIRATORY STATUS

Assessment of respiratory status involves looking at the child's appearance, counting respirations, and listening to lung sounds. A child who is comfortable, breathing normally, and who has pink skin and a healthy appearance most likely has normal respiratory function. A child who is agitated, who appears pale or cyanotic, and who is breathing rapidly may be in respiratory distress. Other signs of respiratory distress include assuming a position of comfort to breathe, wheezes or stridor while breathing, and retractions noted above the sternum, between the ribs, or below the xiphoid process. Auscultation may result in lung sounds with rales or rhonchi, or breath sounds may be diminished or absent.

THORAX AND LUNGS

The **thorax** changes from rounded and boxy in shape during early childhood to longer and thinner at about age 6. An abnormal chest shape in the school age child can indicate cystic fibrosis. A funnel shaped chest (pectus excavatum) is progressive from birth and can affect heart function. Pigeon chest (pectus carinatum) is when the sternum sticks out from the body. It can be congenital in origin. Assess for retractions, which indicated respiratory distress, possibly resulting from pneumonia or asthma. Placing a hand on the chest, the nurse may feel a soft vibration which is normal. If the vibration is pronounced, it may indicate pneumonia. If the vibration is decreased, pulmonary edema or pleural effusion may exist. Percussion can reveal fluid or air trapped in the lungs. Upon auscultation, the lung sounds should be clear and equal. Crackles, wheezes, or rhonchi are abnormal signs of such conditions as bronchiolitis, cystic fibrosis, or asthma. Stridor, a high-pitched sound upon inspiration, can occur with croup and epiglottis.

MUSCULOSKELETAL SYSTEM

Muscles should be symmetrical and firm bilaterally. Spasticity, rigidity, or resistance can indicate cerebral palsy. Muscular dystrophy can cause decreased muscle strength, noted when the child cannot rise to a standing position without using the arms. Check for coordination in gross and fine motor skills. Observe for involuntary movements, such as tics, tremors, or jerking. Lordosis after age 6 is abnormal and can result from dislocation of the hips or congenital kyphosis. Scoliosis is abnormal. Polydactyly (extra digits) and syndactylism (fusion of digits) are signs of congenital syndromes. A knock knee appearance is normal until around 4-6 years of age. Bowlegs are normal until 2 years. If present later, it may indicate rickets. The joints should not be tender or swollen and should be flexible. Painful, swollen, warm joints are indicative of juvenile rheumatoid arthritis. Club foot is a turning in of the foot and toes and is abnormal. Dysplasia of the hips in the infant is abnormal and is associated with birth and familial factors.

ABDOMEN

Observe the child for crying and guarding of areas of the **abdomen** upon palpation, which indicates tenderness or pain. A separation of the rectus muscles in the midline (diastasis recti) is normal in infants. A vertical separation of the stomach muscle is abnormal. If peristalsis can be seen or an olive-shaped mass palpated in the upper right stomach area, pyloric stenosis should be considered. Hirschsprung's disease is indicated by distention of the abdomen by palpable stool and no stool in the rectum. Intussusception can cause pain associated with a sausage-shaped mass in the upper abdomen. Bowel sounds should not be heard in the thorax; this can indicate a diaphragmatic hernia in the newborn. The liver edge should be soft and smooth. If located more than 2 cm below the right rib cage, and hard with a firm border, hepatomegaly should be suspected. Causes can be cardiac failure, tumors, viruses, or bacteria.

GENITALIA

Assess females for discharge, bruising, or scarring of the **genitalia**. A small penis in the clitoral area of the female baby is abnormal. Blood in the diaper in the first two weeks of life are normal (maternal hormones are still present). In males, the urethral meatus should not be located behind or along the underside of the penis (hypospadias), or on the top side of the penis (epispadias). Two testes, round, smooth, and movable, should be felt, although the testes in infants can retract. Cryptorchidism is when the testes do not descend into the scrotal sac. A congenital hydrocele causes enlargement of the scrotum. Assess for inguinal hernias. Assess the anus for bleeding, fissures, skin tags, hemorrhoids, prolapse of the rectum and pinworms. Check for the anal wink (stroking area lightly should produce movement of the anus), the absence of which is abnormal and can result from spinal cord lesions, trauma, or tumors.

CUSTOMIZING ASSESSMENT FOR CHILDREN WITH SPECIAL NEEDS

Children may present in the emergency department with a variety of special needs, so initial assessment should include determining what special needs a child may have and then addressing them.

- **Children with cognitive impairment** (e.g., Down syndrome): Ask the caregiver about the child's level of understanding and comfort measures that might distract or ease the child's anxiety. Talk to the child in a soothing manner.
- **Children with autism**: Ask the caregiver about the things that trigger anxiety/meltdown in the child and ask the caregiver to help support the child. Ask before touching, and touch only as necessary. Explain procedures, especially if the child is high functioning.
- **Children with impaired vision**: Maintain a dialogue explaining activities and procedures, such as "I'm going to feel your tummy." Allow the child to touch equipment, such as a stethoscope, when possible.
- **Children with impaired hearing**: Ask about the degree of hearing loss and methods the child uses to communicate. Use a sign language interpreter if appropriate or ensure hearing aids are in place and functioning. Use pictures of treatments or procedures if possible.

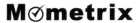

Hold Positions for Assessment and Procedures

Pediatric comfort holding positions for assessments and procedures include the following:

- **Hug hold**: Position an infant or small child facing the caregiver and straddling the caregiver's legs with the caregiver's arms securely hugging the child. Another person should distract the child or secure free arm(s). Good position for injections and venipuncture.
- **Side sitting**: Similar to a hug hold, with the child facing the caregiver, but legs to the side. Good position for older children who want less confinement.
- **Bracing**: Child is held in supine position in the caregiver's arms and braced against the chest or shoulder to prevent movement of the head. Good position for insertion of NG tubes or examination/treatment of mouth or other parts of face.
- **Sitting**: Child sits forward or sideways on caregiver's lap with caregiver's arms around child. Good position for children who want to watch or don't want to be more confined.
- **Supine**: Child lies on table with the caregiver lying behind the child so the child's head lies on the caregiver's lap while the caregiver holds the child or provides distraction.

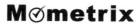

Diagnostic Testing and Screening

SOURCES AND PROCEDURES FOR OBTAINING DIAGNOSTIC STUDIES AND TEST RESULTS

The advent of the electronic health record has somewhat simplified the procedures for obtaining diagnostic studies and test results.

- **Laboratory systems** are typically stand-alone systems that must be interfaced with the electronic health record. The laboratory component of the electronic health record often is utilized as a means to coordinate laboratory orders, laboratory results, and administrative details.
- **Radiology information systems** are typically utilized to enable unification of patient data such as orders, results, and actual images. Radiology information can be accessed using a picture archive and communication system (PACS). PACS can be used to obtain diagnostic medical scans from a variety of imaging devices.

ANALYZING NORMAL AND ABNORMAL TEST RESULTS AND DIAGNOSTIC STUDIES

Knowledge of normal and abnormal values for test results and for diagnostic studies is a vital component of the nursing assessment. Nurses should have a basic knowledge of the purpose and procedures for typical laboratory tests, such as a blood test for complete blood count (CBC), and diagnostic practices, such as X-rays for bone fractures, as well as the specialized tests and studies relevant to their field of expertise. In addition, they should understand accepted standards or **norms**, and how normal values are defined by the facility where they are employed. These norms offer general guidelines for assessing any individual test results or diagnostic studies. Interpreting abnormal test results requires knowing what potential problems may be responsible and what mitigating factors in the patient's history, such as current medications or timing of the last meal, might be influencing these results. Often nurses are the first to review/receive critically abnormal lab results and must be sure to notify the physician immediately in case emergency interventions (such as electrolyte replacement or blood transfusions) must be ordered.

MEDICAL REASONING, DIAGNOSTIC REASONING, THERAPEUTIC REASONING, AND THERAPEUTIC UNCERTAINTY

Medical reasoning refers to the process by which clinicians gather data and information about a patient, and then use those data to arrive at a diagnosis and treatment plan. Diagnostic reasoning and therapeutic reasoning are subsets of medical reasoning. **Diagnostic reasoning** is the process that is used to determine the most likely diagnosis, while **therapeutic reasoning** is the process used to determine what the best treatment is for that particular patient suffering from that particular disease. While the patient is undergoing treatment, it is necessary for the clinician to evaluate the patient's response to treatment on a regular basis. If it is not clear whether the patient is improving, or whether another treatment might be more beneficial, a degree of **therapeutic uncertainty** is introduced. There is also therapeutic uncertainty when the clinician is trying to decide which treatment option to use if the first treatment fails.

IMPORTANCE OF DATA GATHERING TO DIAGNOSTIC REASONING

The gathering and recording of data are of utmost importance to the diagnostic evaluation process. The history and physical section of the patient chart contains a wealth of information (ideally) and should always be taken into consideration when developing a care plan for the patient. Because any number of clinicians can add information to the patient chart (and because all of these clinicians will be reading this information), it is important to record all information clearly and in an organized manner. This can be a daunting task when considering all of the different sources of information, including the patient interview, family member interviews, previous charts, and lab results. By keeping this information clear and concise, errors are minimized, and the differential diagnosis is comprehensive.

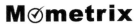

SENSITIVITY AND SPECIFICITY IN RELATION TO DIAGNOSTIC TESTING

Some degree of error is inherent in almost all diagnostic testing. When ordering a diagnostic test for a patient, how confident should the practitioner be that the result will be accurate? The terms **sensitivity and specificity** are used to illustrate the accuracy of diagnostic tests.

- The **sensitivity** of a diagnostic test refers to its ability to correctly identify patients who *do have the disease*. If a test is administered to 1000 patients with diabetes, and all 1000 patients test positive, the test is considered to have a sensitivity of 100%. If only 850 test positive, however, that means that the test has a false-negative rate of 15%, and a sensitivity of 85%.
- The **specificity** of a diagnostic test refers to its ability to identify patients who *do not have the disease*. If 1000 nondiabetic patients are tested for diabetes, and 200 of them test positive, the test has a false-positive rate of 20% and a specificity of 80%.

DIFFERENTIAL DIAGNOSIS PROCESS

The differential diagnosis is an important tool that allows the clinician to familiarize him or herself with the patient's condition, understand the condition, create an effective treatment plan, and follow the progress of the patient. To start, thoroughly examine the patient's chart, making a list of all of the abnormal test results and laboratory values. Add to this list all of the patient's complaints. Once this list is complete, organize the test results, labs, and complaints by anatomic location or organ system. After breaking the list down by organ site, look for any relationships between symptoms and/or results. Create another list of those data that seem to be related, and list all of the diseases or conditions that explain the findings, eliminating any that do not fit.

ANALYTICAL DECISION-MAKING

An **analytical decision** is one that is made after a systematic review and analysis of all factors involved in the decision. Concentration and awareness are important in the analytical decision-making process. In contrast with an intuitive decision, an analytical decision takes longer to make, because it is not automatic. The analysis involves an in-depth look at all factors and is based on scientific evidence (i.e., based on the outcomes of previous similar situations). Because an analytical decision is based on scientific evidence and facts, the outcome of the decision has a high predictive value; this means that by looking at previous outcomes, it is possible to predict the current outcome. Because the clinician has so carefully reviewed all factors, he or she will most likely not experience the emotional anxiety associated with an intuitive decision.

INTUITIVE DECISION-MAKING

When a clinician makes an **intuitive decision**, he or she is making a decision not necessarily based on fact, but more so because it feels like the right decision. Of course, in most cases, one would not want a doctor making decisions this way, although in certain cases (say, a choice between 2 different types of treatment, each of which has the same general risks, or when all other options have been exhausted), it may be necessary. Although these decisions are not based on an analysis of the facts, there is something to be said about the so-called "gut instinct," which years of training and experience can hone. These decisions are made without spending a lot of time on the process of decision-making; though they are based on experience, the clinician may suffer some degree of anxiety about the decision and its outcome.

INFLUENTIAL FACTORS IN CLINICAL DECISION-MAKING PROCESS

Although one would like to think that there isn't much variation in the clinical decision-making process, this simply is not true. The process, of course, will differ depending on the patient, the differential diagnosis, and the clinician. The first variable to consider is the clinician. The way that the clinician conducts the clinical decision-making process is influenced by the knowledge base of the clinician, as well as the level of his experience, the ability he possesses to think both critically and creatively, and the confidence that he has in his ability to make educated decisions. The acuity level of the patient is also a factor in the clinical decision-making process, as is the length of the differential. A time stressor is placed on the clinician when the condition of the patient is critical, and when there are more diseases that must be eliminated from the differential. An element

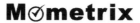

of stress may also exist if the clinician has a high number of patients, especially if he has multiple high-acuity patients.

QUESTIONS TO CONSIDER WHEN DEALING WITH DIAGNOSTIC AND THERAPEUTIC UNCERTAINTY

Diagnosis and subsequent treatment are not easily arrived at for every patient because every patient is different. The clinical presentation of a heart attack, for example, may include severe chest pain, sweating, and nausea for one patient, and may have very mild, almost unnoticeable symptoms in another. **Diagnostic uncertainty** is especially prominent when dealing with diseases that have nonspecific symptoms; in these cases, it is important that the clinician recognize which of the possible diagnoses are life-threatening, and which are not. Ruling out the life-threatening possibilities should be higher on the clinician's list of priorities than the nonlife-threatening ones. Diagnostic testing, and subsequent treatment options, should also be evaluated according to the risks and benefits to the patient.

DEGREE OF CLINICAL UNCERTAINTY

Although the degree of uncertainty is somewhat dependent on the patient, the clinical setting can have an influence on the degree of uncertainty that the clinician is likely to encounter. For example, a clinic, such as a dermatology clinic, is a setting in which the degree of uncertainty is likely to be low; this is because the clinic is nonemergent, and because the clinic treats a specific, limited group of diseases with which the clinicians are very familiar. An urgent care clinic would fall somewhere in the middle because, although there is a wider range of diagnostic possibility, life-threatening emergencies are rarely encountered. An emergency room or a trauma center, on the other hand, sees a high degree of uncertainty because the clinicians see a wide range of diagnostic possibilities, and are expected to work at a fast pace.

PREDICTIVE VALUES IN RELATION TO DISEASE PROBABILITY

Sensitivity and specificity are useful in evaluating the efficacy of a diagnostic test, but the predictive value of a test is more immediately relevant to individual patients. The **positive predictive value (PPV)** of a test is the likelihood that a patient who has *tested positive* truly has the condition that is being tested for. Similarly, the **negative predictive value (NPV)** of a test is the likelihood that a patient who has *tested negative* truly does not have the condition being tested for.

For a given controlled trial, PPV is calculated by dividing the number of true positive results by the number of total positive results (true and false positives). NPV is calculated by dividing the number of true negative results by the number of total negative results. Calculating the PPV and NPV is straightforward, but in order for these values to be applied to an individual patient, the assumption has to be made that the patient's pre-test likelihood of having the tested condition matches that of the trial's population.

SCREENING PROCEDURES FOR CHILDREN THROUGHOUT CHILDHOOD

Many screening procedures are available, including extensive laboratory testing that may be indicated if there is cause for concern that a child may have a disorder. However, some basic screening should be done for all children:

- **Genetic disorders:** Screening is usually done at birth according to state guidelines, and further testing may be indicated if there is concern that a child has a disorder that requires treatment.
- **Hearing:** Testing is usually done with newborns, between ages 3 and 8, and then every 2-3 years until age 18.
- **Height and weight:** These are monitored monthly during the first year and then at least yearly until age 18 to determine if the child's development is within the normal range.
- **Vision:** This is screened at birth, at 3-4 years, and periodically between 5-18. Vision problems may become obvious when the child enters school and can't see the board or has trouble reading.
- **Fasting blood sugar:** Done every 2 years for those at risk.
- **Head circumference:** Measurement is done at birth, 1 year, and 2 years.

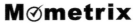

- **Blood pressure:** This is usually checked during infancy (6-12 months) and then periodically throughout childhood.
- **Dental screening:** Bottle fed babies may require earlier screening as they often fall asleep with the bottle in their mouths, leading to infant caries. Dental screening is done periodically throughout childhood, especially after the new teeth come in, to evaluate for malocclusion or other problems.
- **Alcohol/drug use:** Screening may be done periodically for children between 11-18 years, especially if they are at risk.
- **Developmental screening:** There are a number of screening tests that are available and can be used if a child appears to have a developmental delay or abnormality. Screening tests must be age-appropriate. The tests are not diagnostic, but can help to confirm developmental abnormalities. Tests may assess motor skills, language, and cognitive ability.

SCREENING CHILDREN FOR CELIAC DISEASE

Celiac disease is gluten-sensitive enteropathy with a chronic malabsorption syndrome caused by damage to the villi from toxic reactions to gluten in wheat, barley, rye, and oats. Symptoms normally don't appear until the child begins a diet of solid foods and exhibits chronic diarrhea, vomiting, and failure to thrive. A careful family history may indicate a genetic disposition, but these warning symptoms should trigger screening even without such history. Additionally, 4-13% of children with trisomy 21 (Down syndrome) have celiac disease, so screening is recommended for all infants with trisomy 21. Identifying children with celiac disease early and providing dietary counseling for the parents can prevent the damage to the intestines that will otherwise occur. Parents and eventually the child should be taught dietary substitutions and referred to national organizations, such as the American Celiac Society and the Celiac-Sprue Association, which can provide information and support.

SCREENING OF TEENAGERS FOR SCOLIOSIS

Scoliosis is the lateral curvature ≥11° of the spine, usually occurring (in 2-3% of adolescents) during the period between 10-15 when the child goes through a growth spurt, so screening should be done at least twice during this period. Scoliosis is more common in girls than boys. Screening includes:

- Child stands upright and shoulders, waist, and hips are assessed.
- Adams forward bending test, in which the child bends over at the waist (as in toe touching) and the screener observes the hips to determine if there is a difference in height.
- Scoliometer measures the curvature of the spine in the thoracic and lumbar area when the child bends over.
- Moire topography uses a grating positioned near the child so it casts shadows that show contour lines.
- X-rays are used to confirm positive screenings.

Positive findings may include one shoulder lower than another, uneven waistline, prominence of shoulder blade(s), one hip higher than another, or lateral leaning when upright.

COLLECTION OF BLOOD SPECIMENS

COLLECTION OF CAPILLARY BLOOD SAMPLES

The **heel stick** is used in infants up to 6 months of age. The heel is warmed for 5 to 10 minutes, followed by cleaning with an alcohol wipe. Special lancets should be used that ensure the puncture goes no deeper than 2 mm. The outside or inside edge of the heel should be used to prevent osteochondritis. After the specimen is collected, apply pressure until bleeding has stopped and apply a bandage. A colorful bandage will help reassure school age children and keep dirt out of the wound. Pain control should be provided to reduce the pain and stress associated with blood draws.

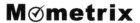

COLLECTION OF VENOUS AND ARTERIAL BLOOD SPECIMENS

The nurse is responsible for overseeing that the **blood specimens** are collected according to protocol, including the timing of collections, the equipment used, and the transportation and storage of the specimens. Venous samples are obtained from an access line (the type of fluid being infused may affect the blood values) or by venipuncture. Pressure is applied after venipuncture to prevent bruising, followed by a bandage. Central lines are the preferred access lines, as peripheral lines are prone to being replaced more often when used to collect blood. Arterial samples are useful for measuring blood gases, using an arterial catheter inserted into the femoral, brachial, or radial arteries or using deep heel stick. Always assess for circulatory problems before attempting an arterial draw. Make sure the child is calm, as crying can affect the values. Heparinized tubes are used to prevent clotting of the blood, and care is taken to ensure that no air bubbles enter the tube. Provide explanations to children according developmental level. Provide pain control as needed.

POSITIONING TECHNIQUES FOR VENIPUNCTURES IN PEDIATRIC PATIENTS

Painful procedures require adequate pain relief. Older children can cooperate and need little restraint. Babies and younger children need good positioning to comfort them and decrease movement. A jugular venipuncture requires that the infant be placed in a mummy restraint (wrapped in a blanket in such a way that restrains the arms and legs) or that the older child's arms and legs are restrained. A small pillow is placed under the neck, the neck is extended, and the head positioned and held still. After the procedure, pressure is applied to the site for 3-5 minutes without compromising breathing or circulation. A femoral venipuncture requires the infant to be supine with the legs turned out. The legs are restrained. For a venipuncture in an extremity, stabilize the arm or leg while another person hugs the child to prevent movement and helps to hold the extremity.

DIAGNOSTIC PURPOSE OF IMAGING TESTS

X-Ray

X-rays are used for diagnosis and evaluation of treatment and to determine correct placement of medical devices. **X-rays** pass more readily through soft tissue than dense tissue, so dense tissue, which has less radiation exposure, appears as white against the darker background of soft tissue. Therefore, x-rays are most commonly used for evaluation of bones, such as for fractures or dislocations. They may also be used for soft tissue when a disease or disorder alters density of tissue, such as with pneumonia in the lungs or gallstones, kidney stones, or tumors although small tumors may go undetected. Different types of tissue have different color gradations. For example, organs with high fluid content (stomach, liver) appear gray while muscles (which have more fat) appear slightly darker. Spaces filled with air (such as the lungs) appear very dark. X-rays may also be used with contrast medium to take images of the cardiovascular or GI systems.

CT Scan

Computerized tomography (CT) involves scanning tissue in successive layers through a narrow-beam x-ray, providing a cross-sectional view. CTs can demonstrate differences in soft-tissue density. CT scans may be done with fluoroscopy or contrast material, such as iodine dye, to evaluate for infections, tumors, or other abnormalities. CT scans can differentiate between cellulitis and formation of abscesses better than a routine x-ray.

MRI

Magnetic resonance imaging (MRI) uses magnetic fields and radiofrequency signals to create a cross-sectional view, and the images are more detailed than with CT. MRI may be done with or without contrast material. MRI uses radio waves and magnetic fields to create images of internal structures, providing information about infections, tumors, or other abnormalities that may not be obvious with x-rays, CT scans, or ultrasounds. MRIs are more expensive than x-rays, CTs, or ultrasounds, so they are often done after other testing has been inconclusive.

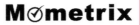

ULTRASOUND

Ultrasound uses ultrasonic sound waves transmitted by a transducer, which picks up reflected sound waves that a computer converts to electronic images. **Ultrasound** can show fluid accumulation, the movement of blood through the organs, masses, malformations (congenital abnormalities), change in size of the organs or other structures, and obstructions.

OVERNIGHT POLYSOMNOGRAM

An overnight polysomnogram (PSG) is a sleep study, which is often used when a child presents with some type of sleep disorder, such as night terrors or sleepwalking. A PSG requires an overnight stay in a sleep lab. Sensors are connected to the child's head to measure brain activity and eye movement during the study. Pulse oximetry may also be used to assess oxygen levels during sleep. The child is connected to the sensors and then goes to sleep in the room. Typically, a parent is allowed to sleep in the same room during the study to reduce the child's fears.

DIFFERENTIAL DIAGNOSIS

PROCESS

The differential diagnosis is an important tool that allows the clinician to become familiar with the patient's condition, understand the condition, create an effective treatment plan, and follow the progress of the patient. To start, thoroughly examine the patient's chart, making a list of all of the abnormal test results and laboratory values. Add to this list all of the patient's complaints. Once this list is complete, organize the test results, labs, and complaints by anatomic location or organ system. After breaking the list down by organ site, look for any relationships between symptoms and/or results. Create another list of those data that seem to be related, and list all of the diseases or conditions that explain the findings, eliminating any that do not fit.

INFLUENCES ON THE CLINICAL DECISION-MAKING PROCESS

Although one would like to think that there isn't much variation in the **clinical decision-making process**, this simply is not true. The process, of course, will differ depending on the patient, the differential diagnosis, and the clinician. Let's start with the clinician. The way the clinician conducts the clinical decision-making process is influenced by the knowledge base of the clinician, as well as the level of his experience, the ability he possesses to think both critically and creatively, and the confidence that he has in his ability to make educated decisions. The acuity level of the patient is also a factor in the clinical decision-making process, as is the length of the differential. A time stressor is placed on the clinician when the condition of the patient is critical, and when there are more diseases that must be eliminated from the differential. An element of stress may also exist if the clinician has a high number of patients, especially if there are multiple high-acuity patients.

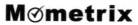

Review of Systems: Cardiovascular

PEDIATRIC CARDIOVASCULAR DYSFUNCTION SIGNS AND RISK FACTORS

The most apparent **clinical signs of cardiovascular dysfunction** will be poor feeding and weight gain, sweating and getting tired during feedings, signs of respiratory distress (rapid breathing, shortness of breath, and cyanosis), always feeling tired and inability to exercise. Children at risk are those whose mothers drank alcohol, smoked, or took medications, were exposed to radiation during pregnancy, had a viral illness during pregnancy, or were over 40 when pregnant. The child may have been premature or have autoimmune or chromosomal disorders. Smoking and alcohol use and medications can increase the risk. Family members who have had cardiovascular problems also increase the child's risk.

The following should be included in cardiac monitoring and maintenance of a child with cardiovascular disease or dysfunction:

- Cardiac monitoring and vital signs are essential.
- Watch for signs of inadequate oxygen intake, such as increased work of breathing, cyanosis, bradycardia or tachycardia, irritability, decreased muscle tone and syncope. Reposition to ease breathing and provide oxygen and medications as prescribed to manage respiratory distress.
- Monitor for respiratory distress (fast RR and HR, retracting, nasal flaring, grunting, coughing, and cyanosis). Thrombosis may present, along with edema, irritability, seizures, paralysis, coma, blood in urine, and decreased urine output.
- Maintain fluid and electrolyte balance.
- Encourage and promote rest.
- Monitor intake and output and provide nutritionally balanced diet with lots of iron and potassium and little sodium.
- Don't overtire with large feedings, and instead feed more often with smaller meals.
- Encourage infection control with hand washing, rest, good nutrition, administration of vaccines, and distancing people with infections from the cardiac patient. Prophylactic antibiotics should be administered before dental procedures to prevent bacterial endocarditis. This illness presents with fever, pale skin, petechiae, weight loss and fatigue.

NORMAL CARDIAC RATES IN THE PEDIATRIC POPULATION

Normal cardiac rates can vary widely from one child to another, so it's important to understand the normal range in order to determine if the child has an abnormal pulse. Rates will also vary depending upon whether the child is awake, asleep, or active. Pulse rate should be taken with a stethoscope because the pulse may be difficult to palpate or count accurately manually, especially for infants and small children. Additionally, this allows assessment for heart murmurs.

	At rest:	Asleep:	Active/sick:
Newborn infant	100–180	80–160	≤220
1–12 weeks	80–205	80–200	≤220
3–24 months	75–190	70–120	≤200
2–10 years	60–150	60–90	≤200
10–adulthood	55–100	50–90	≤200

RELATIONSHIP BETWEEN CO, HR, AND SV

In order to understand the hemodynamics of infants and children, it's important to understand the relationship between cardiac output, stroke volume, and heart rate as the child grows and cardiac size increases:

Age	CO	SV	HR
Newborn	800/mL/ min	5 mL	145
6 months	1,000-1,600 mL/min	10 mL	120
12 months	1,500 mL/min	13 mL	115
4 years	2,700 mL/min	26 mL	105
8 years	3,500 mL/min	42 mL	83
10 years	3,750 mL/min	50 mL	75
15 years (adult levels)	5,000-6,000 mL/min	85 mL	70

ASSESSMENT OF THE CARDIOVASCULAR SYSTEM

Cardiovascular assessment includes questioning the patient for any family history of death at a young age or other cardiovascular diseases. Elderly African-American males are at highest risk for cardiovascular problems. One must question the patient about edema, chest pain, dyspnea, fatigue, vertigo, syncope or other changes in consciousness, weight gain, and leg cramps or pain. If chest pain is a symptom, one must ask about the intensity, timing, location, any radiation, quality, meaning to the patient, factors that aggravate or alleviate the pain, nausea, dyspnea, diaphoresis, or any other accompanying symptoms. Physical assessment includes assessment of vital signs, heart and lung sounds, skin assessment, radial, popliteal, and pedal pulses, circulation and sensation of extremities, and auscultation of the aorta, renal, iliac, and femoral arteries for bruits. Blood should be taken for a lipid profile and electrolytes. The patient must be helped to modify risk factors such as hypertension, smoking, diabetes, obesity, hyperlipidemia, inactivity, and stress.

> **Review Video: Cardiovascular Assessment**
> Visit mometrix.com/academy and enter code: 323076
>
> **Review Video: Circulatory System**
> Visit mometrix.com/academy and enter code: 376581
>
> **Review Video: Heart Blood Flow**
> Visit mometrix.com/academy and enter code: 783139

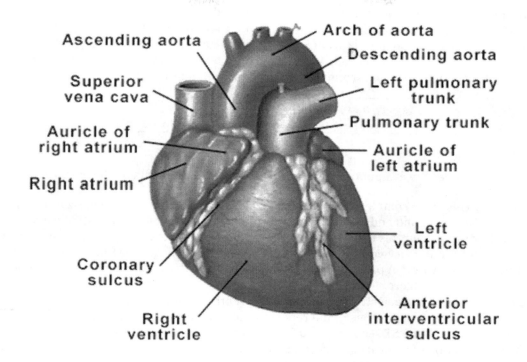

ASSESSMENT OF HEART SOUNDS

Auscultation of heart sounds can help to diagnose different cardiac disorders. Areas to auscultate include the aortic area, pulmonary area, Erb's point, tricuspid area, and the apical area. The **normal heart sounds** represent closing of the valves.

- The **first heart sound** (S1) "lub" is closure of the mitral and tricuspid valves (heard at apex/left ventricular area of the heart).
- The **second heart sound** (S2) "dub" is closure of the aortic and pulmonic valves (heard at the base of the heart). There may be a slight splitting of the S2.

The time between S1 and S2 is systole and the time between S2 and the next S1 is diastole. Systole and diastole should be silent although ventricular disease can cause gallops, snaps, or clicks and stenosis of the valves or failure of the valves to close can cause murmurs. Pericarditis may cause a friction rub.

Additional heart sounds:

- **Gallop rhythms**: S3 commonly occurs after S2 in children and young adults but may indicate heart failure or left ventricular failure in older adults (when heard with patient lying on left side). S4 occurs before S1, during the contracting of the atria when there is ventricular hypertrophy, found in coronary artery disease, hypertension, or aortic valve stenosis.
- **Opening snap**: Unusual high-pitched sound occurring after S2 with stenosis of mitral valve from rheumatic heart disease
- **Ejection click**: Brief high-pitched sound after S1; aortic stenosis

- **Friction rub**: Harsh, grating holosystolic sound; pericarditis
- **Murmur**: Sound caused by turbulent blood flow from stenotic or malfunctioning valves, congenital defects, or increased blood flow. Murmurs are characterized by location, timing in the cardiac cycle, intensity (rated from Grade I to Grade VI), pitch (low to high-pitched), quality (rumbling, whistling, blowing) and radiation (to the carotids, axilla, neck, shoulder, or back).

> **Review Video: Diastolic vs Systolic**
> Visit mometrix.com/academy and enter code: 898934

CARDIAC MONITORING

Cardiac monitoring includes the evaluation of different intervals and segments on the electrocardiogram:

- **QT interval**: This is the complete time of ventricular depolarization and repolarization, which begins with the QRS segment and ends when the Y wave is completed. Typically, duration usually ranges from 0.36 to 0.44 seconds, but this may vary depending on the heart rate. If the heat rate is rapid, the duration is shorter and vice versa. Certain medications can prolong the QT interval, in such cases monitoring this is critical. A prolonged QT interval puts the patient at risk for R-on-T phenomenon, which can result in dangerous arrhythmias.
- **ST segment**: This is an isoelectric period when the ventricles are in a plateau phase, completely depolarized and beginning recovery and repolarization. Deflection is usually isoelectric, but may range from -0.5 to +1mm. If the ST segment is ≥0.5 mm below the baseline, it is considered depressed and may be an indication of myocardial ischemia. Depression may also indicate digitalis toxicity. If the ST segment is elevated ≥1 mm above baseline, this is an indication of myocardial injury.

MAP

The MAP **(mean arterial pressure)** is most commonly used to evaluate perfusion as it shows pressure throughout the cardiac cycle. Systole is one-third and diastole two-thirds of the normal cardiac cycle. The MAP for a blood pressure of 120/60 is calculated as follows:

$$MAP = \frac{Diastole \times 2 + Systole}{3}$$

$$MAP = \frac{60 \times 2 + 120}{3} = \frac{240}{3} = 80$$

Normal range for mean arterial pressure is 70-100 mmHg. A MAP of greater than 60 mmHg is required to perfuse vital organs, including the heart, brain, and kidneys.

OXYGEN SATURATION AS IT RELATES TO HEMODYNAMIC STATUS

Hemodynamic monitoring includes monitoring **oxygen saturation** levels, which must be maintained for proper cardiac function. The central venous catheter often has an oxygen sensor at the tip to monitor oxygen saturation in the right atrium. If the catheter tip is located near the renal veins, this can cause an increase in right atrial oxygen saturation; and near the coronary sinus, a decrease.

- Increased oxygen saturation may result from left atrial to right atrial shunt, abnormal pulmonary venous return, increased delivery of oxygen or decrease in extraction of oxygen.
- Decreased oxygen saturation may be related to low cardiac output with an increase in oxygen extraction or decrease in arterial oxygen saturation with normal differences in the atrial and ventricular oxygen saturation.

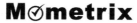

ELECTROCARDIOGRAM

The electrocardiogram records and shows a graphic display of the electrical activity of the heart through a number of different waveforms, complexes, and intervals:

- **P wave**: Start of electrical impulse in the sinus node and spreading through the atria, muscle depolarization
- **QRS complex**: Ventricular muscle depolarization and atrial repolarization
- **T wave**: Ventricular muscle repolarization (resting state) as cells regain negative charge
- **U wave**: Repolarization of the Purkinje fibers

A modified lead II ECG is often used to monitor basic heart rhythms and dysrhythmias:

- Typical placement of leads for 2-lead ECG is 3-5 cm inferior to the right clavicle and left lower ribcage. Typical placement for a 3-lead ECG is (RA) right arm near shoulder, (LA) V_5 position over 5th intercostal space, and (LL) left upper leg near groin.

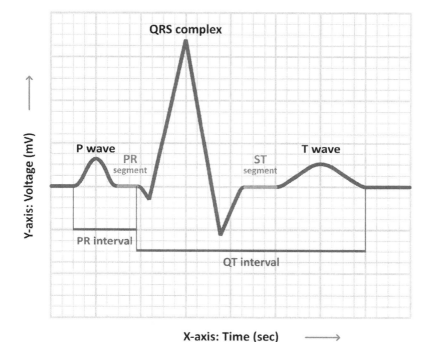

83

ADMINISTRATION OF 12-LEAD ECG

The electrocardiogram provides a graphic representation of the electrical activity of the heart. It is indicated for chest pain, dyspnea, syncope, acute coronary syndrome, pulmonary embolism, and possible MI. The standard **12 lead ECG** gives a picture of electrical activity from 12 perspectives through placement of 10 body leads:

- 4 limb leads are placed distally on the wrists and ankles (but may be placed more proximally if necessary).
- Precordial leads:
    - V1: Right sternal border at 4th intercostal space
    - V2: Left sternal border at 4th intercostal space
    - V3: Midway between V2 and V4
    - V4: Left midclavicular line at 5th intercostal space
    - V5: Horizontal to V4 at left anterior axillary line
    - V6: Horizontal to V5 at left midaxillary line

In some cases, additional leads may be used:

- Right-sided leads are placed on the right in a mirror image of the left leads, usually to diagnose right ventricular infarction through ST elevation.

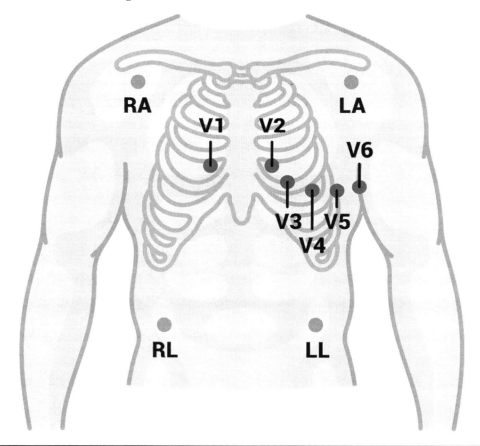

Review Video: 12 Lead ECG
Visit mometrix.com/academy and enter code: 962539

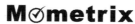

ASSESSMENT OF LOWER EXTREMITIES

Assessment of lower extremities includes a number of different elements:

- **Appearance** includes comparing limbs for obvious differences or changes in skin or nails as well as evaluating for edema, color changes in skin, such as pallor or rubor. Legs that are thin, pale, shiny, and hairless indicate peripheral arterial disease.
- **Perfusion** should be assessed by checking venous filling time and capillary refill, skin temperature (noting changes in one limb or between limbs), bruits (indicating arterial narrowing), pulses (comparing both sides in a proximal to distal progression), ankle-brachial index and toe-brachial index.
- **Sensory function** includes the ability to feel pain, temperature, and touch.
- **Range of motion** of the ankle must be assessed to determine if the joint flexes past 90° because this is necessary for unimpaired walking and aids venous return in the calf.
- **Pain** is an important diagnostic feature of peripheral arterial disease, so the location, intensity, duration, and characteristics of pain are important.

ASSESSMENT OF PULSE AND BRUIT

Evaluation of the pulses of the **lower extremities** is an important part of assessment for peripheral arterial disease/trauma. Pulses should be first evaluated with the patient in supine position and then again with the legs dependent, checking bilaterally and proximal to distal to determine if intensity of pulse decreases distally. Pedal pulses should be examined at both the posterior tibialis and the dorsalis pedis. The pulse should be evaluated as to the rate, rhythm, and intensity, which is usually graded on a 0 to 4 scale:

$$0 = \text{pulse absent}$$
$$1 = \text{weak, difficult to palpate}$$
$$2 = \text{normal as expected}$$
$$3 = \text{full}$$
$$4 = \text{strong and bounding}$$

Pulses may be **palpable** or **absent** with peripheral arterial disease. Absence of pulse on both palpation and Doppler probe does indicate peripheral arterial disease.

Bruits may be noted by auscultating over major arteries, such as femoral, popliteal, peroneal, and dorsalis pedis, indicating peripheral arterial disease.

ASSESSING PERFUSION OF LOWER EXTREMITIES

Assessment of perfusion can indicate venous or arterial abnormalities:

- **Venous refill time**: Begin with the patient lying supine for a few moments and then have the patient sit with the feet dependent. Observe the veins on the dorsum of the foot and count the seconds before normal filling. Venous occlusion is indicated with times greater than 20 seconds.
- **Capillary refill**: Grasp the toenail bed between the thumb and index finger and apply pressure for several seconds to cause blanching. Release the nail and count the seconds until the nail regains normal color. Arterial occlusion is indicated with times of more than 2 to 3 seconds. Check both feet and more than one nail bed.
- **Skin temperature**: Using the palm of the hand and fingers, gently palpate the skin, moving distally to proximally and comparing both legs. Arterial disease is indicated by decreased temperature (coolness) or a marked change from proximal to distal. Venous disease is indicated by increased temperature about the ankle.

ABI
PROCEDURE

The ankle-brachial index **(ABI) examination** is done to evaluate peripheral arterial disease of the lower extremities.

1. Apply BP cuff to one arm, palpate brachial pulse, and place conductivity gel over the artery.
2. Place the tip of a Doppler device at a 45-degree angle into the gel at the brachial artery and listen for the pulse sound.
3. Inflate the cuff until the pulse sound ceases and then inflate 20 mmHg above that point.
4. Release air and listen for the return of the pulse sound. This reading is the brachial systolic pressure.
5. Repeat the procedure on the other arm and use the higher reading for calculations.
6. Repeat the same procedure on each ankle with the cuff applied above the malleoli and the gel over the posterior tibial pulse to obtain the ankle systolic pressure.
7. Divide the ankle systolic pressure by the brachial systolic pressure to obtain the ABI.

Sometimes, readings are taken both before and after 5 minutes of walking on a treadmill.

INTERPRETING RESULTS

Once the ABI examination is completed, the ankle systolic pressure must be divided by the brachial systolic pressure. Ideally, the BP at the ankle should be equal to that of the arm or slightly higher. With peripheral arterial disease the ankle pressure falls, affecting the ABI. Additionally, some conditions that cause calcification of arteries, such as diabetes, can cause a false elevation.

Calculation is simple:

$$ABI = \frac{\text{Ankle systolic}}{\text{Brachial systolic}}$$

The degree of disease relates to the **score**:

- >1.4: Abnormally high, may indicate calcification of vessel wall
- 1.0–1.4: Normal reading, asymptomatic
- 0.9–1.0: Low reading, but acceptable unless there are other indications of PAD
- 0.8–0.9: Likely some arterial disease is present
- 0.5–0.8: Moderate arterial disease
- < 0.5: Severe arterial disease

CARDIAC ENZYMES
CK AND CK-MB

Creatine kinase (CK) and CK-MB levels are evaluated every 6–8 hours in a suspected myocardial injury. Total CK and CK-MB (specific to cardiac cells) initially rise within the first 4–6 hours of an MI. A normal range would be 30 IU/L to 180 IU/L for CK and CK-MB totaling 0–5% of the CK level.

Assuming no further damage is sustained, peak levels (in excess of 6 times the normal range) are reached 12–24 hours after the injury. CK levels will return to normal within 3–4 days of the event. Small spikes in CK level might also occur following invasive cardiac procedures.

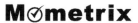

TROPONIN I AND T

Troponin, which is found in cardiac and skeletal muscle, is a type of protein. Both troponin I and T (isolates of troponin) are found in the myocardium, but troponin T is also found in skeletal muscle, so it is less specific than troponin I. Troponin I, therefore, may be used to detect a myocardial infarction after non-cardiac surgery and to detect acute coronary syndrome. Troponin is released into the bloodstream when injury to the tissue (such as the myocardium) occurs and causes damage to the cell membranes, as occurs with myocardial injury.

- **Troponin I** (<0.05 ng/mL): Appears in 2-6 hours, peaks at 15-20 hours and returns to normal in 5-7 days. Exhibits a second but lower peak at 60-80 hours (biphasic).
- **Troponin T** (<0.2 ng/mL): Increases 2-6 hours after MI and stays elevated. Returns to normal in 7 days. (Less specific than troponin I)

ECHOCARDIOGRAPHY

Echocardiography is a non-invasive ultrasound technology that is very useful for assessing and diagnosing anatomic heart abnormalities, blood flow, and valvular lesions:

- The **standard "2D Echo"** is used best for basic structural imaging, such as valvular lesions and assessment of pericardial disorders.
- The **transesophageal (TEE)** probe is an improved version of echocardiography, which allows better visualization of the left atrium and more precise evaluation of the valvular structure. TEE is also the best modality for evaluation of the thoracic aorta in the setting of suspected aortic dissection or aneurysm.
- **Doppler imaging** is used to measure blood flow, often in the context of velocity across a valve and a pressure gradient.
- **Bubble study** is an addition to echocardiography allowing the study to determine if there is right to left blood flow through a patent foramen ovale or a more distal intrapulmonary shunt of blood.

STRESS ECHOCARDIOGRAPHY

Basic **cardiac stress testing** consists of exercise EKG testing (EET) and exercise imaging testing. The exercise imaging testing may be broken down into exercise, or "stress" echocardiography, and exercise myocardial perfusion imaging.

Exercise imaging testing is usually performed with echocardiography. Stress echocardiography is performed similarly to exercise EKG testing and also requires that the patient meet at least 85% maximum heart rate in order to attain optimum sensitivity and specificity. (The maximum heart rate formula is 220 minus the person's age.) Of note, chemicals may substitute for exercise during the "stress" portion of the test. This may be performed with dobutamine (beta-1-agonist: cannot be used after beta-blocker administration) or adenosine (causes diffuse coronary dilatation, leading to decreased perfusion pressure and unmasking of defects, and cannot be used with asthma). Stress imaging allows the study to determine the actual area of ischemia and whether or not this is a reversible defect. Additional information obtained during echocardiography is cardiac output and measurement of viability.

Review of Systems: Respiratory

ASSESSMENT OF THE RESPIRATORY SYSTEM

If significant respiratory distress is present, one must stabilize the patient before doing a **respiratory history** or ask family if available:

- Question the patient about risk factors, such as smoking, exposure to smoke or other inhaled toxins, past lung problems, and allergies.
- Ask the patient about symptoms of respiratory problems, such as dyspnea, cough, sputum production, fatigue, ability to do ADLs and IADLs, and chest pain.
- Determine how long symptoms have been present, the length of periods of dyspnea, aggravating and alleviating factors, and the severity of symptoms.

When performing a **physical assessment**, one should assess vital signs, posture, pulse oximetry, check nails for clubbing, do a skin assessment, listen to lung sounds via auscultation and percussion, and look for accessory muscle use, signs of anxiety, and edema. Depending on condition, blood may be drawn for arterial blood gases, electrolytes, and CBC. Sputum cultures may be obtained.

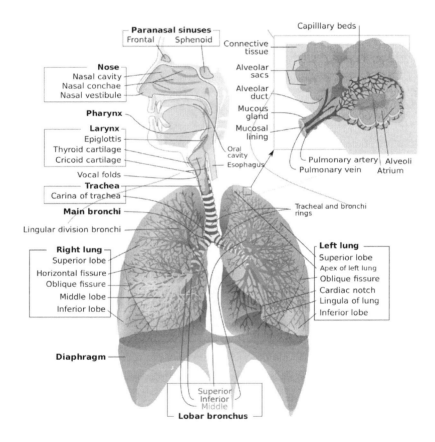

Review Video: Respiratory System
Visit mometrix.com/academy and enter code: 783075

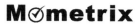

Primary and Secondary Muscles Used for Breathing

Muscles used for breathing are separated into primary and secondary muscle groups.

- The **primary muscle groups** are those that are used in normal, quiet breathing. When patients are in respiratory distress and breathing is more difficult, secondary muscle groups become activated. The muscles considered primary for breathing are the diaphragm and the external intercostal muscles. These muscles act by changing the pressure gradient, allowing the lungs to expand and air to flow in and out.
- The **secondary muscle groups** include the sternocleidomastoid, scaleni, internal intercostals, obliques, and abdominal muscles. These secondary muscle groups work when breathing is difficult, both in inspiration and expiration, in cases such as obstructions or bronchoconstriction. Use of these secondary muscle groups can often be seen on exam and may be described as see-saw or abdominal breathing (when the abdominal muscles are being used during exhalation) or retractions as the muscles activate and can be seen between rigid structures such as bone.

Normal Physiological Airway Clearance

Normal airway clearance is caused by various aspects of the respiratory system. A thin layer of mucus lines the airways as a protective mechanism against debris and helps trap foreign objects before they enter the lower airways. Proper hydration keeps the mucosa adequately moist so it can trap foreign debris. As this debris lands in the mucus, the cilia in the respiratory tract act as an "elevator" to push the debris up to the larynx, where it can either be coughed up or swallowed and digested. An intact cough reflex is necessary for the debris to stimulate the cough, and normal muscle strength and nerve innervation of the diaphragm is required to produce a sufficiently forceful cough.

Ventilation/Perfusion Ratio

In order to maintain homeostasis, the respiratory and cardiac systems need to maintain a careful balance. The **ventilation/perfusion ratio** indicates that ventilation of the lungs and perfusion to the lungs are within a normal balance. A normal ventilation/perfusion ratio is equal to 0.8. A ventilation/perfusion ratio higher than normal is indicative of ventilation that is too high, perfusion that is too low, or some combination of the two. This can occur because of hyperventilation (either physiological or caused by healthcare practitioners due to incorrect ventilator settings), pulmonary embolism, or hypotension. Essentially, a high ventilation/perfusion ratio means that there is more ventilation than perfusion. If the ventilation/perfusion ratio is lower than normal, then ventilation is too low, perfusion is too high, or some combination of the two. This can be caused by atelectasis, pneumonia, or lung disease. Whatever the cause, a low ventilation/perfusion ratio indicates that there is more perfusion than ventilation.

Normal and Abnormal Breath Sound Terms

Normal breath sounds can be divided into three types. Vesicular breath sounds are low, soft sounds that can normally be heard over the peripheral lung space. Bronchovesicular breath sounds are moderate pitch breath sounds that are normally heard in the upper lung fields. Tracheal breath sounds are higher in pitch and heard over the trachea. Abnormal breath sounds are also known as adventitious lung sounds. Wheezes are high-pitched, expiratory sounds caused by air flowing through an obstructed airway. Stridor is also high-pitched, but is usually heard on inspiration in the upper airways. Coarse crackles are caused by an excessive amount of secretions in the airway and can be heard on inspiration and expiration. Fine crackles occur late in the expiratory phase and usually occur when the peripheral airways are being "popped" back open.

> **Review Video: Lung Sounds**
> Visit mometrix.com/academy and enter code: 765616

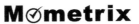

DIAGNOSTIC PROCEDURES AND TOOLS USED DURING PULMONARY ASSESSMENT

The diagnostic procedures and tools used during assessment of **pulmonary and thoracic trauma/disease** will vary according to the type and degree of injury/disease, but may include:

- **Thorough physical examination** including cardiac and pulmonary status, assessing for any abnormalities.
- **Electrocardiogram** to assess for cardiac arrhythmias.
- **Chest x-ray** should be done for all those with injuries to check for fractures, pneumothorax, major injuries, and placement of intubation tubes. X-rays can be taken quickly and with portable equipment so they can be completed quickly during the initial assessment.
- **Computerized tomography** may be indicated after initial assessment, especially if there is a possibility of damage to the parenchyma of the lungs.
- **Oximetry and atrial blood gases** as indicated.
- **12-lead electrocardiogram** may be needed if there are arrhythmias for more careful observation.
- **Echocardiogram** should be done if there is apparent cardiac damage.

CAPNOGRAPHY WITH END-TIDAL CO2 DETECTOR

Capnometry utilizes an **end-tidal CO2 (ETCO) detector** that measures the concentration of CO_2 in expired air, usually through pH sensitive paper that changes color (commonly purple to yellow). Typically, the capnometer is attached to the ETT and a bag-valve-mask (BVM) ventilator attached. The capnogram provides data in the shape of a waveform that represents the partial pressure of exhaled gas. It is often used to confirm placement of endotracheal tubes as clinical assessment is not always sufficient, and it is a noninvasive mode of monitoring carbon dioxide in the respiratory cycle. Information provided by the capnogram includes:

- $PaCO_2$ level
- Type and degree of bronchial obstruction, such as COPD (waveform changes from rectangular to a fin-like)
- Air leaks in the ventilation system
- Rebreathing precipitated by need for new CO_2 absorber
- Cardiac arrest
- Hypothermia or reduced metabolism

The normal capnogram is a waveform that represents the varying CO_2 level throughout the breath cycle:

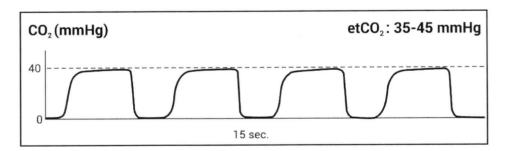

ARTERIAL BLOOD GASES

Arterial blood gases (ABGs) are monitored to assess effectiveness of oxygenation, ventilation, and acid-base status and to determine oxygen flow rates. Partial pressure of a gas is that exerted by each gas in a mixture of gases, proportional to its concentration, based on total atmospheric pressure of 760 mmHg at sea level. Normal values include:

- Acidity/alkalinity (pH): 7.35-7.45
- Partial pressure of carbon dioxide ($PaCO_2$): 35-45 mmHg

90

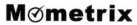

- Partial pressure of oxygen (PaO$_2$): ≥80 mmHg
- Bicarbonate concentration (HCO$_3^-$): 22-26 mEq/L
- Oxygen saturation (SaO$_2$): ≥95%

The relationship between these elements, particularly the PaCO$_2$ and the PaO$_2$ indicates respiratory status. For example, PaCO$_2$ >55 and the PaO$_2$ <60 in a patient previously in good health indicates respiratory failure. There are many issues to consider. Ventilator management may require a higher PaCO$_2$ to prevent barotrauma and a lower PaO$_2$ to reduce oxygen toxicity.

NORMAL RESPIRATORY RATES IN INFANTS AND CHILDREN

Children's vital signs vary considerably according to age, height, and weight. **Normal respiratory rates** are as follows:

- Newborns breathe about 30-60 times per minute and then respirations begin to slow to 30 times per minute by age 1 month, dropping to 24-30 during ages 1-3, and 17-29 by age 6.
- Respiratory rates for children 6-12 are typically 13-23 and then decrease to a rate similar to adults (12-20) between ages 12 and 28.

RESPIRATORY MONITORING WITH PULSE OXIMETRY

Pulse oximetry, continuous or intermittent, utilizes an external oximeter that attaches to the child's foot, toe, or finger (depending on age) to indirectly estimate **arterial oxygen saturation (SPO$_2$)**, the percentage of hemoglobin that is saturated with oxygen. The oximeter also usually attaches to a machine that emits a beep with each heartbeat and indicates the current heart rate and BP. The oximeter uses light waves to determine oxygen saturation (SPO$_2$). Oxygen saturation should be maintained >95% although some patients with cardiovascular or pulmonary disorders may have lower SPO$_2$. Results may be compromised by impaired circulation, excessive light, poor positioning, and fingernail polish. If SPO$_2$ falls, the oximeter should be repositioned, as incorrect position is a common cause of inaccurate readings. Oximetry is often used post-surgically and when patients are on mechanical ventilation. Oximeters do not provide information about carbon dioxide levels, so they cannot monitor carbon dioxide retention. Oximeters cannot differentiate between different forms of hemoglobin, so if hemoglobin has picked up carbon monoxide, the oximeter will not recognize it.

SPIROMETRY/PULMONARY FUNCTION TEST

Spirometry, a form of pulmonary function testing, uses a device to measure the volume of gas and the flow rate. Spirometry measurements can include forced vital capacity (FVC), forced expiratory volume in 1 second (FEV1), multiple forced expiratory flow (FEF) values, forced inspiratory flow (FIFs), and the maximum voluntary ventilation (MVV). Procedure:

1. Explain the procedure and allow the patient to practice taking one or two deep breaths and then exhaling with lips sealed about the mouthpiece, so the patient understands what to do.
2. Gender, age, height, and weight is usually input into the device.
3. The patient should sit because sitting is safer as some may experience dizziness during the test.
4. Secure nose clips.
5. Ask the patient to take a deep breath and then to exhale through the mouthpiece as strongly as possible for as long as possible. (Some computerized devices provide feedback on a computer screen, such as candles that extinguish as the patient breathes out.)
6. Repeat at least 2 more times. The best score out of 3 or more is used.
7. If a patient is to be retested after a bronchodilator, the patient should wait for 15 minutes after receiving the medication before repeating the tests.

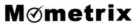

Review of Systems: Neurological

NEUROLOGICAL DYSFUNCTION SYMPTOMS IN CHILDREN

Abnormal neurological symptoms include headaches, dizziness or fainting, loss of consciousness, difficulty with movement or coordination, or delayed development. Factors that put the child at risk include maternal drug/alcohol use, maternal infection, poor maternal nutrition, prematurity, birth trauma, head injury, hypoxia, toxins, meningitis, drug use, chronic disease, child abuse, chromosomal abnormalities, or a family history of neurological disorders. The exam should consist of vital signs (suspect increased ICP if vital signs are abnormal), head circumference (suspect increased ICP if enlarged), level of consciousness (suspect neuro disorder if altered), development, cranial nerve function, senses, cerebellar function (altered gait, balance, or coordination), reflexes, and any abnormal movements. Full fontanels can result from increased ICP. Muscle tone, strength, and sense of position should be assessed. Blood studies will show any infection, toxins, and seizure med levels. UA will show drugs; X-rays will detect any skull fractures; an EEG can detect seizures; echoencephalography, CT scan, MRI, and nuclear brain scan can detect lesions and abnormalities of the brain. A lumbar puncture is used to collect CSF, which can show infection.

A complete neuro check should be done at least every 4 hours: vital signs, LOC, pupil size, equality and reaction to light, vision or reflex abnormalities, motor and sensory function, reflexes, head circumference, fontanels in infants. Assess for changes in developmental level. Provide for proper fluids and monitor I&O. Keep the head above the heart to decrease the ICP. Make sure emergency equipment is nearby. Use seizure precautions: Protective equipment to prevent injury during seizure, do not restrain the child who is seizing or place anything in the child's mouth, keep harmful objects away from the child, maintain a patent airway and turn the child to the side to allow fluids to drain. Note the time and length of the seizure. After the seizure, reorient the child to person, place, and time. Use infection precautions.

CEREBRAL PERFUSION PRESSURE IN CHILDREN

Normal values for cerebral perfusion pressure (CPP) varies based on age:

- Infants and toddlers: 40-50 mmHg
- Children: 50-60 mmHg
- 18 years: 60-100 mmHg

PERIPHERAL NERVE ASSESSMENT OF THE CHILD

A musculoskeletal evaluation should include **peripheral nerve assessment** to determine if injury has impaired nerve function. Nerve function should be assessed for both sensation and movement. Assessment of sensation is done with a sharp or pointed instrument, using care not to prick the skin. The child should feel a slight prick if the sensory function is intact:

- **Median**: The median nerve branches from the brachial plexus, which arises from C5, C6, C7, C8, and T1. The median nerve travels down the arm and forearm, through the carpal tunnel. Sensation is evaluated by pricking the top or distal surface of the index finger. Movement is evaluated by having the child touch the ends of the thumb and little finger together and having the child flex the wrist.
- **Peroneal**: The peroneal nerve branches from the sciatic nerve, which arises from the L4, L5, and S1, S2, and S3 dorsal nerves and travels down the leg. The peroneal nerve enervates the lower leg, foot, and toes. Evaluate sensation by pricking the webbed area between the great and second toe. Evaluate movement by having the child dorsiflex and extend the foot.
- **Radial**: The radial nerve branches from the brachial plexus and enervates the dorsal surface of the arm and hand, including the thumb and fingers 2, 3, and 4. Evaluate sensation by pricking skin in the webbed area between the thumb and the index finger. Evaluate movement by having the child extend the thumb, the wrist, and fingers at the metacarpal joint.

- **Tibial**: The tibial nerve branches from the sciatic nerve. The tibial nerve travels down the back of the leg, through the popliteal fossa at the back of the knee and terminates at the planter surface of the foot. Sensation is evaluated by pricking the medial and lateral aspects of the plantar surface of the foot. Movement is evaluated by having the child plantar-flex the toes and then the ankle.
- **Ulnar**: The ulnar nerve branches from the sciatic nerve and travels down the arm from the shoulder, traveling along the anterior forearm beside the ulna, to the palm of the hand. Sensation is evaluated by pricking the distal fat pad at the end of the small finger. Movement is evaluated by having the child extend and spread all fingers.

EXAMINATION OF THE PUPILS

Note size, shape, symmetry, reaction, and accommodation:

- **Benign anisocoria**: Slight inequality in size with no other abnormalities
- **Horner's syndrome** (impaired sympathetic nerve impulse): Pupil small, regular, reactive to light and accommodation, associated with ptosis
- **Ocular nerve paralysis**: Nonreactive dilated pupil, sometimes associated with lateral deviation and ptosis
- **Tonic pupil**: Large, regular with reduced or absent reaction to light and slow accommodation
- **Argyll Robertson** (usually associated with syphilis): Bilateral small, irregular pupils nonreactive to light but normal accommodation
- **Dilated, fixed**: Brain damage, hypoxia, anticholinergic agents and glutethimide poisoning
- **Small, fixed**: Pontine hemorrhage, glaucoma eye drops, and narcotic drugs
- **Surgical abnormalities**: Iridectomy

CRANIAL NERVES

	Name	Function	PE Test
I	Olfactory	Smell	Test olfaction
II	Optic	Visual acuity	Snellen eye chart; Accommodation
III	Oculomotor	Eye movement/ pupil	Pupillary reflex; Eye/eyelid motion
IV	Trochlear	Eye movement	Eye moves down & out
V	Trigeminal	Facial motor/ sensory	Corneal reflex; Facial sensation; Mastication
VI	Abducens	Eye movement	Lateral eye motion
VII	Facial	Facial expression; Taste	Moves forehead, closes eyes, smile/frown, puffs cheeks; Taste
VIII	Vestibulo-cochlear (Acoustic)	Hearing; Balance	Hearing (Weber/Rinne tests); Nystagmus
IX	Glosso-pharyngeal	Pharynx motor/sensory	Gag reflex; Soft palate elevation
X	Vagus	Visceral sensory, motor	Gag, swallow, cough
XI	Accessory	Sternocleidomastoid and trapezius (motor)	Turns head & shrugs shoulders against resistance
XII	Hypoglossal	Tongue movement	Push out tongue; move tongue from side to side

NEUROLOGICAL MOTOR TESTING AND TESTING FOR NUCHAL RIGIDITY

Neurological motor testing requires careful observation for involuntary or spastic movements and examination of muscles for lack of symmetry or atrophy with observation of gait. Muscle tone is examined by flexing and extending the upper and lower extremities, observing for flaccid or spastic changes. Muscle strength is examined by having the patient press fingers, wrists, elbows, hips, knees, ankles, and plantar area against resistance, graded 0 (no movement) to 5 (normal).

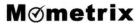

Pronator drift is an indication of disease of the upper motor neurons. The patient stands with eyes closed and both arms extended horizontally in front with the palms facing upwards (supination). The patient should be told to hold the arms still and not move them while the examiner taps downward on the arm. If motor neuron disease is present, the patient's arms will drift downward and hands will drift toward pronation.

Nuchal rigidity is tested by placing the hands behind the patient's head and flexing the neck gently to determine if there is increased resistance.

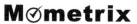

Review of Systems: Endocrine

ASSESSING FOR ENDOCRINE DISORDERS

The **endocrine system** comprises organs that produce hormones that are critical to growth, sexual development, and metabolism, so changes in these areas are suggestive of endocrine disorders. While symptoms may vary widely, there are often generalized symptoms that can be associated with most endocrine disorders. One should question the patient about fatigue and ability to perform ADLs, heat or cold intolerance, changes in sexual libido, sexual functioning, and secondary sexual characteristics, weight fluctuation, sleep problems, decreased concentration and memory, and mood changes. During the physical exam, one should assess the patient for edema, "moon" face or "buffalo hump," exophthalmos, hair loss, female facial hair, enlarged trunk with thin extremities, and enlarged hands and feet. Vital signs should be assessed for hypo or hypertension, and one should assess for changes in skin appearance and vision.

> **Review Video: Endocrine System**
> Visit mometrix.com/academy and enter code: 678939

THYROID IMAGING

Thyroid imaging plays a critical role in assessment of many thyroid diseases. This test may be used to determine the uptake characteristics of the thyroid gland in addition to the size and shape of the gland. In addition, **thyroid imaging** may determine how much iodine-131 is needed in order to safely ablate the gland when necessary. The radioactive iodine uptake scan (RAIU) is basically administration of iodine-123 with imaging performed 8 and 24 hours later:

Uptake of radioactive iodine is increased in disorders such as Graves' disease, "hot" nodules of various etiologies (including toxic multinodular goiter), TSH-secreting pituitary tumor, and iodine deficiency.

Uptake of radioactive iodine is decreased in the setting of thyroiditis and iodine excess.

Ultrasound imaging is used in thyroid disease to determine the size and structure of a thyroid nodule, such as to determine uniformity of shape, irregular contour, solid/cystic structure, and depth.

SIGNS/SYMPTOMS OF PEDIATRIC ENDOCRINE SYSTEM DISORDER

Endocrine disorders may be suspected in a child who is failing to stay within standard growth patterns. This could mean that height may be too tall or too short, that weight could be too heavy or too light, or even that puberty could start too early or too late.

Other signs/symptoms include:

- Developmentally behind peers
- More or less hungry or thirsty
- Vision problems
- Unusual tiredness
- Inability to sweat or too much sweating
- Inability to tolerate changes in temperature
- Behavior and mood swings
- Nausea
- Vomiting
- Sleep problems such as too much or too little sleep

Risk factors include maternal drug use, medication use, illness, or poor diet during pregnancy, prematurity, trauma involving the CNS, infections, chromosomal anomalies, medications, or a family history of endocrine disorders.

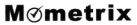

PHYSICAL EXAM, DIAGNOSTIC TESTS, AND NURSE'S ROLE WITH SUSPECTED ENDOCRINE DYSFUNCTION

The physical exam should include assessing the head circumference in children less than 2 years of age, vital signs, mental functioning, skin disorders, vision, facial changes, oral problems or odor, neuromuscular functioning, sexual development, and heart murmurs. Thyroid function tests (thyroid disorders), growth hormone test (inadequate growth hormone), and blood glucose tests (diabetes) are used to diagnose specific disorders. Other tests done may include CBC, blood chemistry levels, urine analysis, x-rays, CT scan, MRI, ultrasound, and genetic studies. The nurse should counsel the family to continue with the treatment prescribed, including medication administration, dietary restrictions, and follow-up appointments.

GLUCOSE LABORATORY TEST

Glucose is manufactured by the liver from ingested carbohydrates and is stored as glycogen for use by the cells. If intake is inadequate, glucose can be produced from muscle and fat tissue, leading to increased wasting. High levels of glucose are indicative of diabetes mellitus, which predisposes people to skin injuries, slow healing, and infection. **Fasting blood glucose levels** are used to diagnose and monitor this condition:

- Normal values: 70–99 mg/dL
- Impaired: 100–125 mg/dL
- Diabetes: ≥126 mg/dL

There are a number of different conditions that can increase glucose levels, including stress, renal failure, Cushing syndrome, hyperthyroidism, and pancreatic disorders. Medications, such as steroids, estrogens, lithium, phenytoin, diuretics, tricyclic antidepressants, may increase glucose levels. Other conditions, such as adrenal insufficiency, liver disease, hypothyroidism, and starvation can decrease glucose levels.

HEMOGLOBIN A1C LABORATORY TEST

Hemoglobin A1c comprises hemoglobin A with a glucose molecule because hemoglobin holds onto excess blood glucose, so it shows the average blood glucose levels over a 3-month period and is used primarily to monitor long-term diabetic therapy:

- Normal value: <6%
- Elevation: >7%

BASIC THYROID FUNCTION TESTING AND ANTIBODY TESTING

Thyroid stimulating hormone (TSH) is produced by the pituitary as a result of thyrotropin releasing hormone (TRH) from the hypothalamus. TSH stimulates the thyroid to produce T4 (mostly) and T3. T4 is deiodinated to T3 (active hormone), and the free hormone is active while the majority is bound to albumin and thyroxine-binding globulin. The best testing of thyroid function is the free T4 (unbound). Free T4 and TSH testing allows appropriate screening for thyroid disease.

Additionally, certain antibodies are used to screen for thyroid disease. Thyroglobulin antibodies are found in 50% of patients with Graves' disease and about 90% of those with Hashimoto's thyroiditis. Thyroid peroxidase antibodies are detected in >90% of those with Hashimoto's thyroiditis. TSH receptor antibodies (TSHR) may be either thyroid stimulating immunoglobulin (TSI) which stimulate the receptor to produce thyroid hormone (found in Graves' disease), or TSHR-blocking antibodies, which may inhibit production of thyroid hormone.

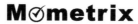

Lab values to consider include:

- **Thyroid stimulating hormone (TSH)** (0.4-6.15 mIU/L). Increase in TSH indicates hypothyroidism and decrease indicates hyperthyroidism.
- **Free thyroxine**: (FT4) (0.9-2.4 ng/dL). FT4 is used to confirm TSH abnormalities. Serum T3 (80-180 ng/dL) and T4 (4.5-11.5 mcg/dL). These usually increase together, but T3 more accurately diagnoses hyperthyroidism. T3 resin uptake (25-35%). Increases with hyperthyroidism and decreases with hypothyroidism.

ADDITIONAL ENDOCRINE FUNCTION STUDIES

There is a wide range of endocrine function studies:

- **Pituitary:** Serum levels of pituitary hormones and hormones of target organs, dependent on stimulation by pituitary hormones, are measured to determine abnormalities.
- **Parathyroid:** Parathyroid hormone (PTH) level (10-65 ng/L) and serum calcium levels (8.5-10.2 mg/dL) both increase with hyperparathyroidism. Calcium levels decrease with hypoparathyroidism, and phosphate levels (2.5-4.5 mg/dL) increase.
- **Adrenal**: Catecholamine (urine and serum) levels: Epinephrine (<75 ng/L) and norepinephrine (<100-550 ng/mL) elevate with pheochromocytoma. Electrolyte and glucose levels.
- **ACTH** and **serum cortisol levels** and **ACTH stimulation test** to evaluate for Addison's. Dexamethasone suppression test for Cushing's disease.

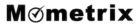

Review of Systems: Immunologic/Oncologic

ASSESSING FOR INFECTION

ERYTHROCYTE SEDIMENTATION RATE

Erythrocyte sedimentation rate (sed rate) measures the distance erythrocytes fall in a vertical tube of anticoagulated blood in 1 hour. Because fibrinogen, which increases in response to infection, also increases the rate of the fall, the sed rate can be used as a non-specific test for inflammation when infection is suspected. The sed rate is sensitive to osteomyelitis and may be used to monitor treatment response. Normal values:

- Neonates: 0-2 mm/hr
- Infant through puberty: 3-13 mm/hr

The sed rate increases with many disorders, including collagen disease, acute myocardial infarction (MI), carcinoma, pregnancy, rheumatic fever, rheumatoid arthritis, lymphoma, heavy metal poisoning, Crohn's disease, anemia, infections, pulmonary embolism, temporal arteritis, and tuberculosis (TB). It decreases with high blood glucose or conditions causing increased red blood cells (RBC) or hemoglobin count. Rates may be falsely elevated during menses.

COLLECTION OF BODY FLUIDS

Collection of various body fluids can be used to assess for infection:

- **Nasopharyngeal secretions**: Collect with swab of nasopharyngeal area. Place swab in tube with transport medium.
- **Saliva**: Collect in a sterile container after the patient rinses their mouth and waits a few minutes. Test immediately (point of care) or freeze for hormone tests to maintain stability.
- **Sputum**: First morning production of sputum is preferred because a larger volume is likely to be produced after sleeping. Transport at room temperature and process immediately.

NASOPHARYNGEAL WASH

Nasopharyngeal wash obtains a diagnostic specimen for diagnosis of influenzae A and B, RSV, adenovirus, and parainfluenzae types I, II, and III. Contraindications include thrombocytopenia (<20,000), respiratory distress (oximetry ≤90%), epistaxis, and lesions or nasopharyngeal trauma. The procedure for a nasopharyngeal wash is as follows:

1. Don personal protective equipment and exam gloves.
2. Fill two 3–5 mL syringes with 1–4 mL of normal saline (nonbacteriostatic), depending on the patient's age and size. Attach soft catheter (6 Fr for neonate, 8 Fr for infants and toddlers, and 10 Fr for school-age children).
3. Estimate the length of catheter necessary to reach the nasopharynx (usually about 1.5 to 2 inches).
4. Tilt the patient's head into sniff position and hold one nostril closed while inserting NS into the other nostril. Do not apply lubricant to the catheter.
5. Gently aspirate fluid while removing the catheter.
6. Inject aspirant into a sterile container.
7. Repeat this procedure with the other nostril.

RAPID STREP TEST

The rapid strep test is done using a kit, such as the Rapid Response Strep A kit. Procedure:

1. Gather supplies, including a timer, gloves, mask and kit (sterile swab, test strip, test tubes, reagent A, reagent B, positive and negative controls, and work station to hold test tubes).
2. Carry out hand hygiene and don PPE.

98

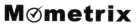

3. Place test tube in work station and add 4 drops of reagent A and 4 drops of reagent B. Swirl tube 10 times to mix the reagents.
4. Ask the child to open their mouth, stick out their tongue, and say "ahhhh."
5. Swab both tonsils or tonsil areas and the posterior pharynx with the sterile swab.
6. Place swab into the tube with reagents, agitate the swab by rotating at least 10 times, and leave for one minute.
7. Remove swab, squeezing it with the sides of the flexible tube to retain as much fluid as possible.
8. Place test strip into the tube with reagents and leave in place for 5 minutes (must be read between 5 and 10 minutes after immersion).
9. Each test strip has a T (test) zone and a C (control zone). Check results: one rose-pink band in the C zone indicates a negative test. One rose-pink band in the T zone and one in the C zone indicate a positive test for strep. Note: if no band appears or if a T band occurs with no C band, these tests are invalid and the specimen should be retested.
10. Positive and negative control tests are done similarly and should be carried out periodically.

INCIDENCE AND PREVALENCE OF MAJOR CHILDHOOD CANCERS

While childhood cancer is a relatively rare occurrence overall, it is the leading cause of disease-related mortality in the pediatric population. **Cancer incidence in children** is generally divided into those aged 0-14 and those aged 15-19. Within these subsets, different types of cancer predominate as do their outcomes. In the US, the younger subset reaches about 10,500 new diagnoses annually while the older group accounts for roughly 3,800 new cases annually. Combined, cancer is diagnosed in those younger than 20 years old at a rate of 14.9/100,000. Among those in the 0-14 age group, it is a major cause of death, second only to accidents. In those aged 15-19, it ranks fourth after accidents, homicide, and suicide. In the younger group, ALL is by far the most common type of cancer diagnosed, accounting for nearly 24% of the group's diagnoses. In the older subset, Hodgkin's (16.4%) and germ-cell tumors (12.8%) are the most common forms of cancer.

GENERAL RISK FACTORS, SYMPTOMS, AND PRESENTATION OF CANCER

The child with **cancer** may present with a lump, swelling or mass, lethargy, pale skin, a limp, unexplained bruising or bleeding, unexplained persistent pain, persistent fever with no known cause, headaches and vomiting, visual disturbances, or weight loss. Maternal exposure to medication, drugs, infection, or radiation can put the child at risk for cancer. A personal history of radiation or toxin exposure, chromosomal anomalies, frequent medication use, allergies, or a previous malignancy, as well as a family history of cancer can increase the child's risk of cancer. The exam should consist of assessment of: vital signs (fever, high, or low BP), weight (loss), skin lesions or bleeding/bruising, bleeding from the nose or mouth, skin and eyes for color changes, gait for limping, reflexes, an infection that doesn't produce pus, enlarged lymph nodes, abdomen for masses or enlarged organs, tenderness anywhere on the body, and lung and heart sounds (murmurs).

DIAGNOSTIC TOOLS AND NURSING CARE OF A CHILD WITH CANCER

The following tests may be done to **diagnose cancer**: CBC, UA and blood chemistries (assess health), peripheral blood smears (type of cancer cell), chest x-ray, ultrasound, bone scan (bone lesions), bone marrow aspiration (leukemia), lumbar puncture (abnormal cells in the CSF), CT scan, ultrasonography, and MRI (tumors), and biopsies (stage of cancer). Treatment may include chemotherapy, radiation, and bone marrow transplantation. During chemotherapy, the nurse should observe for infiltration at the IV site (some agents can cause serious tissue damage). If signs of irritation are found, the IV must be stopped and restarted elsewhere. Watch for signs of allergic reaction during the first 20 minutes of the infusion. Emergency medications should be close at hand. Adverse reactions to chemotherapy can include bleeding, infection, nausea, vomiting, anemia, inability to eat, mouth ulcers, or loss of hair. Adverse reactions to radiation can include the above reactions and dry mouth, sore throat, inability to taste, and inflammation of the parotid glands (appear as mumps).

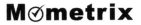

CANCER

Cancer is a potentially life-threatening disease that occurs due to irregular cell growth and reproduction. These cells can develop into a tumor that can occupy an area where normal body cells are usually found. **Cancer cells** also have the ability to metastasize, or extend, into other areas of the body. Cells within the body are constantly being replaced by normal cells. During this process, an abnormality in a cell's DNA can occur which causes it to become a malignant cancer cell. The body's immune system will usually attack and destroy this cell, but sometimes there can be a failure of the immune system to do this or the immune system is not able to destroy the cell. When this happens, the cancer cell can continue to reproduce itself until a tumor is formed. Some cancers can even attack normal, healthy cells within the body and alter their DNA so they will begin to reproduce as cancer cells.

> **Review Video: Cancer Classifications and Metastasis**
> Visit mometrix.com/academy and enter code: 878417

STAGES OF CANCER DEVELOPMENT

There are three stages of the development of cancer:

- **Initiation** is the action of a cancer-causing substance entering the body, reacting with DNA, and causing DNA mutation. Examples include cigarette smoke, radiation exposure, etc. The effects of initiation are irreversible; it results in permanent genetic change. Any daughter cells produced from the division of the mutated cell will also carry the mutation.
- **Promotion** is the process in which the body is repeatedly exposed to the cancer-causing substance. This repeats the process mentioned above and increases the likelihood of cancer cells being reproduced.
- **Progression** occurs when the malignant cancer cells begin to outnumber the normal, healthy cells because of continued replication within the body. At this point, the body is no longer able to attempt to repair the damage done to DNA by the cancer-causing agents and the normal cells continue to replicate as cancer cells.

CAUSES OF CANCER

There are five main causes of cancer:

- **Radiation** can cause cancer by altering a cell's DNA. If the body is not able to repair the damages, the cell can reproduce as a cancer cell. Radiation exposure can be accidental or from diagnostic testing. UV light exposure is a form of radiation, also, and it causes skin cancer. Asbestos is considered a form of radiation, also, and causes mesothelioma tumors within the lungs.
- **Chemical carcinogens** can alter a cell's DNA to cause cancer. An example of this is cigarette smoke and exposure to tar within cigarettes.
- **Viruses** can cause cancer. Viruses that alter a cell's genetic material can stimulate the production of cancer cells.
- **The immune system** may be unsuccessful in repairing or destroying cells with altered DNA, which can lead to cancer. Certain cancer cells have the ability to alter the immune system so that it cannot recognize the formation of malignant cells within normal tissues.
- Cancer can also occur because of **inherited factors**. A person can inherit oncogenes responsible for causing certain types of cancer.

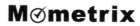

TUMOR STAGING AND TUMOR GRADING

Tumor staging and grading are two types of tumor severity assessment. They are assigned by the surgical pathologist. Tumor staging is a measurement of the size or extent of spread of a tumor. It is based on three parameters, known collectively as **TNM**. T stands for the size of the original local tumor, N specifies whether there is regional lymph node involvement, and M indicates whether there is distant metastatic spread. There is also a distinction between clinical staging prior to treatment and pathological staging after surgical resection. On the other hand, tumor grading is a histopathologic evaluation of the extent of differentiation of the tumor. Grading assesses the difference between the tumor and the surrounding tissues. Grade 1 tumors do not differ much in appearance from the normal tissue and are said to be well-differentiated. When the histopathological variation between normal and tumor tissues is large, graded as 3 or 4, the tumors are considered poorly differentiated (and more aggressive).

IMPORTANT TERMS

- **Invasion** is the process in which cancer cells continue to reproduce and effectively take over an area of the body's normal, healthy tissue.
- **Angiogenesis** is the process in which a tumor causes the body to produce blood vessels that enable the tumor to survive and grow.
- **Metastasis** is the extension of cancer cells to other parts of the body. This occurs when the cancer cells continue to reproduce and spread into other tissues in the area where the original cancer started. It can also occur through the blood or lymph stream by carrying cancer cells to other tissues within the body. Certain cancers have a propensity for metastasizing to specific areas of the body. For example, prostate and breast cancers are more likely to metastasize to the spine.
- **Tumor heterogeneity** is the term used to describe the dissimilarities found between cancer cells within a tumor. The more heterogeneous a tumor is, the more difficult it can be to treat and the more types of treatments may be required to treat it.
- **Hyperplasia** is the process in which the quantity of cells within a certain tissue multiplies. This occurs in healthy tissue and in cancerous tissue.
- **Metaplasia** is when one type of cell is interchanged with another within a specific tissue. This occurs in response to chronic damage inflicted on a certain type of cell.
- **Dysplasia** is a change in normal cells. This can involve a change in any of the cell's characteristics.
- **Anaplasia** is used to explain cancer cells. It means that certain cells hold the characteristics that are seen with cancer cells.

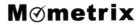

Review of Systems: Hematologic

HEMATOLOGIC SYSTEM

The hematologic system comprises the blood and those areas involved in the production of blood, such as the bone marrow and the reticuloendothelial system. Blood is a tissue that circulates through the heart and vascular system. Blood consists of a serous liquid, plasma (78%) and solids (22%), such as platelets, red blood cells, and white blood cells. Blood has a number of functions:

- Transporting nutrients, ions, and hormones
- Providing a defense system (white blood cells)
- Transporting agents of immune responses
- Maintaining temperature
- Removing waste products such as urea and carbon dioxide

Blood cells are formed in the bone marrow. Bone marrow appears yellow in areas with fatty deposits but red in areas producing blood (hematopoiesis). In children, most of the marrow is red, but as bones age, more and more of the red marrow is replaced by yellow marrow. The health of the bone marrow is critical to blood production.

Blood cells are produced in the bone marrow from stem cells, which can replicate throughout life to produce new cells. Stem cells are stimulated, according to the needs of the body, to differentiate into 2 types of stem cells:

- **Lymphoid cells**, which produce T and B lymphocytes, which are integral to both the cell-mediated and the antibody-mediated immune response.
- **Myeloid cells**, which produce all other types of blood cells (RBCs, WBCs, and platelets).

Most blood cells have a life span that is relatively short, so there is a need for constant hematopoiesis to replenish the supply.

The reticuloendothelial system comprises tissue macrophages derived from monocytes, produced in the marrow. The monocytes circulate in the blood for the first 24 hours and then enter the tissues where they mature and differentiate into macrophages, which defend against pathogenic microorganisms through phagocytosis.

SPLEEN AND THYMUS

The spleen and the thymus are important to the reticuloendothelial system and the circulatory system:

- **Spleen:** This small organ contains small areas of white pulp (lymphoid tissue and B and T lymphocytes), red pulp (RBCs and macrophages), and cavities for storage of red blood cells (5%) and platelets (20-40%). Lymphocytes and other cells of the immune system are produced and stored in the spleen. The lymphoid tissue filters the blood as it circulates through, removing worn out cells and platelets and breaking down hemoglobin into bilirubin, which is then removed from circulation by the liver and kidneys. Blood circulating through the spleen can activate the lymphocytes. The spleen can produce some blood cells if the bone marrow malfunctions.
- **Thymus:** This organ is where T lymphocytes begin to mature. Then, they migrate to the spleen and lymph nodes where they continue to mature, after which they circulate between the lymph system and the blood.

ABNORMALLY FUNCTIONING HEMATOLOGIC SYSTEM

Major symptoms of abnormal function of the hematologic system can include bone/joint pain, numerous infections, abnormal bleeding or bruising, weight loss, tiredness, headache, crankiness and dizziness. Assess for maternal-fetal blood incompatibility, prematurity, low birth weight, dietary factors (low iron intake, inadequate nutrition), or excess bleeding (menstruation). Increased heart rate or rapid breathing may be noted, along with blood spots on the skin, pallor or flushed skin, yellow sclera, retinal hemorrhage, blurry vision, pale mucus membranes, cyanosis, enlarged lymph nodes, apathy, swollen joints, blood in urine, or heavy menstrual bleeding. Abdominal organs may be enlarged. Small muscle mass and tenderness over joints or bones may be noted. Listen for heart murmurs and abnormal lung sounds. The following lab studies may be indicated (what they can detect): RBC count, WBC counts with differential (infection, deficiencies), Hgb (anemia), Hct (anemia), mean corpuscular volume (RBC size), Hgb, Hgb concentration, platelet count (bleeding disorders), retics (anemia), coagulation and hemostasis studies (hemorrhagic disorders), total iron-binding capacity, ferritin, iron, and transferring levels (anemia), and bone marrow aspiration (aplastic anemia, leukemia).

Monitor for infection (steroids increase risk of infection) and use precautions as needed. Adequate nutrition and rest can decrease risk of infection. Assess skin color and vital signs to monitor tissue oxygenation. Provide O_2 (severe tissue hypoxia) and blood transfusions as prescribed. Watch for signs of bleeding (petechiae, bruising, blood in stool or urine). If a bleeding problem exists, limit activities, do not give aspirin or take rectal temps, and avoid IM injections. Teach parents and patients the signs of bleeding: swelling, tingling, tenderness, pain, warmth, and petechiae. Teach the family ways to prevent bleeding: choose activities not likely to cause physical injury, avoid aspirin, tobacco, alcohol and drugs, and use protective gear for high-risk activities.

PEDIATRIC WHITE BLOOD CELL COUNT

White blood cell (leukocyte) count is used as an indicator of bacterial and viral infection. **WBC** is reported as the total number of all white blood cells.

- Neonate: 9000-30,000 per mm^3
- 1-2 months: 5000-19,500 per mm^3
- 3 months-1 year: 6000-17,500 per mm^3
- 1-2 years: 6000-17,000 per mm^3
- 2-6 years: 5500-15,500 per mm^3
- 6-18 years: 4500-10,800 per mm^3
- >18 years: 4500-10,500 per mm^3

The differential provides the percentage of each different type of leukocyte. An increase in the white blood cell count is usually related to an increase in one type of leukocyte and often an increase in immature neutrophils, known as bands, which is referred to as a "shift to the left," an indication of an infectious process.

Cells	Normal value	Changes
Immature neutrophils (bands)	0-5%	Increase with infection
Segmented neutrophils (segs)	40-60%	Increase with acute, localized, or systemic bacterial infections
Eosinophils	0-1%	Decrease with stress and acute infection
Basophils	0-1%	Decrease in acute stage of infection
Lymphocytes	20-40%	Increase in some viral and bacterial infections
Monocytes	0-2%	Increase in recovery stage of acute infection

RED BLOOD CELLS

Red blood cells (RBCs or erythrocytes) are biconcave disks that contain **hemoglobin** (95% of mass), which carries oxygen throughout the body. The heme portion of the cell contains **iron**, which binds to the oxygen. RBCs live about 120 days, after which they are destroyed and their hemoglobin is recycled or excreted. Normal values of **red blood cell count** vary by gender:

- Males >18 years: 4.7-6.1 million per mm^3
- Females >18 years: 4.2-5.4 million per mm^3

The most common **disorders of RBCs** are those that interfere with production, leading to various types of **anemia**:

- Blood loss
- Hemolysis
- Bone marrow failure

The **morphology** of RBCs may vary depending upon the type of anemia:

- Size: Normocytes, microcytes, macrocytes
- Shape: Spherocytes (round), poikilocytes (irregular), drepanocytes (sickled)
- Color (reflecting concentration of hemoglobin): Normochromic, hypochromic

LABORATORY TESTS

A number of different tests are used to evaluate the condition and production of red blood cells in addition to the red blood cell count.

Hemoglobin: Carries oxygen and is decreased in anemia and increased in polycythemia. Normal values:

- Males >18 years: 14.0-17.46 g/dL
- Females >18 years: 12.0-16.0 g/dL

Hematocrit: Indicates the proportion of RBCs in a liter of blood (usually about 3 times the hemoglobin number). Normal values:

- Males >18 years: 40-50%
- Females >18 years: 35-45%

Mean corpuscular volume (MCV): Indicates the size of RBCs and can differentiate types of anemia. For adults, <80 is microcytic and >100 is macrocytic. Normal values:

- Males >18 years: 84-96 μm^3
- Females >18 years: 76-96 μm^3

Reticulocyte count: Measures marrow production and should rise with anemia. Normal values: 0.5-1.5% of total RBCs.

WBC COUNT AND DIFFERENTIAL

White blood cell (leukocyte) count is used as an indicator of bacterial and viral infection. WBC count is reported as the total number of all white blood cells.

- Normal WBC for adults: 4,800-10,000
- Acute infection: 10,000+; 30,000 indicates a severe infection
- Viral infection: 4,000 and below

The **differential** provides the percentage of each different type of leukocyte. An increase in the white blood cell count is usually related to an increase in one type, and often an increase in immature neutrophils (bands), referred to as a "shift to the left," is an indication of an infectious process:

- Normal immature neutrophils (bands): 1-3%, increases with infection
- Normal segmented neutrophils (segs) for adults: 50-62%, increases with acute, localized, or systemic bacterial infections
- Normal eosinophils: 0-3%, decreases with stress and acute infection
- Normal basophils: 0-1%, decreases during acute stage of infection
- Normal lymphocytes: 25-40%, increases in some viral and bacterial infections
- Normal monocytes: 3-7%, increases during recovery stage of acute infection

C-REACTIVE PROTEIN AND ERYTHROCYTE SEDIMENTATION RATE

C-reactive protein is an acute-phase reactant produced by the liver in response to an inflammatory response that causes neutrophils, granulocytes, and macrophages to secrete cytokines. Thus, levels of C-reactive protein rise when there is inflammation or infection. It is helpful to measure the response to treatment for pyoderma gangrenosum ulcers:

- Normal values: 2.6-7.6 µg/dL

Erythrocyte sedimentation rate (sed rate) measures the distance erythrocytes fall in a vertical tube of anticoagulated blood in one hour. Because fibrinogen, which increases in response to infection, also increases the rate of the fall, the sed rate can be used as a non-specific test for inflammation when infection is suspected. The sed rate is sensitive to osteomyelitis and may be used to monitor treatment response. Values vary according to gender and age:

- <50: Males 0-15 mm/hr; females 0-20 mm/hr
- >50: Males 0-20 mm/hr; females 0-30 mm/hr

ELEMENTS OF THE COAGULATION PROFILE

The coagulation profile measures clotting mechanisms, identifies clotting disorders, screens preoperative patients, and diagnoses excessive bruising and bleeding. Values vary depending on lab:

- **Prothrombin time (PT)**: 10-14 seconds
  - Increases with anticoagulation therapy, vitamin K deficiency, decreased prothrombin, DIC, liver disease, and malignant neoplasm. Some drugs may shorten PT.
- **Partial thromboplastin time (PTT)**: 25-35 seconds
  - Increases with hemophilia A and B, von Willebrand disease, vitamin deficiency, lupus, DIC, and liver disease.
- **Activated partial thromboplastin time (aPTT)**: 21-35 seconds
  - Similar to PTT, but decreases in extensive cancer, early DIC, and after acute hemorrhage. Used to monitor heparin dosage.
- **Thrombin clotting time (TCT) or Thrombin time (TT)**: 7-12 seconds
  - Used most often to determine the dosage of heparin. Prolonged with multiple myeloma, abnormal fibrinogen, uremia, and liver disease.
- **Bleeding time**: 2-9.5 minutes
  - (Using the IVY method on the forearm) Increases with DIC, leukemia, renal failure, aplastic anemia, von Willebrand disease, some drugs, and alcohol.

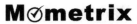

- **Platelet count**: 150,000-400,000 per μL
  - Increased bleeding <50,000 (transfusion required) and increased clotting >750,000.

Review Video: <u>The Coagulation Profile</u>
Visit mometrix.com/academy and enter code: 423595

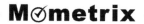

Review of Systems: Gastrointestinal

GASTROINTESTINAL ABNORMALITIES IN CHILDREN

Abnormal GI findings would include the child who is anorexic or has a recent large weight gain or loss. Nausea, vomiting, diarrhea, constipation, pain in the abdomen, and blood in the stool are all cause for concern. Assess the family and child history for drugs or medications taken during pregnancy, any problems during or after birth, possible poisoning or drug use, or GI disorders. Assess the diet for deficiencies and assess growth for failure to thrive. Fever may reveal dehydration or infection. Assess the mouth for cavities, infection or cleft palate/lip. Palpate the palate for defects. The skin should not be pale, jaundiced, or orange (check the sclera). Assess the stomach for distention, masses, tenderness, rigidity, enlarged organs, umbilical hernia, or visible peristalsis. The bowel sounds should be audible without being excessive. The anus should be patent with no bleeding. Percuss for gas, fluid, and masses or enlarged organs.

DIAGNOSTIC TESTS WHEN GASTROINTESTINAL ABNORMALITY IS SUSPECTED

An ultrasound or CT scan can show cysts, tumors, abscesses, gallstones, biliary duct obstruction, and appendicitis. GI studies (upper, lower, esophagus, stomach, small bowel), such as a barium enema, help find lesions, obstructions and problems with movement of the system. Esophagogastroduodenoscopy, endoscopy, and gastroscopy examine the upper GI tract, detecting bleeding, ulcers, and tissue problems. Colonoscopy, proctoscopy, anoscopy, sigmoidoscopy, and proctosigmoidoscopy examine the lower GI tract, detecting bleeding, IBD, diarrhea, and allowing for biopsies.

STOOL COLLECTION

Collecting stool specimens may be indicated to identify what organisms are causing gastrointestinal disturbances or to assess for blood in the stool. Infants in diapers may need a urine bag to separate stool from urine. Toilet trained children can be told to urinate first, flush, and then helped to collect the stool in a bedpan or toilet. Plastic wrap can be placed over the toilet bowl to catch the stool. The specimen is collected and placed in the appropriate container, labeled, and delivered to the laboratory. If the sample cannot be delivered to the laboratory immediately, it may be refrigerated. Time limits for refrigeration exist and must be adhered to per laboratory orders. Take care not to contaminate the specimen.

PEDIATRIC ABDOMINAL PRESSURE MONITORING

Abdominal pressure monitoring is indicated for ascites, abdominal trauma, major fluid resuscitation, and abdominal/retroperitoneal bleeding. Intra-abdominal pressure is measured by attaching a pressure transducer or water-column manometer to a Foley catheter in the bladder, because bladder pressure correlates with abdominal pressure. The patient should be in supine flat position if possible. The bladder must be empty for accurate measurement. The catheter should be clamped, and the transducer should be zeroed at the iliac crest along the midaxillary line. Then, 1 mL/kg (usually about 10 mL for critically ill patients) of fluid is injected into the bladder and left in place for 30-60 seconds before reading the pressure following a patient expiration. Abdominal cavity pressure should be 0 mmHg in a well child, and 1-8 mmHg in a critically ill child. Intraabdominal pressure may also be checked with an indwelling NG tube. If risk for compartment syndrome exists, the wound should not be closed. Sudden release of pressure and reperfusion may cause acidosis, vasodilation, and cardiac arrest, so the patient should be given crystalloid solutions before decompression.

ASSESSMENT OF THE GASTROINTESTINAL SYSTEM

Assessment of the gastrointestinal system includes:

- Ask about personal and family history of gastrointestinal problems and risk factors, such as alcoholism, smoking, drug and medicine use, and poor dietary habits.
- Ask about symptoms, such as GI discomfort, flatus, nausea, vomiting, diarrhea, and abdominal pain.
- Determine the defecation pattern and ask about weight fluctuations.

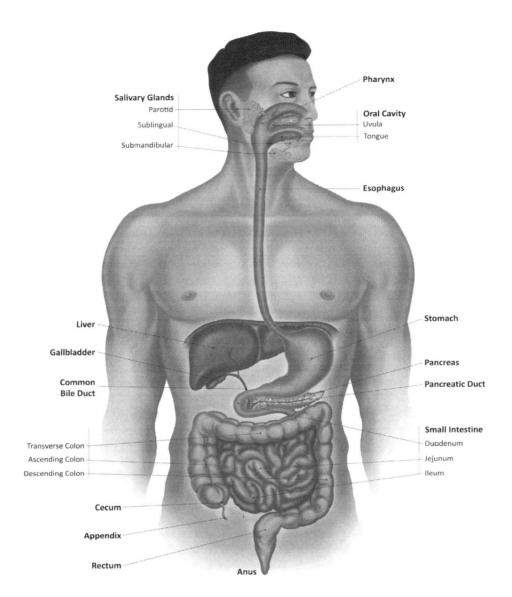

When performing a **physical assessment**, one must assess oral mucosa, tongue, teeth, pharynx, thyroid and parathyroid glands, skin color, moisture, turgor, nodules or lesions, bruises, scars, abdominal shape, and bowel sounds, assessing the abdomen in all 4 quadrants using the stethoscope diaphragm. The number of sounds heard determine if the intestines are functioning:

- **Absent**: no sounds in 3-5 minutes
- **Hypoactive**: only one sound in 2 minutes
- **Normal**: sounds heard every 5-20 seconds
- **Hyperactive**: 5-6 sounds in <30 seconds

One should examine the anal region for fissures, inflammation, tears, and dimples. Blood may be drawn for liver function studies, lipid profile, iron studies, CBC.

Review Video: <u>Gastrointestinal System</u>
Visit mometrix.com/academy and enter code: 378740

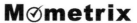

ASSESSMENT FOR GALLBLADDER AND PANCREATIC DISEASE

Gallbladder and pancreatic assessments are prompted by the appearance of symptoms. Symptoms of gallbladder disease include epigastric discomfort following fatty food intake, abdominal distension, right upper quadrant pain, which may be colicky, nausea, and vomiting. Pain may occur intermittently.

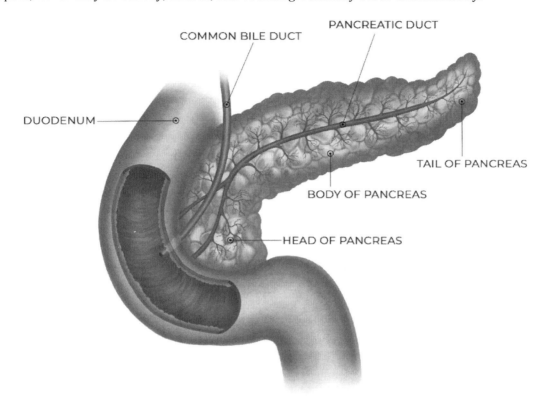

The patient with pancreatitis may have acute onset of severe abdominal pain, back pain, extensive vomiting, and dyspnea. Pancreatitis is most often related to gallstones or alcoholism, so history of alcohol use and examination for gallstones must be done:

- Assess for RUQ tenderness and mass, bowel sounds, and abdominal guarding.
- Assess the vital signs for hypotension, tachycardia, or fever and note any anxiety, agitation, or confusion.
- Note signs of hypoxia.
- Assess the skin for jaundice and bruising on the flanks and near the umbilicus.
- Blood is drawn to assess amylase and lipase, CBC, calcium, glucose, and bilirubin.

ASSESSMENT FOR LIVER DISEASE

The liver must be 70% damaged before lab tests show abnormalities. Assessment of risk factors and early symptoms are important to identify early disease. Risk factors for liver disease include alcoholism and drug abuse, risky sexual practices, exposure to infection or environmental toxins, and travel to countries with poor sanitation. One should question the patient about symptoms of liver disease, such as fatigue, itching, abdominal pain, anorexia, weight gain, fever, blood in stools or black stools, sleep problems, lack of menstruation, and lack of libido. Physical assessment includes checking vital signs and skin for scratches, pallor, jaundice, dryness, bruising, petechiae, abdominal veins and spider angiomas, and red palms:

- Assess for gynecomastia, abdominal distension, fluid waves, bowel sounds, liver margins, tenderness, consistency, and hardness and sharpness of the edge.
- Examine extremities for wasting, edema, and weakness.
- Assess neurological system for cognitive status, tremors, balance problems, slurred speech.
- Identify testicular atrophy.
- Blood should be drawn for serum enzymes and proteins, bilirubin, ammonia, clotting factors, and lipid profile.

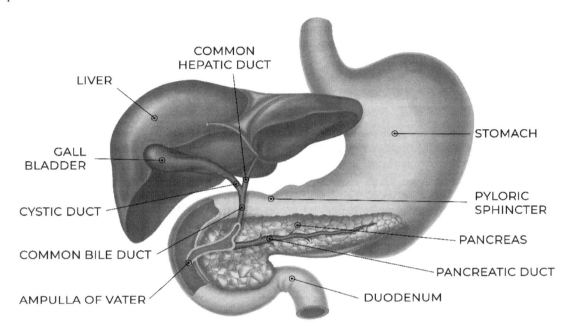

ASSESSMENT OF NUTRITIONAL STATUS

Assessment of nutritional status begins with an assessment of the patient's intake. The patient is asked to report intake for the previous 24 hours. This may indicate the need for a **food diary** over a period of time:

- Compare the patient's nutritional intake with the requirements of the USDA's MyPlate.
- Measure height and weight and check against a BMI table to help determine nutritional status.
- Measure waist circumference.
- Assess the patient for physical signs of poor nutrition such as muscle wasting, obesity, hair breakage and loss, poor skin turgor, ulcers, bruising, and loss of subcutaneous tissue.
- Assess mucous membranes and condition of teeth, abdomen, extremities, and thyroid gland.

Nutritional status is connected to endocrine disease, infections, other acute and chronic diseases, digestion, absorption, excretion, and storage of nutrients, so these areas must also be assessed. Blood testing should include proteins, transferrin, electrolytes, vitamins A and C, carotene, and CBC. Test urine for creatinine, thiamine, riboflavin, niacin, albumin, and iodine.

> **Review Video: Transferrin**
> Visit mometrix.com/academy and enter code: 267479

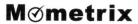

ASSESSING NUTRITIONAL STATUS OF HOSPITALIZED PATIENTS

Assessing the nutritional status of the hospital inpatient is an important part of forming a care plan. The two screening tools that are most commonly used are the **Subjective Global Assessment (SGA)** and the **Prognostic Nutritional Index (PNI)**. The SGA provides a nutritional assessment based on both the patient history and current symptoms. The patient is asked about any changes in weight and is also asked questions about his or her diet. The presence of symptoms that may lead to weight loss and poor nutritional status, such as diarrhea, nausea, and vomiting, as well as water retention (edema) and muscle wasting (cachexia), is also included in the SGA. The PNI is also used as an indicator of malnutrition and is especially helpful in determining how well a patient will recover from surgery. The PNI assesses nutritional status through the measurement of serum proteins such as albumin and transferrin combined with a skinfold measurement and a cutaneous hypersensitivity test as an indicator of immune function.

LIVER FUNCTION STUDIES

Liver function studies are described below:

- **Bilirubin:** Determines the ability of the liver to conjugate and excrete bilirubin, direct 0.0–0.3 mg/dL, total 0.0–0.9 mg/dL, and urine bilirubin, which should be 0
- **Total protein:** Normal: 6.0–8.0 g/dL (Albumin: 4.0–5.5 g/dL, Globulin: 1.7–3.3 g/dL); normal albumin/globulin (A/G) ratio: 1.5:1 to 2.5:1, measured by serum protein electrophoresis
- **Prothrombin time (PT):** 100% or clot detection in 10-14 seconds; PT increases with liver disease
  - International normalized ratio (PT result/normal average): <2 for those not receiving anticoagulation, 2-3 for those receiving anticoagulation, critical value >3 in patients receiving anticoagulation therapy
- **Alkaline phosphatase:** 36–93 units/L in adults (normal values vary with method); indicates biliary tract obstruction if no bone disease
- **AST (SGOT):** 10–40 units (increases with liver cell damage)
- **ALT (SGPT):** 5–35 units (increases with liver cell damage)
- **GGT, GGTP:** 5–55 μ/L females, 5–85 μ/L males (increases with alcohol abuse)
- **LDH:** 100–200 units (increases with alcohol abuse)
- **Serum ammonia:** 150–250 mg/dL (increases with liver failure)
- **Cholesterol:** Increases with bile duct obstruction and decrease with parenchymal disease

NUTRITIONAL LAB MONITORING

TOTAL PROTEIN AND ALBUMIN

Total protein levels can be influenced by many factors, including stress and infection, but it may be monitored as part of an overall nutritional assessment. Protein is critical for general health and wound healing, and because metabolic rate increases in response to a wound, protein needs increase:

- Normal values: 6–8 g/dL
- Diet requirements for wound healing: 1.25–1.5 g/kg/day

Albumin is a protein that is produced by the liver and is a necessary component for cells and tissues. Levels decrease with renal disease, malnutrition, and severe burns. Albumin levels are the most common screening to determine protein levels. Albumin has a half-life of 18–20 days, so it is sensitive to long-term protein deficiencies more than short-term.

- Normal values: 3.5–5.5 g/dL
- Mild deficiency: 3.0–3.5 g/dL
- Moderate deficiency: 2.5–3.0 g/dL
- Severe deficiency: <2.5 g/dL

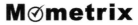

Levels below 3.2 correlate with increased morbidity and death. Dehydration (poor intake, diarrhea, or vomiting) elevates levels, so adequate hydration is important to ensure meaningful results.

PREALBUMIN

Prealbumin (transthyretin) is most commonly monitored for acute changes in nutritional status because it has a half-life of only 2–3 days. Prealbumin is a protein produced in the liver, so it is often decreased with liver disease. Oral contraceptives and estrogen can also decrease levels. Levels may rise with Hodgkin's disease or the use of steroids or NSAIDS. Prealbumin is necessary for transportation of both thyroxine and vitamin A throughout the body, so if **prealbumin levels** fall, both thyroxine and vitamin A utilization are also affected:

- Normal values: 16–40 mg/dL
- Mild deficiency: 10–15 mg/dL
- Moderate deficiency: 5–9 mg/dL
- Severe deficiency: <5 mg/dL

Prealbumin is a good measurement because it quickly decreases when nutrition is inadequate and rises quickly in response to increased protein intake. Protein intake must be adequate to maintain levels of prealbumin. Death rates increase with any decrease in prealbumin levels.

TRANSFERRIN

Transferrin, which transports about one-third of the body's iron, is a protein produced by the liver. It transports **iron** from the intestines to the bone marrow where it is used to produce **hemoglobin**. The half-life of transferrin is about 8–10 days. It is sometimes used as a measure of nutritional status; however, transferrin levels are sensitive to many factors. Levels rapidly decrease with protein malnutrition. Liver disease and anemia can also depress levels, but a decrease in iron, commonly found with inadequate protein, stimulates the liver to produce more transferrin, which increases transferrin levels but also decreases production of albumin and prealbumin. Transferrin levels may also increase with pregnancy, use of oral contraceptives, and polycythemia. Thus, **transferrin levels** alone are not always reliable measurements of nutritional status:

- Normal values: 200–400 mg/dL
- Mild deficiency: 150–200 mg/dL
- Moderate deficiency: 100–150 mg/dL
- Severe deficiency: <100 mg/dL

EGD

Esophagogastroduodenoscopy (EGD) with a flexible fiberscope equipped with a lighted fiberoptic lens allows direct inspection of the mucosa of the esophagus, stomach, and duodenum. The scope has a still or video camera attached to a monitor for viewing during the procedure. The scope may be used for biopsies or therapeutically to dilate strictures or treat gastric or esophageal bleeding. The patient is positioned on the left side (head supported) to allow saliva drainage. Conscious sedation (midazolam, propofol) is commonly used along with a topical anesthetic spray or gargle to facilitate placing the lubricated tube through the mouth into the esophagus. Atropine reduces secretions. A bite guard in the mouth prevents the patient from biting the scope. The airway must be carefully monitored through the procedure (which usually takes about 30 minutes), including oximeter to measure oxygen saturation. While perforation, bleeding, or infection may occur, most complications are cardiopulmonary in nature and relate to drugs (conscious sedation) used during the procedure, so reversal agents (flumazenil, naloxone) should be available.

> **Review Video: GI Diagnostic Procedures**
> Visit mometrix.com/academy and enter code: 645436

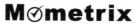

Review of Systems: Genitourinary

GENITOURINARY SYSTEM DYSFUNCTION IN CHILDREN

A newborn experiencing genitourinary system dysfunction may eat poorly, lose weight, excrete excess urine, cry when urinating, become dehydrated, possibly convulse, and develop a fever. An infant may strain while urinating, the urine may smell foul, and he may develop a diaper rash. The older child may complain of being thirsty and urinating all the time, incontinence, vomiting, bloody or foul-smelling urine, being tired, lack of appetite, fever, and pain in the side, stomach or back. Risk factors for a GU problem can include young or old maternal age during pregnancy, multiparity, frequent UTIs, catheterizations, problems with toilet training, diabetes, poor immune system, sexual activity, strep infections, and a family history of GU problems. Assess growth, temperature (elevated), BP (elevated or low), signs of respiratory distress (tachypnea, cyanosis, increased work of breathing, edema), abdomen (distention), any congenital abnormalities, bladder (distention), and kidneys (tender, enlarged).

Maintain strict I&O and daily weights. Provide fluids that the child likes to encourage intake. Avoid caffeine. Assess for dehydration. Assess for overhydration by checking BP frequently and monitoring respiratory status for signs of pulmonary edema. If prescribed, keep the child on a low-sodium diet. Offer meals with foods that are healthy and that the child likes to encourage adequate nutrition. Avoid infection with good hand washing, having the child avoid those with illnesses, making sure the child gets good nutrition and plenty of rest, and using good aseptic technique with invasive procedures.

DIAGNOSTIC TOOLS AND FINDINGS

The following are diagnostic tools used for a child with suspected genitourinary dysfunction and what the findings may show:

- **Urinalysis**: Assesses renal function.
- **Urine culture and sensitivity**: Tests for the presence of bacteria (allowing for the provider to identify which antibiotic will work against it).
- **Blood urea nitrogen**: Will be elevated due to impaired renal filtration and rapid protein catabolism.
- **Creatinine**: Will be elevated due to reduced creatinine excretion.
- **Ultrasonography**: A noninvasive exam of the urinary tract.
- **Voiding cystourethrography**: X-rays of the bladder and urethra with contrast medium.
- **Computed tomography scan**: Visualizes cross sections of the kidney.
- **Intravenous pyelography**: X-rays of the kidneys and ureters with contrast medium.
- **Cystoscopy**: Visualizes the urinary tract through an inserted tube.
- **Renal biopsy**: The removal of renal tissue that is then examined to determine types of nephrotic syndrome.
- **Renal scan**: Serial films of the kidneys after injecting them with radioactive materials.
- **Urodynamics**: Tests both bladder and urethral function and innervation.

URINALYSIS

Elements assessed in a **urinalysis** include the following:

- **Color**: Urine is normally a pale yellow/amber and darkens when urine is concentrated or other substances (such as blood or bile) are present.
- **Appearance**: Normally urine appears clear but may be slightly cloudy.
- **Odor**: Slight odor is normal. Bacteria may give urine a foul smell, depending upon the organism. Some foods, such as asparagus, change the odor of urine.
- **Specific gravity**: Normal range is 1.015-1.025. This may increase if protein levels increase or if there is fever, vomiting, or dehydration.
- **pH**: Normally ranges from 4.5 to 8.0 with an average of 5-6.

- **Sediment**: Sediment results from various casts. Red cell casts result from acute infections, broad casts from kidney disorders, and white cell casts from pyelonephritis. Leukocytes > 10 per mL^3 are present with urinary tract infections.
- **Glucose, ketones, protein, blood, bilirubin, and nitrate**: A negative result for these elements is normal. Urine glucose may increase with infection (with normal blood glucose). Frank blood may be caused by some parasites and diseases but also by drugs, smoking, excessive exercise, and menstrual fluids. Increased red blood cells may result from lower urinary tract infections.
- **Urobilinogen**: 0.1-1.0 units

URINE COLLECTION IN INFANTS

Obtaining **urine specimens** from infants requires a special collection bag. The perineal area is cleaned and dried, and then the bag, with an adhesive outer portion, is attached. Urine should be aspirated directly from the bag as soon as possible after voiding. Urine can also be obtained from disposable diapers if using a urine dipstick. If the urine must be saved, it requires refrigeration. Older children and adolescents can collect their urine in a cup, with help as needed. If it is a clean-catch specimen, they should be taught how to clean themselves (females wipe front to back three times with a separate wipe each time, males clean the tip of the penis) and then void a small amount into the toilet before collecting any urine in the cup. Answer any questions the school age child has and ask the adolescent female if she is menstruating (the collection may be delayed or documentation made about the presence of red blood cells). Toddlers may need support from parents and a "potty chair."

CATHETERIZATION AND SUPRAPUBIC ASPIRATION OF PEDIATRIC PATIENTS

When a urine specimen is needed quickly, the child cannot void, or if kidney failure or obstruction is suspected, **bladder catheterization** may be indicated. In seriously ill infants, suprapubic aspiration is used to confirm a diagnosis of urinary tract infection.

Some birth defects preclude the use of a catheter, and using **suprapubic aspiration** decreases the risk of contamination. The doctor will insert a needle above the pubic bone when the bladder is full. It is a painful procedure and pain management is essential, such as using lidocaine cream at the insertion site

MICROSCOPIC ANALYSES OF URINE

Microscopic analyses of urine involve placing the urine specimen in a centrifuge to separate out the **sediment**, which is then examined under a microscope:

- **Erythrocytes** should not be in the urine and may indicate inflammation, injury, or slight bleeding from strenuous exercise.
- **Leukocytes** in the urine usually are indicative of infection, cancer, or kidney disorders.
- **Casts** are caused from kidney disease that causes tiny tube-like plugs of material (red or white cells, protein, fatty substances) to be flushed from the kidneys to the urine. The type of cast may help with diagnosis.
- **Crystals** should appear in small numbers. Some types of crystals or large numbers of crystals may be a sign of kidney stones or a metabolic disorder.
- **Bacteria** in the urine indicate an infection.
- **Fungi** in the urine indicate a yeast infection
- **Parasites** may migrate to the urinary system in some types of infestation.

VOIDING CYSTOURETHROGRAM

A **voiding cystourethrogram (VCUG)** is a type of radiologic test, often with contrast, that is performed on the urinary system. The test takes a series of pictures of the child's bladder to determine how the contrast moves through the urinary system and to ensure that the bladder, ureters, and urethra are intact and that there are no blockages. When the child voids during the test, it also monitors the flow of urine exiting the body in a

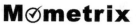

normal pattern. A VCUG can detect the presence of urinary reflux, or if a child is having frequent urinary tract infections, it may detect the presence of urinary abnormalities that are causing the condition.

ASSESSMENT OF KIDNEYS AND URINARY TRACT

Assessment of kidneys and urinary tract includes:

- Assess the health history for family urinary system disease and risk factors, such as previous urinary disease, increased age, immobility, hypertension, diabetes, chemical exposure, chronic disease, radiation to the pelvis, STDs, alcohol or drug use, and complications of pregnancy and delivery.
- Determine daily fluid intake.
- Question symptoms such as flank or abdominal pain, hesitancy, urgency, difficulty or straining with voiding, difficulty emptying the bladder, urinary incontinence, fatigue, SOB, exercise intolerance from anemia, fever, chills, blood in the urine, and GI symptoms.

Physical assessment includes vital signs, kidney and bladder palpation, and percussion over the bladder after urination:

- Palpate for ascites and edema.
- Measure the DTRs and check gait and ability to walk heel-to-toe.
- Examine the genitalia and check the urethra and vagina for herniation, irritation, or tears.

Urine specimen is obtained via clean catch midstream technique for analysis and culture if indicated. Blood is taken for a CBC, and in males, prostate-specific antigen (PSA) levels will also be measured via blood specimen.

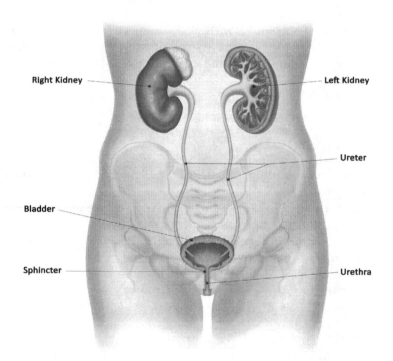

Review Video: Urinary System
Visit mometrix.com/academy and enter code: 601053

KIDNEY REGULATORY FUNCTIONS REGARDING FLUID BALANCE

Kidney regulatory functions include maintaining **fluid balance**. Fluid excretion balances intake with output, so increased intake results in a large output and vice versa:

- **Osmolality** (the number of electrolytes and other molecules per kg/urine) measures the concentration or dilution. With dehydration, osmolality increases; with fluid retention, osmolality decreases. With kidney disease, urine is dilute and the osmolality is fixed.
- **Specific gravity** compares the weight of urine (weight of particles) to distilled water (1.000). Normal urine is 1.010-1.025 with normal intake. High intake lowers the specific gravity, and low intake raises it. In kidney disease, it often does not vary.
- **Antidiuretic hormone** (ADH/vasopressin) regulates the excretion of water and urine concentration in the renal tubule by varying water reabsorption. When fluid intake decreases, blood osmolality rises, and this stimulates the release of ADH, which increases reabsorption of fluid to return osmolality to normal levels. ADH is suppressed with increased fluid intake, so less fluid is reabsorbed.

ASSESSING SEXUAL HEALTH AND PREFERENCES

Bringing up the topic of sex gives a patient permission to ask questions and openly discuss **sexual concerns**:

- Ask for permission to ask questions about sexual health and preferences during the gynecological/urological portion of the health history.
- If the patient refuses, go on with the rest of the health history, otherwise continue.
- Ask first if the person has sex with men, women, or both.
- Be nonjudgmental and do not assume that those who are elderly or disabled do not have sex. Use layman terms according to the patient's age and education level.
- Ask if the person is having any problems with relationships or sexual intercourse.
- Ask if the person has ever been forced to have sex or if is afraid of anyone close to them.
- End by asking if there are any questions about expression of sexual feelings, contraception, safe sex practices, or risky behavior.
- Refer those with problems to their doctor, or a gynecologist, urologist, or sex therapist.

RENAL FUNCTION STUDIES

Renal function studies are described below:

- **Osmolality (urine):** Normal: 350-900 mOsm/kg/day. Shows early changes when the kidney has difficulty concentrating urine.
- **Osmolality (serum):** Normal: 275-295 mOsm/kg. Gives a picture of the amount of solute in the blood.
- **Uric acid:** Normal: 3.0-7.2 mg/dL. Increases with renal failure.
- **Creatinine clearance (24-hour):** Normal: 75-125 mL/min. Evaluates the amount of blood cleared of creatinine in 1 minute. Approximates the GFR.
- **Serum creatinine:** Normal: 0.6-1.2 mg/dL. Increase with decreased renal function, urinary tract obstruction, and nephritis.
- **Urine creatinine:** Normal: 11-26 mg/kg/day. Product of muscle breakdown. Increase with decreased renal function.
- **Blood urea nitrogen (BUN):** Normal: 7-8 mg/dL (8-20 mg/dL if age >60). An increase indicates impaired renal function, as urea is the end product of protein metabolism.
- **BUN/creatinine ratio:** Normal: 10:1. Increases with hypovolemia. With intrinsic kidney disease, the ratio is increased.
- **Urinalysis:** Tests various qualities of a urine sample that are reflective of kidney function and other disease processes.

URINALYSIS

Urinalysis components and normal findings are described below:

- **Color:** Pale yellow/amber and darkens when urine is concentrated or other substances (such as blood or bile) are present.
- **Appearance:** Clear but may be slightly cloudy.
- **Odor:** Slight. Bacteria may give urine a foul smell, depending upon the organism. Some foods, such as asparagus, change the odor.
- **Specific gravity:** Normal: 1.005-1.025. May increase if protein levels increase or if there is fever, vomiting, or dehydration.
- **pH:** Usually ranges from 4.5-8 with an average of 5-6.
- **Sediment:** Red cell casts from acute infections, broad casts from kidney disorders, and white cell casts from pyelonephritis. Leukocytes >10 per mL^3 are present with urinary tract infections.
- **Glucose, ketones, protein, blood, bilirubin, and nitrate:** Negative. Urine glucose may increase with infection (with normal blood glucose). Frank blood may be caused by some parasites and diseases but also by drugs, smoking, excessive exercise, and menstrual fluids. Increased red blood cells may result from lower urinary tract infections.
- **Urobilinogen:** 0.1-1.0 units.

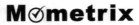

Review of Systems: Integumentary

GENERAL SKIN ASSESSMENT

Skin color varies according to ethnicity. Color changes should be assessed to determine if they are local or extend over the entire body, and if they are permanent or transient. Pallor may indicate stress, impaired oxygenation, and vasoconstriction. Erythema may indicate vasodilation, local inflammation, and blushing. Cyanosis indicates impaired oxygenation, and jaundice indicates increased bilirubin.

Temperature is typically assessed by touching the skin with the back of the hand. Skin should be warm and equal bilaterally. Hypothermia may indicate impaired circulation, intravenous infusion, and immobilized limb (such as in a cast). Hyperthermia may indicate fever, infection, and excessive exercise.

> **Review Video: Skin Assessment**
> Visit mometrix.com/academy and enter code: 794925

EFFECTS OF AGE ON SKIN

Age is an important consideration when evaluating the skin because the characteristics of the skin change as people age.

- An **infant's** skin is thinner than an adult's because, while the epidermis is developed, the dermis layer is only about 60% of that of an adult and continues to develop after birth. The skin of premature infants is especially friable, allowing for transepidermal water loss and evaporative heat loss.
- During **adolescence**, the hair follicles activate, the thickness of the dermis decreases about 20%, and epidermal turnover time increases, so healing slows.
- As people **continue to age**, Langerhans' cells decrease in number, making the skin more prone to cancer, and the inflammatory reactions decrease. The sweat glands, vascularity, and subcutaneous fat all decrease, interfering with thermoregulation and contributing to dryness and irritation of the skin. The epidermal-dermal junction flattens, resulting in skin that is prone to tearing. The elastin in the skin degrades with age and solar exposure. The thinning of the hypodermis can lead to pressure ulcers.

> **Review Video: Integumentary System**
> Visit mometrix.com/academy and enter code: 655980

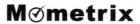

BRADEN SCALE

The Braden scale is a risk assessment tool that has been validated clinically as predictive of the risk of patient's developing pressure sores. It was developed in 1988 by Barbara Braden and Nancy Bergstrom and is in wide use. The scale scores six different areas with five areas scored 1-4 points, and one area 1-3 points. The lower the score, the greater the risk.

Area	Score of 1	Score of 2	Score of 3	Score of 4
Sensory perception	Completely limited	Very limited	Slightly limited	No impairment
Moisture	Constantly moist	Very moist	Occasionally moist	Rarely moist
Activity	Bed	Chair	Occasional walk	Frequent walk
Mobility	Immobile	Limited	Slightly limited	No limitations
Nutritional pattern	Very poor	Inadequate	Adequate	Excellent
Friction and shear	Problem	Potential problem	No apparent problem	

EVALUATING WOUNDS FOR ETIOLOGY

Wounds should be evaluated for **etiology** during the initial assessment to ensure proper treatment. Wounds can arise from a number of different causes:

- **Pressure**: Wounds that occur over bony prominences, such as the heels and coccyx, may be related to pressure, shear, or friction. The skin should be carefully examined for discolorations or changes in texture that might indicate compromise.
- **Arterial**: Arterial insufficiency is associated with a decrease in pedal pulses, and cool atrophic (shiny, dry) skin. It may result in small punctate-type ulcers, frequently on the dorsum of foot.
- **Venous stasis**: A decrease in venous circulation often results in hemoglobin leaking into the tissues of the lower leg, giving a brown discoloration. Tissue is often edematous, and ulcers are most common near the medial malleolus.
- **Diabetic neuropathy/ischemia**: Neuropathy can result in a lack of sensation to pain so that injuries to the feet may go unnoticed. Diabetes may also cause damage to small vessels, resulting in ischemia that can lead to ulcerations.
- **Trauma**: Injuries resulting from accidents or other types of trauma may vary considerably with some resulting in extensive damage to bones, tissues, organs, and circulation. Additionally, the wounds may be contaminated. Each wound must be assessed individually for multiple factors.
- **Burns**: Burn wounds may be chemical or thermal and should be assessed according to the area, the percentage of the body burned, and the depth of the burn. First-degree burns are superficial and affect the epidermis only. Second-degree burns extend through the dermis. Third degree burns affect underlying tissue, including vasculature, muscles, and nerves.
- **Infection**: An infected surgical or wound site can result in pain, edema, cellulitis, drainage, erosion of the sutures and ulceration of the tissue. Surgical sites must be assessed carefully and laboratory findings reviewed.

ELEMENTS OF WOUND ASSESSMENT

LOCATION AND SIZE

Wound location should be described in terms of anatomic position using landmarks (such as sternal notch, umbilicus, lateral malleolus), correct medical terminology, and directional terms:

- Anterior (in front)
- Posterior (behind)
- Superior (above)
- Inferior (below)

Wound size should be carefully described through actual measurement rather than association (the size of a dime). Measurements should be done with a disposable ruler in millimeters or centimeters. The current standard for measurement:

$$\text{Length} \times \text{width} \times \text{depth} = \text{dimension}$$

However, a clear description requires more detail. The measurement should be done at the greatest width and greatest length. More than two measurements may be needed if the wound is very irregularly shaped. The depth of the wound should be measured by inserting a sterile applicator and grasping or marking the applicator at skin level and then measuring the length below. Ideally, the wound should be photographed as well, following protocols for photography.

WOUND BED TISSUE

Wound bed tissue should be described as completely as possible, including color and general appearance:

- **Granulation tissue** is slightly granular in appearance and deep pink to bright red and moist, bleeding easily if disturbed.
- **Clean non-granular tissue** is smooth and deep pink or red and is not healing.
- **Hypergranulation** is excessive, soft, flaccid granulating tissue that is raised above the level of the periwound tissue, preventing proper epithelization, and may reflect excess moisture in the wound.
- **Epithelization** should appear at wound edges first and then eventually cover the wound. It is dry and light pink or violet in color.
- **Slough** is necrotic tissue that is viscous, soft, and yellow-gray in appearance and adheres to the wound.
- **Eschar** is hard dark brown or black leathery necrotic tissue that accumulates with death of the tissue.

WOUND MARGINS

Wound margins and the tissue surrounding the wound should be described carefully and with correct terminology:

- **Color** should be described using color descriptions and such terms as blanched, erythematous (red), or ecchymosed (purple, green, yellow).
- **Skin texture** may be normal, indurated (hardened), or edematous (swollen). Note if there is cellulitis or maceration evident.
- **Wound edges** may be diffuse (without clear margins), well defined, or rolled. A healing ridge may be evident if granulation has begun. Note if the wound is closed (as with a surgical incision) or open (as with dehiscence or ulcerations). Note if wound edges are attached or unattached (indicating undermining or tunneling).
- **Tunneling or undermining** should be assessed by probing the wound margins with a moist sterile cotton applicator, using clock face locators (toward the head is 12 o'clock, for example). Tunneling may be described as extending from 3 o'clock to 4 o'clock. A large area is usually described as undermining. The size should be measured or estimated as closely as possible.

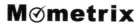

DISTRIBUTION, DRAINAGE, AND ODOR

Distribution of lesions should be clearly delineated if there is more than one lesion over an area. The arrangement of the lesions can be helpful for diagnosis and treatments.

- Linear (in a line)
- Satellites (small lesions around a larger one)
- Diffuse (scattered freely over an area)

Drainage may vary considerably from nothing at all to copious outpourings of discharge.

- Serous drainage is usually clear to slightly yellow.
- Serosanguineous drainage is a combination of serous drainage and blood.
- Sanguineous drainage is bloody.
- Purulent discharge may be thick and milky, yellow, brownish, or green, depending upon the infective agent.

Odor requires more subjective assessment, but the odor and type of discharge together can provide useful information. Some infective agents, such as *Pseudomonas*, produce distinctive odors, which may be described in various ways: musty, foul, sweet.

ASSESSMENT CHARACTERISTICS OF ARTERIAL, NEUROPATHIC, AND VENOUS ULCERS

The assessment process is important in delineating between the arterial, neuropathic, or venous origin of the ulcer. Characteristics of each must be known and closely examined:

Location

- **Arterial**: Ends of toes, pressure points, traumatic nonhealing wounds
- **Neuropathic**: Plantar surface, metatarsal heads, toes, and sides of feet
- **Venous**: Between knees and ankles, medial malleolus

Wound Bed

- **Arterial**: Pale, necrotic
- **Neuropathic**: Red (or ischemic)
- **Venous**: Dark red, fibrinous slough

Exudate

- **Arterial**: Slight amount, infection common
- **Neuropathic**: Moderate to large amounts, infection common
- **Venous**: Moderate to large amounts

Wound Perimeter

- **Arterial**: Circular, well-defined
- **Neuropathic**: Circular, well-defined, often with callous formation
- **Venous**: Irregular, poorly-defined

Pain

- **Arterial**: Very painful
- **Neuropathic**: Pain often absent because of reduced sensation
- **Venous**: Pain varies

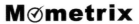

Skin

- **Arterial**: Pale, friable, shiny, and hairless, with dependent rubor and elevational pallor
- **Neuropathic**: Ischemic signs (as in arterial) may be evident with comorbidity
- **Venous**: Brownish discoloration of ankles and shin, edema common

Pulses

- **Arterial**: Weak or absent
- **Neuropathic**: Present and palpable, diminished in neuroischemic ulcers
- **Venous**: Present and palpable

PEDIATRIC FLUORESCEIN STAINING

Fluorescein staining is used with a Wood's light, which converts ultraviolet light into visible light and is used to diagnose skin lesions and injuries to the eye. The procedure must be carried out in a room that can be darkened, and the procedure should be explained to the child and/or parent beforehand so that they are aware the room will be dark.

- **Skin**: The skin must be clean and dry prior to application of the dye. For the skin, the chemical is applied directly to the lesion and surrounding tissue or area of concern. The affected area will have a different color from the surrounding tissue although not all types of lesions fluoresce.
- **Eye**: A strip of blotting paper containing the fluorescein dye is touched lightly to the surface of the eye and the patient asked to blink in order to spread the dye about the corneal surface. Once the dye is applied, the room light is turned off, and the Wood's light is turned on and used to scan the area. If the cornea or sclera has been disrupted, this area will uptake more of the dye and the injured area will appear bright yellow-green.

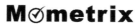

Review of Systems: Musculoskeletal

MUSCULOSKELETAL DYSFUNCTION IN CHILDREN

The first sign of musculoskeletal dysfunction may be a delay in gross motor skills, such as walking. There may be limited range of motion, stiffness, or pain. The mother may have taken drugs or medications, experienced trauma, or had an infection during pregnancy. Other risk factors are hypoxia or a strange position in the womb, a multiple birth, breech delivery, or a genetic problem, obesity, sports, steroids, delayed development, or family history of skeletal or muscular disorders. Chart the height and weight of the child. Assess the child's walk, posture, spinal alignment (scoliosis), and any discrepancies in symmetry. Inspect for any deformities, masses, lesions, tenderness, or warmth. Assess joint range of motion, strength of muscles (symmetry), and any lack of muscle mass. Diagnostic tools that may be used include x-rays, ultrasound, arthroscopy (see inside the joints), arthrography, bone scans (find tumors and inflammation), CT scans, MRI (find tumors and assess muscles, ligaments, and bones), joint aspiration (aspirate excess fluid), and blood tests (check for certain enzymes that aid in the diagnosis).

LIMB ASSESSMENT AND CAST CARE

If a limb is affected, assess the **vascular and nerve status**. Check the color, temperature, capillary refill, sensation, and if the child can move it. Help with physical therapy to maintain proper movement, muscle tone and bone health. Prevent injury and skin breakdown by turning the child frequently, using special mattresses, applying lotion to healthy skin, and protecting pressure points.

For **cast care**, assess the skin under the cast for odor and pain or warmth and keep the cast clean and dry. Use stool softeners, fluids, and a high fiber diet to help prevent constipation. Encourage frequent urination and a low calcium diet to prevent UTIs. Teach deep breathing techniques and assess for pulmonary or cardiac dysfunction related to bed rest. Give pain meds as needed, but use positioning and diversion to help with pain. Provide a proper diet and adequate fluids. Encourage as much physical activity as the child can tolerate and help the child to do as much as possible for herself.

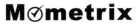

Review of Systems: EENT

NORMAL HEARING DEVELOPMENTAL CHARACTERISTICS USED TO ASSESS HEARING DEFICITS IN INFANTS AND TODDLERS

Hearing deficits may be identified very early if developmental characteristics are carefully observed in infants and children. **Normal hearing** responses include:

- **≤3 months**: Positive Moro (startle) reflex to sound. Noise disturbs sleep and the infant reacts to sounds by opening eyes or blinking.
- **3-6 months**: The infant is comforted at the sound of their parent's voice and tries to emulate sounds. The infant looks in the direction of sound.
- **6-12 months**: The infant begins to vocalize more with cooing and gurgling with different inflections. The infant responds to their name and simple words and looks in the direction of sound.
- **12-18 months**: The toddler begins first words about 12-15 months and imitates sounds, follows vocal directions, and points to familiar items when asked.
- **18-24 months**: The toddler is more verbal with about half of vocabulary understandable and knows about 20-50 words. The toddler points to body parts of familiar objects with asked.

AUDIOMETRY

Audiometry is used to test hearing in pediatric patients 6 months or older. Testing requires an audiometry tool that tests for decibel frequencies between 500 and 4000 Hz and an earpiece in the appropriate size for the child so that it seals the opening of the ear canal. Impacted cerumen should be removed prior to testing, and testing should be done in a quiet area.

Procedure:

1. Position the child in a sitting position on the table or their mother's lap. If the child is able to cooperate, ask the child to raise a hand if hearing a sound or watch the child for a response.
2. Activate the probe and insert into the ear (procedure may vary depending on the type of audiometry). For handheld models, pull the pinna back for young children and up and back for adolescents when inserting the earpiece.
3. Test according to the procedure manual for the device.
4. Note the results for the different decibel settings.
5. Compare the child's results to those for normal hearing.
6. If the child's hearing is outside of normal limits, the test may be repeated at another time.
7. If the results show that the child's hearing is persistently outside the normal range after 2 or 3 tests, then the child should be referred to an audiologist for more comprehensive testing.

VISUAL ACUITY TESTING

Visual acuity testing uses the **Snellen eye chart**, which has various letters and numbers in decreasing sizes. The alternate **Illiterate/Tumbling Eye chart** with the letter E facing in various directions and in three different sizes can also be used. Testing is done with the child standing or sitting 20 feet from a chart, so charts are usually placed at the end of a long hallway, but lighting must be adequate. In some cases, mirrors are used to simulate 20 feet.

Procedure:

1. Place the child in the appropriate position and ask the child to cover one eye.
2. Ask the child to read the smallest line that the child is able to see well enough to read. If using the E chart, the child uses a finger to point in the direction the E is facing.
3. Repeat the test with the opposite eye and then both eyes.

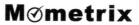

4. Record the results. If there is a difference of 2 or more levels between the eyes, this may be an indication of amblyopia. The normal vision (20/20) line is usually considered the fourth line from the bottom of the Snellen chart.

Note: A measurement of 20/30 means that at 20 feet the person can read what a person with normal vision can read at 30 feet.

CERUMEN IMPACTION AND REMOVAL

Cerumen impaction may involve partial or complete obstruction of the ear canal and may cause pain, tinnitus, feeling of fullness, itching, loss of hearing, odor, and cough. Begin by examining the ear with an otoscope to determine the location and amount of cerumen. **Methods of removal** include:

- **Curettage:** A special loop instrument is used with an otoscope (for visualization) to scoop out cerumen, but this method may result in trauma. A lighted curette is also available.
- **Suction:** A special suction tube is used with an otoscope (for visualization) to remove the cerumen.
- **Cerumenolytic agent:** An agent (such as Cerumenex) is instilled into the ear with the child lying on the opposite side. An earplug is used to keep the solution in place for 15 to 30 minutes. This is followed by irrigation.
- **Irrigation:** With the child sitting upright or lying flat, hold an emesis basin below the ear to catch solution. Use an ear irrigating syringe with warm water and gently squirt water into the ear canal to loosen the cerumen. Check periodically with the otoscope and catch loose material with the loop instrument or crocodile forceps if necessary. The irrigation may be used with or without a cerumenolytic agent but is usually more effective if the cerumen has been softened.

Note that if the cerumen is very hard or thick, first softening may work best with all different approaches. In some cases, a combination of methods may be used.

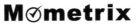

Pain Assessment

PATHOPHYSIOLOGY OF PAIN

NOCICEPTORS

Nociceptors are the primary neurons, or **sensory receptors**, responding to stimuli in the skin, muscle, and joints, as well as the stomach, bladder, and uterus. These neurons have specialized responses for mechanical, thermal, or chemical stimuli. The **neuron stimulation** is a direct result of tissue injury and follows four stages: **transduction** where a change occurs, **transmission** where the impulse is transferred along the neural path, **modulation** or translation of the signal, and **perception** by the patient. When injury occurs, the nociceptors initiate the process that begins **depolarization of the peripheral nerve**. Nociceptors may consist of either A-fiber axons or C-fiber axons. The message travels along the neural pathway and creates a perception of pain. A-fiber axons carry these pain messages at a much faster rate than C-fiber axons.

NOCICEPTIVE PAIN

Nociceptive pain is an umbrella term for pain caused by **stimulation of the neuroreceptor**. This stimulation is a direct result of tissue injury. The severity of pain is proportionate to the extent of the injury. Nociceptive pain can be subdivided into two classifications: somatic and visceral pain. **Somatic pain** is located in the cutaneous tissues, bone joints, and muscle tissues. **Visceral pain** is specific to internal organs protected by a layer of viscera, such as the cardiovascular, respiratory, gastrointestinal, or genitourinary systems. Both types are treatable with opioids.

VISCERAL PAIN

Visceral pain is associated with the internal organs. It can be very different depending on the affected organ. Not all internal organs are sensitive to pain (some lack **nociceptors**, such as the spleen, kidney, and pancreas), and may withstand a great deal of damage without causing pain. Other internal organs, such as the stomach, bladder, and ureters, can create significant pain from even the slightest damage. Visceral pain generally has a **poorly defined area**. It is also capable of referring pain to other remote locations away from the area of injury. It is described as a squeezing or cramping: a deep ache within the internal organs. The patient may complain of a generalized sick feeling or have nausea and vomiting. Visceral pain generally responds well to treatment with **opioids**.

SOMATIC PAIN

Somatic pain refers to messages from pain receptors located in the **cutaneous or musculoskeletal tissues**. When the pain occurs within the musculoskeletal tissue, it is referred to as **deep somatic pain**. Metastasizing cancers commonly cause deep somatic pain. **Surface pain** refers to pain concentrated in the **dermis and cutaneous layers** such as that caused by a surgical incision. Deep somatic pain is generally described as a dull, throbbing ache that is well focused on the area of trauma. It responds well to **opioids**. Surface somatic pain is also directly focused on the injury. It is frequently described as sharper than deep somatic pain. It may also present as a burning or pricking sensation.

> **Review Video: Somatic Pain**
> Visit mometrix.com/academy and enter code: 982772

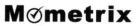

NEUROPATHIC PAIN

Neuropathic pain results from injury to the **nervous system**. This can result from cancer cells compressing the nerves or spinal cord, from actual cancerous invasion into the nerves or spinal cord, or from chemical damage to the nerves caused by chemotherapy and radiation. Other causes include diabetes- and alcohol-related damage, trauma, neuralgias, or other illnesses affecting the neural path either centrally or peripherally. When the nerves become damaged, they are unable to carry accurate information. This results in more severe, distinct **pain messages**. The nerves may also relay pain messages long after the original cause of the pain is resolved. It can be described as sharp, burning, shooting, shocking, tingling, or electrical in nature. It may travel the length of the nerve path from the spine to a distal body part such as a hand, or down the buttocks to a foot. NSAIDs and opioids are generally ineffective against neuropathic pain, though adjuvants may enhance the therapeutic effect of opioids. Nerve blocks may also be used.

> **Review Video: Neuropathic Pain**
> Visit mometrix.com/academy and enter code: 780523

ADVERSE SYSTEMIC EFFECTS OF PAIN

Acute pain causes adverse systemic effects that can negatively affect many body systems.

- **Cardiovascular**: Tachycardia and increased blood pressure is a common response to pain, causing increased cardiac output and systemic vascular resistance. In those with pre-existing cardiovascular disease, such as compromised ventricular function, cardiac output may decrease. The increased myocardial need for oxygen may cause or worsen myocardial ischemia.
- **Respiratory**: Increased need for oxygen causes an increase in minute ventilation and splinting due to pain, which may compromise pulmonary function. If the chest wall movement is constrained, tidal volume falls, impairing the ability to cough and clear secretions. Bed rest further compromises ventilation.
- **Gastrointestinal**: Sphincter tone increases and motility decreases, sometimes resulting in ileus. There may be an increased secretion of gastric acids, which irritates the gastric lining and can cause ulcerations. Nausea, vomiting, and constipation may occur. Reflux may result in aspiration pneumonia. Abdominal distension may occur.
- **Urinary**: Increased sphincter tone and decreased motility result in urinary retention.
- **Endocrine**: Hormone levels are affected by pain. Catabolic hormones such as catecholamine, cortisol, and glucagon increase, and anabolic hormones such as insulin and testosterone decrease. Lipolysis increases along with carbohydrate intolerance. Sodium retention can occur because of increased ADH, aldosterone, angiotensin, and cortisol. This in turn causes fluid retention and a shift to extracellular space.
- **Hematologic**: There may be reduced fibrinolysis, increased adhesiveness of platelets, and increased coagulation.
- **Immune**: Leukocytosis and lymphopenia may occur, increasing risk of infection.
- **Emotional**: Patients may experience depression, anxiety, anger, decreased appetite, and sleep deprivation. This type of response is most common in those with chronic pain, who usually have different systemic responses from those with acute pain.

CORE PRINCIPLES OF PAIN ASSESSMENT AND MANAGEMENT

According to the Joint Commission, assessing pain should be a priority in patient care, and organizations must establish **policies** for assessment and treatment of pain and must educate staff members about these policies. The Joint Commission considers a **plan of care** regarding pain control an essential patient right. Hospitals should be consistent in the use of the same assessment tools throughout the organization, specific to different patient populations (for example, pediatrics and geriatrics). The latest standards (2018) of evidence-based practice include the following:

- Organizations must establish a clinical leadership team to oversee pain management and safe prescription of opioids.
- Patients must be involved in planning and setting goals and should receive education regarding safe use of opioid and non-opioid medications.
- Patients should be screened for pain in all assessments, including visits to the emergency department.
- Patients at high risk for opioid misuse or adverse effects must be identified and monitored.
- Healthcare providers should have access to prescription drug monitoring safety databases, such as the prescription databases provided by most states.
- Organizations must provide performance improvement educational programs regarding pain assessment and management and must collect and analyze data on its pain assessment and management.

AREAS ADDRESSED WHEN ASSESSING PAIN

Information concerning a patient's pain can be gathered from a variety of sources, including observations, interviews with the patient and family, medical records, and observations of other health care providers. However, it is important to remember that each patient's pain is **subjective** and **personal**. Pain is defined as whatever the patient says it is. Having the patient give parameters of quality, location, duration, speed of onset, and intensity can all be beneficial in forming a treatment plan based on the patient's needs. Pain is also influenced by psychological, social, and spiritual factors. Behavioral, psychological, and subjective assessment information such as physical demeanor and vital signs can be helpful in further defining a patient's pain parameters.

PHYSICAL SIGNS OF PAIN

The best assessment of the patient's pain is **the patient's own report**. All other information is assessed as supporting this report. However, when this method is restricted or unavailable, **physical signs and symptoms** can help the nurse's assessment capabilities. It is important to be familiar with the patient's **baseline** or resting information to give a clear picture of the changes the body may go through when experiencing significant pain. Systolic blood pressure, heart rate, and respirations may all increase above the patient's normal parameters. Tightness or tension may be felt in major muscle groups. Posturing can also occur: the patient may guard areas of the body, curl themselves up into a fetal position, or hold only certain body portions rigid. Calling out, increased volume in speech, and moaning can also be indicators. Facial expressions, such as flat affect or grimacing, and distraction from their surroundings also indicate a significant increase in stressful stimuli.

IMPORTANCE OF PAIN ASSESSMENTS IN ADVANCED DISEASE

As many as 90% of all **advanced disease patients** will experience some level of pain. The hospice and palliative care philosophy focuses on the relief of pain and provision for comfort measures for all patients who desire it to improve quality of life. Each patient has the right to accept or refuse treatment for their pain. This becomes difficult when the patient is unable to **communicate** their desires and pain level. It can be assumed that if a patient was experiencing pain when able to communicate, they will continue to experience pain when the ability to communicate has been compromised—pain will be present even in an unconscious state. Changes from previous behavioral, psychological, and subjective and objective assessment data provide the supporting information for continued pain assessments in a nonverbal patient.

PAIN ASSESSMENT TOOLS

ABCDE MNEMONIC APPROACH TO PAIN ASSESSMENT

The Agency for Healthcare Policy and Research recommends use of the **ABCDE method** for assessing and managing pain:

- **A**sking the patient about the extent of pain and assessing systematically.
- **B**elieving that the degree of pain the patient reports is accurate.
- **C**hoosing the appropriate method of pain control for the patient and circumstances.
- **D**elivering pain interventions appropriately and in a timely, logical manner.
- **E**mpowering patients and family by helping them to have control of the course of treatment.

The **5 key elements of pain assessment** include:

- **Quality**: Words are used to describe pain, such as *burning*, *stabbing*, *deep*, *shooting*, and *sharp*. Some may complain of pressure, squeezing, and discomfort rather than pain.
- **Intensity**: Use of a 0-10 scale or other appropriate scale to quantify the degree of pain.
- **Location**: Where does the patient indicate pain?
- **Duration**: Is it constant; does it come and go; is there breakthrough pain?
- **Aggravating/alleviating factors**: What increases the intensity of pain and what relieves the pain?

> **Review Video: Assessment Tools for Pain**
> Visit mometrix.com/academy and enter code: 634001
>
> **Review Video: How to Accurately Assess Pain**
> Visit mometrix.com/academy and enter code: 693250

UNIDIMENSIONAL TOOLS FOR PAIN ASSESSMENT

Unidimensional tools for pain assessment focus on one aspect only: the patient's level of pain. Tools include:

- **Visual analog/numeric rating scale**: A 1-10 rating scale presented visually or verbally from which the patient chooses a number to describe the degree of pain the patient is experiencing. Zero represents no pain, 1 very mild pain, and 10 the most severe pain the patient can imagine.
- **Descriptive**: Pain is described in simple terms that a patient can choose from: mild, moderate, or severe. This may be especially helpful for patients from other countries or cultures where the 1-10 scale is not generally used.
- **FACES**: A chart shows a facial expression scale of simple drawings showing faces with different emotions, such as happiness, fear, and pain. Used primarily for children over age 3 and for nonverbal adults, although both a child's and an adult's version are available. A revised version applies numeric values to expressions so that pain can be assessed according to a numeric rating scale as well.

MULTIDIMENSIONAL TOOLS FOR PAIN ASSESSMENT

Multidimensional tools used for pain assessment include:

- **Multidimensional pain inventory**: The patient begins by identifying a significant other and then answering 20 questions (rating scale 0-6) about the current rate of pain, the degree of interference in daily life, the ability to work, satisfaction from social/recreational activities, support level of the significant other, mood, pain during the previous week, changes brought about by pain, concerns of the significant other, ability to deal with pain, irritability, and anxiety.
- **Brief pain inventory**: Patients are assessed on the severity of pain (on a 1-10 scale), location of pain, impact of pain on daily function, pain medication, and amount of pain relief in the past 24 hours or the past week. They are asked if the pain interferes with general activity, walking, normal work, mood, interpersonal relations, sleep, or enjoyment of life.

- **McGill pain questionnaire**: The patient marks areas of internal and external pain on body diagrams and selects appropriate adjectives for 20 different sections regarding sensory, affective, and evaluative perceptions. For example, the questionnaire allows the patient to indicate if the pain is "flickering, quivering, pulsing, throbbing, beating, or pounding." The patient also rates present pain intensity (PPI) from 0 (none) to 5 (excruciating).

PAIN ASSESSMENT OF NEONATES/INFANTS

Pain assessment of neonates and infants depends on careful observation of a number of characteristics. The Neonate/Infant Pain Scale (NIPS) assesses 6 areas with a score >3 indicating pain. Five areas are scored 0-1, depending upon the degree of stress. Crying, which is often the most indicative of pain, is scored 0-2:

Characteristic	0	1	2
Expression on face	Rested, normal	Negative, tightened muscles, grimace	
Crying	None	Intermittent, moaning, whimper	Loud, shrill continuous crying
Respiratory patterns	Relaxed, normal	Changes include irregular breathing, tachypnea, holding breath, gagging	
Upper extremities	Relaxed, random movement	Tense, rigid, or rapid extending and flexing.	
Lower extremities	Relaxed, random movement	Tense, rigid, or rapid extending and flexing.	
Arousal state	Quiet, awake or asleep with random leg movements	Restless, fussing, thrashing about.	

ASSESSING PAIN IN PEDIATRIC PATIENTS

When assessing the pediatric patient, the nurse must take into consideration the **chronological and developmental age** of the child. These factors help determine which measure the child might use to express pain, as well as treatments that might prove most successful. Assessment parameters must also include the presence of and parameters surrounding chronic illness, as well as neurological impairment. The nurse must identify the underlying cause of the pain, what nonpharmacological measures have been tried for pain control, and what methods can be used to deliver pharmacological interventions. The weight of the child in kilograms determines the appropriate dosages of medications. If the child is able to speak, do the child and the parents speak the same language as the health care provider, and are there any other obvious barriers to communication or pain relief measures?

> **Review Video: How to Properly Assess Pediatric Pain**
> Visit mometrix.com/academy and enter code: 264352

PRETEEN/ADOLESCENT PAIN SCALE

Pain is subjective and may be influenced by the individual's pain sensation threshold (the smallest stimulus that produces the sensation of pain) and tolerance threshold (the maximum degree of pain that a person can tolerate). The most common current pain assessment tool for preteens and adolescents is the 1-10 pain scale:

- 0 = no pain
- 1-2 = mild pain
- 3-5 = moderate pain
- 6-7 = severe pain
- 8-9 = very severe pain
- 10 = excruciating pain

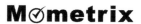

However, assessment also includes information about onset, duration, and intensity. Identifying pain triggers and what relieves the pain is essential when developing a pain management plan. Children may show very different behaviors when they are in pain. Some may cry and moan with minor pain, and others may seem indifferent even when they are truly suffering. Thus, judging pain by behavior alone can lead to the wrong conclusions.

NON-COMMUNICATING CHILDREN'S PAIN CHECKLIST

The **Non-Communicating Children's Pain Checklist** (NCCPC) is designed for children ages 3-8 who are cognitively impaired, but a modified version may be used for children recovering from anesthesia. The checklist contains 7 categories with sub-listings that are each scored: 0 (not occurring), 1 (occurring occasionally), 2 (occurring fairly often), 3 (occurring frequently), and NA (not applicable).

- **Vocal**: Moaning, whining, crying, screaming, yelling, or using a specific word for pain
- **Social**: Uncooperative, unhappy, withdrawn, seeking closeness, or can't be distracted
- **Facial**: Furrowed brow, eye changes, not smiling, lips tight or quivering, or clenching or grinding teeth.
- **Activity**: Not moving and quiet or agitated and fidgety.
- **Body and limbs**: Floppy, tense, rigid, spastic, pointing to a part of body that hurts, guarding part of the body, flinching, or positioning body to show pain.
- **Physiological**: Shivering, pallor, increased perspiration, tears, gasping, or holding breath
- **Eating and sleeping**: Eating less or sleeping significantly more or less than usual

The child is usually observed for 2 hours and then scored. All scores are then added together. A score of ≥7 indicates pain.

QUESTT PEDIATRIC PAIN ASSESSMENT TOOL

QUESTT is designed to focus on assessment, action, and consequent reassessment for results.

- **Question** both the child and parent about the pain experience.
- **Use** assessment tools and rating scales that are appropriate to the developmental stage and situation and understanding of the child.
- **Evaluate** the patient for both behavioral and physiological changes.
- **Secure** the parent's participation in all stages of the pain evaluation and treatment process.
- **Take the cause of the pain into consideration** during the evaluation and choice of treatment methods.
- **Take action** to treat the pain appropriately, and then evaluate the results on a regular basis.

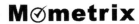

Psychosocial Assessment

ELEMENTS OF THE PSYCHOSOCIAL ASSESSMENT

A psychosocial assessment should provide additional information to the physical assessment to guide the patient's plan of care and should include:

- Previous hospitalizations and experience with healthcare
- Psychiatric history: Suicidal ideation, psychiatric disorders, family psychiatric history, history of violence and/or self-mutilation
- Chief complaint: Patient's perception
- Complementary therapies: Acupuncture, visualization, and meditation
- Occupational and educational background: Employment, retirement, and special skills
- Social patterns: Family and friends, living situation, typical activities, support system
- Sexual patterns: Orientation, problems, and sex practices
- Interests/abilities: Hobbies and sports
- Current or past substance abuse: Type, frequency, drinking pattern, use of recreational drugs, and overuse of prescription drugs
- Ability to cope: Stress reduction techniques
- Physical, sexual, emotional, and financial abuse: Older adults are especially vulnerable to abuse and may be reluctant to disclose out of shame or fear
- Spiritual/Cultural assessment: Religious/Spiritual importance, practices, restrictions (such as blood products or foods), and impact on health/health decisions

COGNITIVE ASSESSMENT

Individuals with evidence of dementia, delirium, or short-term memory loss should have cognition assessed. The **mini-mental state exam (MMSE)** or the **mini-cog test** are both commonly used. These tests require the individual to carry out specified tasks and are used as a baseline to determine change in mental status.

MMSE:

- Remembering and later repeating the names of 3 common objects
- Counting backward from 100 by 7s or spelling "world" backward
- Naming items as the examiner points to them
- Providing the location of the examiner's office, including city, state, and street address
- Repeating common phrases
- Copying a picture of interlocking shapes
- Following simple 3-part instructions, such as picking up a piece of paper, folding it in half, and placing it on the floor

A score of ≥24/30 is considered a normal functioning level.

Mini-cog:

- Remembering and later repeating the names of 3 common objects
- Drawing the face of a clock, including all 12 numbers and the hands, and indicating the time specified by the examiner

A score of 3-5 (out of 5) indicates a lower chance of dementia but does not rule it out.

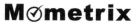

CONFUSION ASSESSMENT METHOD

The Confusion Assessment Method is an assessment tool intended to be used by those without psychiatric training in order to assess the progression of delirium in patients. The tool covers 9 factors, some factors have a range of possibilities, and others are rated only as to whether the characteristic is present, not present, uncertain, or not applicable. The tool also provides room to describe abnormal behavior. Factors indicative of delirium include:

- **Onset**: Acute change in mental status
- **Attention**: Inattentive, stable, or fluctuating
- **Thinking**: Disorganized, rambling conversation, switching topics, illogical
- **Level of consciousness**: Altered, ranging from alert to coma
- **Orientation**: Disoriented (person, place, and time)
- **Memory**: Impaired
- **Perceptual disturbances**: Hallucinations, illusions
- **Psychomotor abnormalities**: Agitation (tapping, picking, moving) or retardation (staring, not moving)
- **Sleep-wake cycle**: Awake at night and sleepy in the daytime

The Confusion Assessment Method indicates delirium if there is an acute onset, fluctuating inattention, and disorganized thinking OR altered level of consciousness.

HAMILTON ANXIETY SCALE

The Hamilton Anxiety Scale (HAS or HAMA) is utilized to evaluate the anxiety related symptomatology that may be present in adults as well as children. It provides an evaluation of overall **anxiety** and its degree of severity. This includes **somatic anxiety** (physical complaints) and **psychic anxiety** (mental agitation and distress). This scale consists of 14 items based on anxiety produced symptoms. Each item is ranked 0-4 with 0 indicating no symptoms present and 4 indicating severe symptoms present. This scale is frequently utilized in psychotropic drug evaluations. If performed before a particular medication has been started and then again at later visits, the HAS can be helpful in adjusting medication dosages based in part on the individual's score. It is often utilized as an outcome measure in clinical trials.

BECK DEPRESSION INVENTORY

The Beck Depression Inventory (BDI) is a widely utilized, self-reported, multiple-choice questionnaire consisting of 21 items, which measures the **degree of depression**. This tool is designed for use in adults ages 17-80. It evaluates physical symptoms such as weight loss, loss of sleep, loss of interest in sex, fatigue, and attitudinal symptoms such as irritability, guilt, and hopelessness. The items rank in four possible answer choices based on an increasing severity of symptoms. The test is scored with the answers ranging in value from 0 to 3. The total score is utilized to determine the degree of depression. The usual ranges include: 0-9 no signs of depression, 10-18 mild depression, 19-29 moderate depression, and 30-63 severe depression.

EVALUATION FOR SUICIDAL OR HOMICIDAL THOUGHTS

During a risk assessment two of the most important areas to evaluate are the patient's **risk for self-harm or harm to others**. The staff member performing the assessment should very closely evaluate for any descriptions or thoughts the patient may have concerning these risks. Direct questioning on these subjects should be performed and documented. Close evaluation of any delusional thoughts the patient may be having should be carefully evaluated. Does the patient believe he or she is being instructed by others to perform either of these acts? Safety of the patient and others needs to be a top priority and carefully documented. If the patient indicates that they are having these thoughts or ideas, they must be placed in either suicidal or assault precautions with close monitoring per facility protocol.

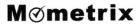

SUICIDE RISK ASSESSMENT

A suicide risk assessment should be completed and documented upon admission, with each shift change, at discharge, or any time suicidal ideations are suggested by the patient. This risk assessment should evaluate some of the following criteria:

- Would the patient sign a contract for safety?
- Is there a suicide plan? How lethal is the plan?
- What is the elopement risk?
- How often are the suicidal thoughts, and have they attempted suicide before?

Any associated symptoms of hopelessness, guilt, anger, helplessness, impulsive behaviors, nightmares, obsessions with death, or altered judgment should also be assessed and documented. The higher the score the higher the risk for suicide.

ALCOHOL USE ASSESSMENT

The **Clinical Instrument for Withdrawal for Alcohol (CIWA)** is a tool used to assess the severity of alcohol withdraw. Each category is scored 0-7 points based on the severity of symptoms, except #10, which is scored 0-4. A score <5 indicates mild withdrawal without need for medications; for scores ranging 5-15, benzodiazepines are indicated to manage symptoms. A score >15 indicates severe withdrawal and the need for admission to the unit.

1. Nausea/Vomiting
2. Tremor
3. Paroxysmal Sweats
4. Anxiety
5. Agitation
6. Tactile Disturbances
7. Auditory Disturbances
8. Visual Disturbances
9. Headache
10. Disorientation or Clouding of Sensorium

The **CAGE** tool is used as a quick assessment to identify problem drinkers. Moderate drinking, (1-2 drinks daily or one drink a day for older adults) is usually not harmful to people in the absence of other medical conditions. However, drinking more can lead to serious psychosocial and physical problems. One drink is defined as 12 ounces of beer/wine cooler, 5 ounces of wine, or 1.5 ounces of liquor.

- **C** – *Cutting Down*: "Do you think about trying to cut down on drinking?"
- **A** – *Annoyed at Criticism*: "Are people starting to criticize your drinking?"
- **G** – *Guilty feeling*: "Do you feel guilty or try to hide your drinking?"
- **E** – *Eye opener*: "Do you increasingly need a drink earlier in the day?"

"Yes" on one question suggests the possibility of a drinking problem. "Yes" on ≥2 indicates a drinking problem

SCREENING FOR RISK-TAKING BEHAVIOR

The ability to assess outcomes and respond appropriately to risks are part of the decision-making process. Decision making can be impaired in patients with mental health disorders such as depression, anxiety, bipolar disorder, and personality disorders, as well as in patients who have experienced a brain injury or have a dependence on drugs or alcohol. Health care providers should screen patients for the presence of high-risk behaviors. This may be accomplished through a self-administered questionnaire or through a patient interview with a trained clinician. Examples of **high-risk behaviors** include substance use/abuse, high risk sexual behaviors, high risk driving behaviors such as drinking and driving, speeding or riding with a drunk driver, and

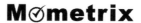

violence related behaviors. Patients with an increased response to risk taking may exhibit signs of impulsivity and sensation seeking. Conversely, other patients may exhibit abnormally cautious behavior.

ASSESSMENT OF UNIQUE NEEDS OF VETERANS

Assessment of **veterans** must include not only the standard assessments appropriate for the patient's age and gender but also assessment of combat-associated injuries and illnesses:

- Shrapnel and/or gunshot injuries: Associated physical limitations, pain
- Amputations: Mobility and prosthesis issues; body image issues
- PTSD: Extent, frequency of attacks, limiting factors, triggers
- Depression, suicidal ideation
- Substance abuse: Type and extent

Because a large number of veterans are among the homeless population, the veteran's living arrangements should be explored and appropriate referrals made if the patient is in need of housing. Veterans may be unaware of programs offered through the US Department of Veterans Affairs and should be provided information about these programs as appropriate for the patient's needs.

IDENTIFYING AND REPORTING NEGLECT OR LACK OF SUPERVISION IN CHILDREN

While some children may not be physically or sexually abused, they may suffer from profound **neglect** or **lack of supervision** that places them at risk. Indicators include the following:

- Appearing dirty and unkempt, sometimes with infestations of lice, and wearing ill-fitting or torn clothes and shoes
- Being tired and sleepy during the daytime
- Having untended medical or dental problems, such as dental caries
- Missing appointments and not receiving proper immunizations
- Being underweight for stage of development

Neglect can be difficult to assess, especially if the nurse is serving a homeless or very poor population. Home visits may be needed to ascertain if adequate food, clothing, or supervision is being provided; this may be beyond the care provided by the nurse, so suspicions should be reported to appropriate authorities, such as child protective services, so that social workers can assess the home environment.

Planning and Management

Respiratory Pathophysiology

ACUTE RESPIRATORY FAILURE

CARDINAL SIGNS

The cardinal signs of respiratory failure include:

- Tachypnea
- Tachycardia
- Anxiety and restlessness
- Diaphoresis

Symptoms may vary according to the cause. An obstruction may cause more obvious respiratory symptoms than other disorders.

- Early signs may include changes in the depth and pattern of respirations with flaring nares, sternal retractions, expiratory grunting, wheezing, and extended expiration as the body tries to compensate for hypoxemia and increasing levels of carbon dioxide.
- Cyanosis may be evident.
- Central nervous depression, with alterations in consciousness occurs with decreased perfusion to the brain.
- As the hypoxemia worsens, cardiac arrhythmias, including bradycardia, may occur with either hypotension or hypertension.
- Dyspnea becomes more pronounced with depressed respirations.
- Eventually stupor, coma, and death can occur if the condition is not reversed.

HYPOXEMIC AND HYPERCAPNIC RESPIRATORY FAILURE

Hypoxemic respiratory failure occurs suddenly when gaseous exchange of oxygen for carbon dioxide cannot keep up with demand for oxygen or production of carbon dioxide:

- PaO_2 <60 mmHg
- $PaCO_2$ >40 mmHg
- Arterial pH <7.35

Hypoxemic respiratory failure can be the result of low inhaled oxygen, as at high elevations or with smoke inhalation. The following ventilatory mechanisms may be involved:

- Alveolar hypotension
- Ventilation-perfusion mismatch (the most common cause)
- Intrapulmonary shunts
- Diffusion impairment

Hypercapnic respiratory failure results from an increase in $PaCO_2$ >45-50 mmHg associated with respiratory acidosis and may include:

- Reduction in minute ventilation, total volume of gas ventilated in one minute (often related to neurological, muscle, or chest wall disorders, drug overdoses, or obstruction of upper airway)
- Increased dead space with wasted ventilation (related to lung disease or disorders of chest wall, such as scoliosis)

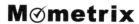

- Increased production of CO_2 (usually related to infection, burns, or other causes of hypermetabolism)
- Oxygen saturation normal or below normal

UNDERLYING CAUSES

There are a number of underlying causes for respiratory failure:

- **Airway obstruction:** Obstruction may result from an inhaled object or from an underlying disease process, such as cystic fibrosis, asthma, pulmonary edema, or infection.
- **Inadequate respirations:** This is a common cause among adults, especially related to obesity and sleep apnea. It may also be induced by an overdose of sedation medications such as opioids.
- **Neuromuscular disorders:** Those disorders that interfere with the neuromuscular functioning of the lungs or the chest wall, such as muscular dystrophy or spinal cord injuries can prevent adequate ventilation.
- **Pulmonary abnormalities:** Those abnormalities of the lung tissue, found in pulmonary fibrosis, burns, ARDS, and reactions to drugs, can lead to failure.
- **Chest wall abnormalities:** Disorders that impact lung parenchyma, such as severe scoliosis or chest wounds can interfere with lung functioning.

Nursing interventions to help prevent respiratory issues:

- Turn, position, and ambulate the patient.
- Have the patient cough and breathe deeply.
- Use vibration and percussion treatments.
- Hydrate the patient to help hydrate the airway secretions, and incentive spirometry.

MANAGEMENT

Respiratory failure must be **treated** immediately before severe hypoxemia causes irreversible damage to vital organs.

- **Identifying and treating** the underlying cause should be done immediately because emergency medications or surgery may be indicated. Medical treatments will vary widely depending upon the cause; for example, cardiopulmonary structural defects may require surgical repair, pulmonary edema may require diuresis, inhaled objects may require surgical removal, and infections may require aggressive antimicrobials.
- **Intravenous lines/central lines** are inserted for testing, fluids, and medications.
- **Oxygen therapy** should be initiated to attempt to reverse hypoxemia; however, if refractory hypoxemia occurs, then oxygen therapy alone will not suffice. Oxygen levels must be titrated carefully.
- **Intubation and mechanical ventilation** are frequently required to maintain adequate ventilation and oxygenation. Positive end expiratory pressure (PEEP) may be necessary with refractory hypoxemia and collapsed alveoli.
- **Respiratory status** must be monitored constantly, including arterial blood gases and vital signs.

CLINICAL INDICATIONS OF ACUTE RESPIRATORY INFECTIONS

FEVER, LYMPH NODES, AND MENINGEAL IRRITATION

Children with acute respiratory infections may manifest a wide range of symptoms:

- **Fever** is usually absent in neonates but is highest in those from 6 months to 3 years of age, and may reach 103-105 °F. Sudden temperature rises to 104 °F may result in seizures in children <4 years of age. Fever may result in some children being listless and others hyperactive.
- **Cervical lymph nodes** may be tender and enlarged.

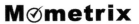

- **Meningeal irritation** occurs in some children without meningitis in the presence of an abrupt increase in fever and may manifest with headaches, nuchal rigidity and pain, as well as positive Kernig and Brudzinski signs.
  - Kernig's sign: Flex each hip and then try to straighten the knee while the hip is flexed. Spasm of the hamstrings makes this painful and difficult.
  - Brudzinski's sign: With the child lying supine, flex the neck by pulling head toward chest. The neck stiffness causes the hips and knees to pull up into a flexed position.

NASAL AND RESPIRATORY SYMPTOMS

Nasal and respiratory symptoms are indicative of acute respiratory infection:

- **Nasal symptoms** may include swelling of nasal passages, causing obstruction that can interfere with feeding in small infants. Exudate may be thin and watery or thick and purulent, depending on the type of infection. Irritation about the nares and upper lip related to exudate is common in infants and small children.
- **Sore throat** is usually a complaint of older children. Small infants and children may have an inflamed throat but appear to suffer less discomfort.
- **Cough** is a common symptom that may occur only during the acute phase of the respiratory infection or may persist for months after initial infection.
- **Change in respiratory sounds** may include wheezing and hoarseness in addition to cough. On auscultation, abnormal sounds may occur, such as hyperresonance, fine to coarse rales, wheezing, or absence of breath sounds in areas of the lungs.

GASTROINTESTINAL SYMPTOMS

Children with respiratory infections may initially manifest with gastrointestinal symptoms:

- **Poor appetite** or poor feeding is often the initial symptom and may persist throughout the febrile and convalescent period. This is a common symptom of acute infection in children.
- **Nausea and vomiting** may occur before other symptoms by several hours and usually subsides fairly quickly although it may persist with some children. It is most common in small children.
- **Diarrhea** is common with respiratory infections, especially those of viral origin. In most children it is mild and short lasting, but in others it may be severe and increase dehydration.
- **Abdominal pain** may be related to muscle spasms from vomiting or lymphadenitis of mesentery, especially if the child is very tense. The type of pain may be similar to or indistinguishable from pain associated with appendicitis.

BRONCHIOLITIS

Bronchiolitis is inflammation of the bronchiolar level and is usually caused by the **respiratory syncytial virus (RSV)** although adenoviruses, parainfluenza and *M. pneumoniae* have also been implicated. It is most common in very small children between the ages of 2 months and 2 years and rarely occurs after that age. Most children who require hospitalization are infants under 6 months of age. The infection is usually seasonal and mild although it can result in severe respiratory complications, so children should be observed carefully. Symptoms include dyspnea, a paroxysmal cough that is non-productive, tachypnea, and wheezing. The infection is usually self-limiting and runs its course in 8-15 days but is highly contagious.

Treatment is aimed at symptom management and includes:

- **Antipyretics**, such as acetaminophen
- **Oxygen therapy** with intubation and mechanical ventilation may be required in the presence of severe disease and respiratory compromise
- **Ribavirin aerosol** is used for severe disease

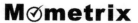

BACTERIAL PHARYNGITIS AND BACTERIAL TONSILLITIS

Bacterial pharyngitis and bacterial tonsillitis are caused by group A beta-hemolytic *streptococci*.

Bacterial pharyngitis presents as a sore throat, lethargy, high fever, headache, stomachache and possibly trouble swallowing. The throat is red, the tonsils are enlarged, red, and may have a white discharge, and the soft palate may have petechiae on it.

Bacterial tonsillitis presents with headache, sudden high fever, vomiting, and aches. A throat culture is needed to determine a bacterial infection. Antibiotics (penicillin) are used for 10 days. Follow care guidelines for upper respiratory infection. Tonsillectomy may be indicated if there are recurrent infections, abscess or chronic enlargement of tonsils. Pre-op care involves teaching the family and child about what to expect post-surgery. Post-op care includes watching for increased bleeding, taking vital signs, watching for signs of respiratory distress and cyanosis, and encouraging fluids. Administer pain meds as indicated, discourage coughing (prevent bleeding), and apply ice as directed.

SPREAD AND SYMPTOMS OF TONSILLITIS AND INDICATIONS FOR TONSILLECTOMY

Tonsillitis is a contagious disease that is typically caused by a virus or infection with group A *Streptococcus* bacterium. Tonsillitis is treated with antibiotics if the cause of the condition is a bacterial infection; a viral infection is typically treated with rest and fluids. Recommendations vary among physicians, but children who get this condition more than five times in a year may be candidates for a tonsillectomy.

POST-TONSILLECTOMY COMPLICATIONS

A tonsillectomy, often combined with adenoidectomy, may be performed by a variety of different methods, with some posting more risk of postoperative bleeding than others. Hemorrhage may occur in the initial 24-hour postoperative period (primary) or after 7–10 days (secondary) when the scar begins to slough. Indications of bleeding include evidence of bright red blood in the mouth, spitting up of blood, or excessive swallowing as blood runs down the back of the child's throat. The first indication the child has been swallowing blood may be hematemesis. Bleeding may occur from either the tonsillectomy or adenoidectomy site. Other indications include pallor, restlessness, thirst, hypotension, and tachycardia (>100 bpm). Initial treatment includes starting IV-line, blood sample for type and crossmatch, and gentle suctioning of large clots. Small bleeding sites or those slowly oozing may be cauterized. The child should sit upright with an ice collar. Uncontrollable bleeding requires immediate surgical intervention with rapid sequence induction. Blood transfusions may be necessary with severe bleeding.

ACUTE LTB AND SPASMODIC CROUP

Acute laryngotracheobronchitis (LTB) is a narrowing of the throat and trachea, with inflammation, and is caused by a virus. It starts after a URI moves down the respiratory tract into the trachea. The symptoms come on gradually and include a hoarse voice, stridor, fever, crankiness, retractions, wheezing, crackles, rales and diminished breath sounds in some areas of the lungs, cyanosis and severe respiratory distress.

Spasmodic croup is not viral, but may have genetic or allergic origins. It begins suddenly in the middle of the night when the child wakes with a barking cough and difficulty breathing. Assess the child for signs of respiratory distress and treat with oxygen, humidity, and medications (bronchodilator, anti-inflammatory). The parents should be taught, when the child wakes up with a barking cough, to take the child into the bathroom, close the door, and run a hot shower to create warm humidity. This will help open the child's airway.

TREATMENT FOR CROUP

Croup occurs when the structures of the upper airway become inflamed; it is typically caused by a viral infection. The most common symptom of croup is a barky cough, although a child also develops a hoarse voice, congestion, and fever. Untreated, the condition can lead to respiratory distress and cyanosis. The most common form of treatment is providing moist air, which eases breathing. Children may sit with their parents in a steam-filled area, such as a bathroom while running a hot shower. A steam tent is also used for treatment. Pain relievers may help to reduce symptoms of pain or fever. Severe inflammation may require a steroid injection to reduce swelling if the airway passages become so inflamed that breathing is difficult.

PNEUMONIA

Pneumonia is inflammation of the lung parenchyma, filling the alveoli with exudate. It is common throughout childhood and adulthood. Pneumonia may be a primary disease or may occur secondary to another infection or disease, such as lung cancer. Pneumonia may be caused by bacteria, viruses, parasites, or fungi. Common causes for community-acquired pneumonia (CAP) include:

- *Streptococcus pneumoniae*
- *Legionella* species
- *Haemophilus influenzae*
- *Staphylococcus aureus*
- *Mycoplasma pneumoniae*
- Viruses

Pneumonia may also be caused by chemical damage. Pneumonia is characterized by **location**:

- **Lobar** involves one or more lobes of the lungs. If lobes in both lungs are affected, it is referred to as bilateral or double pneumonia.
- **Bronchial/lobular** involves the terminal bronchioles, and exudate can involve the adjacent lobules. Usually, the pneumonia occurs in scattered patches throughout the lungs.
- **Interstitial** involves primarily the interstitium and alveoli where white blood cells and plasma fill the alveoli, generating inflammation and creating fibrotic tissue as the alveoli are destroyed.

> **Review Video: Pneumonia**
> Visit mometrix.com/academy and enter code: 628264

HOSPITAL-ACQUIRED PNEUMONIA

Hospital-acquired pneumonia (HAP) is defined as pneumonia that did not appear to be present on admission that occurs at least 48 hours after admission to a hospital. **Healthcare-associated pneumonia (HCAP)** is defined as pneumonia that occurs in a patient within 90 days of being hospitalized for 2 or more days at an acute care hospital or LTAC. **Ventilator-associated pneumonia (VAP)** is one type of hospital acquired pneumonia that a patient acquires more than 48 hours after having an ETT placed. The most common way that the patient is infected is via aspiration of bacteria that is colonized in the upper respiratory tract. It is estimated that close to 75% of patients that are critically ill will be colonized with multidrug resistant bacteria within 48 hours of entering an ICU. Aspiration occurs at a rate of about 45% in patients with no health problems and the rate is much higher in those with HAP, HCAP, and VAP. The frequency of patients developing these types of pneumonia is increasing, with those at highest risk being those with immunosuppression, septic shock, currently hospitalized for more than five days, and those who have had antibiotics for another infection within the previous three months. These types of pneumonia should be considered if a patient already hospitalized has purulent sputum or a change in respiratory status such as deoxygenating, in combination with a worsening or new chest x-ray infiltrate.

Treatment includes:

- Antibiotic therapy
- Using appropriate isolation and precautions with infected patients
- Preventive measures including maintaining ventilated patients in 30° upright positions, frequent oral care for vent patients, and changing ventilator circuits as per protocol

Antibiotic treatment options for HAP, HCAP, and VAP should take into account many factors, including culture data (when available), patient's comorbidities, flora in the unit, any recent antibiotics by the patient, and whether the patient is at high risk for having multidrug resistant bacteria. As most critical care patients are at high risk, due to factors such as being in an ICU setting, ventilators, and comorbidities, antibiotic recommendations to follow are for coverage for patients with risk factors for multidrug resistant bacteria.

One of the following:

- Ceftazidime 2 g every 8 hours IV **OR**
- Cefepime 2 g every 8 hours IV **OR**
- Imipenem 500 mg every 6 hours IV **OR**
- Piperacillin-tazobactam 4.5 g every 6 hours IV

AND one of the following:

- Ciprofloxacin 400 mg every 8 hours IV **OR**
- Levaquin 750 mg every 24 hours IV

ASPIRATION PNEUMONITIS/PNEUMONIA

Aspiration pneumonitis/pneumonia may occur as the result of any type of aspiration, including foreign objects. The aspirated material creates an inflammatory response, with the irritated mucous membrane at high risk for bacterial infection secondary to the aspiration, causing pneumonia. Gastric contents and oropharyngeal bacteria are commonly aspirated. Gastric contents can cause a severe chemical pneumonitis with hypoxemia, especially if the pH is <2.5. Acidic food particles can cause severe reactions. With acidic damage, bronchospasm and atelectasis occur rapidly with tracheal irritation, bronchitis, and alveolar damage with interstitial edema and hemorrhage. Intrapulmonary shunting and V/Q mismatch may occur. Pulmonary artery pressure increases. Non-acidic liquids and food particles are less damaging, and symptoms may clear within 4 hours of liquid aspiration or granuloma may form about food particles in 1-5 days. Depending upon the type of aspiration, pneumonitis may clear within a week, ARDS or pneumonia may develop, or progressive acute respiratory failure may lead to death.

There are a number of risk factors that can lead to **aspiration pneumonitis/pneumonia:**

- Altered level of consciousness related to illness or sedation
- Depression of gag, swallowing reflex
- Intubation or feeding tubes
- Ileus or gastric distention
- Gastrointestinal disorders, such as gastroesophageal reflux disorders (GERD)

Diagnosis is based on clinical findings, ABGs showing hypoxemia, infiltrates observed on x-ray, and elevated WBC if infection is present.

Symptoms: Similar to other pneumonias:

- Cough often with copious sputum
- Respiratory distress, dyspnea
- Cyanosis
- Tachycardia
- Hypotension

Treatment includes:

- Suctioning as needed to clear upper airway
- Supplemental oxygen
- Antibiotic therapy as indicated after 48 hours if symptoms not resolving
- Symptomatic respiratory support

FOREIGN BODY ASPIRATION

Foreign body aspiration can cause obstruction of the pharynx, larynx, or trachea, leading to acute dyspnea or asphyxiation, and the object may also be drawn distally into the bronchial tree. With adults, most foreign bodies migrate more readily down the right bronchus. Food is the most frequently aspirated, but other small objects, such as coins or needles, may also be aspirated. Sometimes the object causes swelling, ulceration, and general inflammation that hampers removal.

Symptoms include:

- **Initial**: Severe coughing, gagging, sternal retraction, wheezing. Objects in the larynx may cause inability to breathe or speak and lead to respiratory arrest. Objects in the bronchus cause cough, dyspnea, and wheezing.
- **Delayed**: Hours, days, or weeks later, an undetected aspirant may cause an infection distal to the aspirated material. Symptoms depend on the area and extent of the infection.

Treatment includes:

- Removal with laryngoscopy or bronchoscopy (rigid is often better than flexible)
- Antibiotic therapy for secondary infection
- Surgical bronchotomy (rarely required)
- Symptomatic support

ACUTE EPIGLOTTITIS

Acute epiglottitis (supraglottitis) occurs in children primarily from 1–8 years of age although it can occur at any age. It requires immediate medical attention as it can rapidly become obstructive. The onset is usually very sudden and often occurs during the night. The child may awaken suddenly with a fever but usually does not have a cough. The **symptoms** include:

- **Tripod position**: Child sits upright, leaning forward with chin out, mouth open, and tongue protruding.
- **Agitation**: The child appears restless, tense, and agitated.
- **Drooling**: Excess secretions combined with pain or dysphagia and mouth open position cause drooling.
- **Voice**: The child is not hoarse, but their voice sounds thick and "froglike."
- **Cyanosis**: Color is usually pale and sallow initially but may progress to frank cyanosis.
- **Throat**: On examination, the epiglottis appears bright red and swollen.
  NOTE: the child's throat should not be examined with a tongue blade unless intubation and tracheostomy equipment are immediately available as the examination can trigger obstruction.

AIR LEAK SYNDROMES

Air leak syndromes may result in significant respiratory distress. Leaks may occur spontaneously or secondary to some type of trauma (accidental, mechanical, iatrogenic) or disease. As pressure increases inside the alveoli,

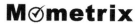

the alveolar wall pulls away from the perivascular sheath and subsequent alveolar rupture allows air to follow the perivascular planes and flow into adjacent areas. There are two categories:

- **Pneumothorax:**
  - Air in the pleural space causes a lung to collapse.
- **Barotrauma/volutrauma** with air in the interstitial space (usually resolve over time):
  - Pneumoperitoneum is air in the peritoneal area, including the abdomen and occasionally the scrotal sac of male infants.
  - Pneumomediastinum is air in the mediastinal area between the lungs.
  - Pneumopericardium is air in the pericardial sac that surrounds the heart.
  - Subcutaneous emphysema is air in the subcutaneous tissue planes of the chest wall.
  - Pulmonary interstitial emphysema (PIE) is air trapped in the interstitium between the alveoli.

PNEUMOTHORAX

Pneumothorax occurs when there is a leak of air into the pleural space, resulting in complete or partial collapse of a lung.

PNEUMOTHORAX

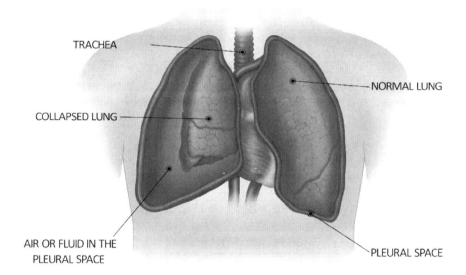

Symptoms: Vary widely depending on the cause and degree of the pneumothorax and whether or not there is an underlying disease. Symptoms include acute pleuritic pain (95%), usually on the affected side, and decreased breath sounds. In a *tension pneumothorax*, symptoms include tracheal deviation and hemodynamic compromise.

Diagnosis: Clinical findings; radiograph: 6-foot upright posterior-anterior; ultrasound may detect traumatic pneumothorax.

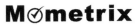

Treatment: Chest-tube thoracostomy with underwater seal drainage is the most common treatment for all types of pneumothorax.

- Tension pneumothorax: Immediate needle decompression and chest tube thoracostomy
- Small pneumothorax, patient stable: Oxygen administration and observation for 3-6 hours. If no increase is shown on repeat x-ray, patient may be discharged with another x-ray in 24 hours.
- Primary spontaneous pneumothorax: Catheter aspiration or chest tube thoracostomy

> **Review Video: <u>Pneumothorax</u>**
> Visit mometrix.com/academy and enter code: 186841

BRONCHOPULMONARY DYSPLASIA

Bronchopulmonary dysplasia (**BPD**) is a chronic lung disease characterized by alveolar damage resulting from abnormal development with inflammation and development of scar tissue. Risk factors include:

- Prematurity of >10 weeks prior to due date
- Birthweight <2.5 lb or 1000 g
- Hyaline membrane disease or respiratory distress syndrome (RDS) at birth
- Long-term ventilatory support/oxygen

Most of the infants with BPD have immature lungs with inadequate surfactant to allow the lungs to expand properly, so they cannot breathe without assistance. **Symptoms** include severe respiratory distress and cyanosis. Their lungs often have fewer but enlarged alveoli with inadequate blood supply. BPD is usually diagnosed if respiratory symptoms do not improve after 28 days.

Supportive **treatment** provides oxygenation, protects vital organs, and allows the lungs to mature. Treatment includes:

- Surfactant
- Nasal continuous positive airway pressure (NCPAP)
- Mechanical ventilation or high-frequency jet ventilation (HFJV)
- Supplemental oxygen
- Bronchodilators (albuterol) to open airways
- Furosemide (Lasix) to reduce pulmonary edema
- Antibiotics as indicated
- Gastric/enteral feedings or total parenteral nutrition (TPN)

Complications: Most infants are hospitalized for about 4 months but may need treatment for months or years at home. Most will eventually develop nearly normal lung function as new lung tissue grows and takes over the function of the scarred tissue. Some long-term complications may occur:

- Increased risk of bacterial and viral infections, such as RSV and pneumonia
- Chronic or recurrent pulmonary edema
- Pulmonary hypertension
- Side effects related to long-term use of diuretics, such as hearing deficits, renal calculi, and electrolyte imbalances
- Slow growth patterns

CONGENITAL DIAPHRAGMATIC HERNIA

Congenital diaphragmatic hernia (**CDH**) may cause severe respiratory distress. The primary CDHs that affect children are posterolateral (Bochdalek):

- Left sided (85%) includes herniation of the large and small intestine and intraabdominal organs into the thoracic cavity.
- Right sided (13%) may be asymptomatic. It usually involves just liver herniation or part of the large intestine.

Symptoms	Treatment
• Neonates with left CDH may exhibit severe respiratory distress and cyanosis. The lungs may be underdeveloped because of pressure exerted from displaced organs during fetal development. • There may be a left hemothorax with a mediastinal shift and the heart pressing on the right lung, which may be hypoplastic. • Bowel sounds are heard over the chest area. • Pulmonary hypertension and cardiopulmonary failure may occur.	• Immediate surgical repair. • HFOV and nitric oxide for pulmonary hypoplasia. • Extracorporeal membrane oxygenation (ECMO) for cardiopulmonary dysfunction. • Despite treatment, mortality rates are 50%, and children who survive may have emphysema, with larger volume but inadequate numbers of alveoli.

PULMONARY HYPOPLASIA

Pulmonary hypoplasia occurs when the lungs and component parts are present but severely underdeveloped with less volume, decreased alveoli, fewer airway generations, and decreased pulmonary arteries. Pulmonary hypoplasia may result from congenital diaphragmatic hernia or embryologic defect that may include various other anomalies, such as prune-belly or Potter syndrome. Fetal urine in the amniotic fluid is necessary for development of fetal lungs, so renal agenesis or obstruction results in pulmonary hypoplasia. Hypoplasia is usually a secondary rather than primary disorder. If the hypoplasia is the result of compression caused by a diaphragmatic hernia, then after surgical repair, the lung will partially recover. Mortality rates range from 70-95%, depending upon severity and other anomalies. Preventive methods include providing amnioinfusions for preterm ruptured membranes <32 weeks to reduce hypoplasia. After birth, **treatment** includes:

- Respiratory support: supplemental oxygen or ventilation (HFOV and EMCO)
- Surfactants (Survanta) to improve ventilation and oxygenation
- Surgical repair as indicated
- Vasodilators and/or bronchodilators as indicated

CHOANAL ATRESIA

If the nurse is unable to pass a suctioning tube through the nares of the newborn, the infant may have choanal atresia, a rare condition that occurs in approximately 1 in 10,000 live births. It occurs in females twice as often as males. The choana are the two openings in the posterior nares that connect the nasal passages with the nasopharynx. Newborns are obligate nasal breathers. Successful nose breathing requires air to pass through the choana, so if these openings fail to form during fetal development, the infant must become a mouth breather. If atresia occurs only on one side (unilaterally), the infant may have no symptoms at birth. The infant with bilateral choanal atresia has periods of respiratory distress and cyanosis that are alleviated by crying. Bilateral choanal atresia often becomes a medical emergency requiring intubation, but definitive treatment requires surgical perforation of the atresia to create an opening, sometimes with insertion of a stent.

ESOPHAGEAL ATRESIA

Esophageal atresia often occurs with **tracheoesophageal fistula (TEF)**. In esophageal atresia, the esophagus has a blind pouch and does not completely pass to the stomach. In TEF, an abnormal connection is present between the trachea and the esophagus. A congenital tracheoesophageal fistula (TEF) may be associated with genetic anomalies, such as trisomy 13, 18, or 21 and various other anomalies. TEF is often associated with polyhydramnios, as esophageal atresia prevents the fetus from swallowing amniotic fluid. Acquired TEF may be secondary to intubation trauma or neoplasms.

Symptoms	Treatment
• Fine, white, frothy bubbles of mucous in the mouth and nose • Copious secretions, despite suctioning • Episodes of coughing, choking, and cyanosis, which worsen with feeding	• Enteral feedings or gastrostomy feedings • Mechanical ventilation and a cuffed endotracheal tube (preventing reflux until the child stabilizes enough for surgical repair) • Maintaining cuff pressures <25 mmHg (helps prevent traumatic TEF)

CHILDHOOD ASTHMA

Asthma is a chronic reversible or partially reversible inflammation of the airway (especially the lower airways) that results in obstruction associated with genetic predisposition, environmental exposures, viral illnesses, and allergens. Children usually experience their first asthma attack between ages 3 and 8. In some cases, children may complain of a prodromal itch in the neck or upper part of the back prior to an episode. Childhood asthma is characterized by increased airway reactivity with obstruction related to inflammation and edema of mucous membranes, accumulation of secretions, and spasms of the smooth muscles of the bronchi and bronchioles. This bronchial constriction increases airway resistance that results in forced expiration through the constricted lumens. Symptoms may include dyspnea, inspiratory and expiratory high-pitched wheezing, cough, prolonged expiration, anxiety, sweating, and cyanosis. Wheezing and crackles may be heard throughout lung fields. Older children often sit upright with shoulders hunched over. Initial cough is usually hacking and nonproductive but then becomes productive of frothy gelatinous sputum. The three primary symptoms of asthma are cough, wheezing, and dyspnea.

GUIDELINES FOR DIAGNOSIS AND TREATMENT

The National Institutes of Health (NIH) and National Heart Blood and Lung Institute (NHBLI) have developed guidelines for the diagnosis and treatment of asthma. Component 1 of these guidelines addresses the assessment and monitoring of asthma.

The severity of the disease (including degree of impairment and risks), the degree of control, and the responsiveness to therapy must be assessed. Assessment is emphasized for initial diagnosis and monitoring for continued care. **Diagnosis** is based on:

- **History**: Cough, wheeze, triggers (precipitating factors or co-morbid conditions), and time of day variations.
- **Physical exam**: Hyperexpansion of thorax, wheezing, increased nasal secretions, polyps, swelling, and allergic skin conditions.
- **Spirometry** (for those 5 and older): Episodic symptoms of airflow obstruction that are at least partially reversible and not caused by other conditions. Responsiveness to therapy is demonstrated by FEV1 increase ≥12% from baseline or ≥10% of predicted FEV1 after inhalation of a short-acting bronchodilator. Additional pulmonary function studies, bronchoprovocation, chest x-ray, allergy testing, and biomarkers for inflammation may be assessed.

ASSESSMENT CRITERIA BASED ON SEVERITY OF ASTHMA ATTACKS

Assessment criteria for the severity of asthma attacks is as follows:

Mild	Moderate	Severe
• Peak expiratory flow rate (PEFR) 70–90% of normal • Respiratory rate ≤30% above average • Remains alert and no cyanosis or pallor • Dyspnea: Mild or absent with no or mild intercostal retractions • Pulsus paradoxus <10 mmHg • Oxygen saturation >95% and PCO_2 <35 • End expiratory wheeze only on auscultation	• PEFR 50–70% of normal • Respiratory rate 30–50% above average • Remains alert but pale • Moderate dyspnea but can speak in phrases • Moderate intercostal retractions with tracheosternal retractions and use of accessory muscles • Pulsus paradoxus 10–20 mmHg • Oxygen saturation 90–95% and PCO_2 <40 • Inspiratory and expiratory wheeze on auscultation	• PEFR <50% of normal • Respiratory rate >50% above average • Less alert and may be cyanotic • Severe dyspnea with difficulty speaking and severe retractions with nasal flaring and hyperinflation of chest • Pulsus paradoxus 20–40 mmHg • Oxygen saturation <90% and PCO_2 <40 • Breath sounds increasingly inaudible

EXERCISE-INDUCED ASTHMA

Exercise-induced asthma (bronchospasm) is especially a risk for those with pre-existing asthma or allergies, especially with high pollen counts, high levels of smog, and cold dry weather. Children usually begin to cough, wheeze, and complain of shortness of breath and chest tightness after about 5 minutes of exercise. The symptoms may increase 5 to 10 minutes after exercise ceases, but symptoms usually recede by 30 minutes. Children should be cautioned to regularly take all prescribed preventive medications and warm up for 5 to 10 minutes before doing strenuous exercise. Additionally, they should breathe through their noses to warm the air and learn to monitor their own breathing. Immediate care includes stopping activity, positioning the person in an upright position, and having them use an inhaled bronchodilator. If symptoms are severe and do not begin to subside after ceasing activity and using bronchodilator, the child may require emergent treatment.

GINA TREATMENT RECOMMENDATIONS CHILDREN AGES 12+ WITH ASTHMA

In 2019, the **Global Initiative for Asthma (GINA)** updated their recommendations for asthma treatment and management due to compiling evidence of the ineffectiveness of a short-acting bronchodilator alone (SABA) approach to asthma management. Years of research supported their recommendation that daily low dose inhaled corticosteroids (ICS) significantly reduce asthma exacerbations in individuals (age 12 and older) with moderate to severe asthma, but it was also recommended for mild asthma. The SABA recommendation only remains for those with exacerbations twice a month or less with no risk factors for asthma exacerbations. GINA acknowledged that the likelihood of patient adherence to a daily ICS may be a barrier to improved outcomes in the population with mild asthma, but maintained this recommendation regardless. GINA breaks their recommendations down into 5 steps:

- **Step 1 (Less than two exacerbations a month)**: Low dose ICS-formoterol as needed is the preferred controller.
- **Step 2 (Two or more exacerbations a month OR those with risk factors for exacerbations)**: Daily low dose ICS or low dose ICS-formoterol as needed are the preferred methods of control.
- **Step 3 (Moderate asthma; two or more exacerbations despite daily low dose ICS/low dose ICS-formoterol as needed)**: Daily low dose ICS-long acting β_2 agonist (LABA) is the preferred controller.

- **Step 4 (Severe asthma not controlled by low dose ICS-LABA)**: Medium dose daily ICS-LABA is the preferred controller.
- **Step 5 (Severe asthma not controlled by medium dose ICA-LABA)**: High dose daily ICS-LABA with a referral for phenotypic assessment and potential add-on therapies.

Cardiovascular Pathophysiology

CONGENITAL HEART DEFECTS IN CHILDREN

Congenital heart defects occur when the heart and/or great vessels develop with deformities in utero. Most cases have an unknown cause, but the following may contribute to the development of CHD: maternal infection during the first trimester, maternal alcohol or drug use during pregnancy, a mom who is over 40 years of age or who has insulin dependent diabetes, poor diet in pregnancy, an immediate family member has CHD, or the baby has a chromosomal disorder. CHD can include defects which lead to increased pulmonary blood flow (patent ductus arteriosus, atrial or ventricular septal defect, atrioventricular canal defect), defects which are obstructive (coarctation of aorta, aortic stenosis, pulmonic stenosis), defects that decrease pulmonary blood flow (tricuspid atresia, tetralogy of Fallot), and mixed defects (transposition of the great vessels, hypoplastic left heart syndrome, truncus arteriosus).

ACYANOTIC AND CYANOTIC CONGENITAL HEART DISEASE

Congenital heart disease is one of the leading causes of death in children within the first year of life. There are two main types of congenital heart disease: Acyanotic and cyanotic. They may also be classified according to hemodynamics related to the blood flow pattern.

ACYANOTIC

Increased pulmonary blood flow	Atrial septal defect Atrioventricular canal defect Patent ductus arteriosus Ventricular septal defect
Obstructed ventricular blood flow	Aortic stenosis Coarctation of aorta Pulmonic stenosis

CYANOTIC

Decreased pulmonary blood flow	Tetralogy of Fallot Tricuspid atresia
Mixed blood flow	Hypoplastic left heart syndrome Total anomalous pulmonary venous return Transposition of great arteries Truncus arteriosus. Ebstein's anomaly

ACYANOTIC CONGENITAL DEFECTS

ATRIAL SEPTAL DEFECT

An atrial septal defect (ASD) is an abnormal opening in the septum between the right and left atria. Because the left atrium has higher pressure than the right atrium, some of the oxygenated blood returning from the lungs to the left atrium is shunted back to the right atrium where it is again returned to the lungs, displacing deoxygenated blood.

Symptoms	Treatment
• Asymptomatic (some infants) • Congestive heart failure • Heart murmur • Increased risk for dysrhythmias and pulmonary vascular obstructive disease over time	Treatment may not be necessary for small defects, but larger defects require closure: • Open-heart surgical repair may be done. • Heart catheterization and placing of closure device (Amplatz device) across the atrial septal defect.

VENTRICULAR SEPTAL DEFECT

Ventricular septal defect is an abnormal opening in the septum between the right and left ventricles. If the opening is small, the child may be asymptomatic, but larger openings can result in a left to right shunt because of higher pressure in the left ventricle. This shunting increases over 6 weeks after birth with symptoms becoming more evident, but the defect may close within a few years.

Symptoms	Treatment
• Congestive heart failure with peripheral edema • Tachycardia • Dyspnea • Difficulty feeding • Heart murmur • Recurrent pulmonary infections • Increased risk for bacterial endocarditis and pulmonary vascular obstructive disease	• Diuretics, such as furosemide (Lasix) may be used for heart failure • ACE inhibitor (Captopril) to decrease pulmonary hypertension • Surgical repair includes pulmonary banding or cardiopulmonary bypass repair of the opening with suturing or a patch, depending upon the size.

ATRIOVENTRICULAR CANAL DEFECT

Atrioventricular canal defect is often associated with Down syndrome and involves a number of different defects, including openings between the atria and ventricles as well as abnormalities of the valves. In partial defects, there is an opening between the atria and mitral valve regurgitation. In complete defects, there is a large central hole in the heart and only one common valve between the atria and ventricles. The blood may flow freely about the heart, usually from left to right. Extra blood flow to the lungs causes enlargement of the heart. Partial defects may go undiagnosed for 20 years.

Symptoms	Treatment
Typical congestive heart failure signs: • Weakness and fatigue • Cough and/or wheezing with production of white or bloody sputum • Peripheral edema and ascites • Dysrhythmia and tachycardia • Dyspnea • Poor appetite • Failure to thrive, low weight • Cyanosis of skin and lips	• Symptom management as indicated. • Open-heart surgery to patch holes in the septum and valve repair or replacement.

PDA

Patent ductus arteriosus (PDA) is failure of the ductus arteriosus that connects the pulmonary artery and aorta to close after birth, resulting in left to right shunting of blood from the aorta back to the pulmonary artery. This increases the blood flow to the lung and causes an increase in pulmonary hypertension that can result in damage to the lung tissue.

Symptoms	Treatment
• Essentially asymptomatic (some infants) • Cyanosis • Congestive heart failure • Machinery-like murmur • Frequent respiratory infections and dyspnea, especially on exertion	• Indomethacin (Indocin) given within 10 days of birth is successful in closing about 80% of defects • Surgical repair with ligation of the patent vessel

COARCTATION OF THE AORTA

Coarctation of the aorta is a stricture of the aorta, proximal to the ductus arteriosus intersection. The increased blood pressure caused by the heart attempting to pump the blood past the stricture causes the heart to enlarge. Blood pressure to the head and upper extremities also increases, while blood pressure decreases to the lower body and extremities. With severe stricture, symptoms may not occur until the ductus arteriosus closes, causing sudden loss of blood supply to the lower body.

Symptoms	Treatment
• Difference in blood pressure between upper and lower extremities • Congestive heart failure symptoms in infants • Headaches, dizziness, and nosebleeds in older children • Increased risk of hypertension, ruptured aorta, aortic aneurysm, bacterial endocarditis, and brain attack	• Prostaglandin (alprostadil), such as Prostin VR Pediatric, to reopen the ductus arteriosus for infants • Balloon angioplasty • Surgical resection and anastomosis or graft replacement (usually at 3-5 years of age unless condition is severe). Infants who have surgery may need later repair

PULMONIC STENOSIS

Pulmonic stenosis is a stricture of the pulmonic valve that controls the flow of blood from the right ventricle to the lungs, resulting in right ventricular hypertrophy as the pressure increases in the right ventricle and resulting in decreased pulmonary blood flow. The condition may be asymptomatic, or symptoms may not be evident until the child enters adulthood, depending upon the severity of the defect. Pulmonic stenosis may be associated with a number of other heart defects.

Symptoms	Treatment
• Loud heart murmur • Congestive heart murmur • Mild cyanosis • Cardiomegaly • Angina • Dyspnea • Fainting • Increased risk of bacterial endocarditis	• Balloon valvuloplasty is used to separate the cusps of the valve for children. • Surgical repair includes the (closed) transventricular valvotomy (Brock) procedure for infants and the cardiopulmonary bypass pulmonary valvotomy for older children.

AORTIC STENOSIS

Aortic stenosis is a stricture (narrowing) of the aortic valve that controls the flow of blood from the left ventricle, causing the left ventricular wall to thicken as it increases pressure to overcome the valvular resistance, increasing afterload, and increasing the need for blood supply from the coronary arteries. This condition may result from a birth defect or childhood rheumatic fever and tends to worsen over the years as the heart grows. Treatment in children may be done before symptoms develop because of the danger of sudden death.

Symptoms	Treatment
<ul><li>Chest pain on exertion and intolerance of exercise.</li><li>Heart murmur.</li><li>Hypotension on exertion may be associated with sudden fainting.</li><li>Sudden death can occur.</li><li>Tachycardia with faint pulse.</li><li>Poor feeding.</li><li>Increased risk for bacterial endocarditis and coronary insufficiency.</li><li>Increases mitral regurgitation and secondary pulmonary hypertension.</li></ul>	<ul><li>Balloon valvuloplasty is used to dilate the valve non-surgically.</li><li>Surgical repair of the valve or replacement of the valve, depending upon the extent of stricture.</li></ul>

CYANOTIC CONGENITAL DEFECTS

TRICUSPID ATRESIA

Tricuspid atresia is lack of tricuspid valve between the right atrium and right ventricle. This causes blood to flow through the foramen ovale or an atrial defect to the left atrium and then through a ventricular wall defect from the left ventricle to the right ventricle and out to the lungs, causing oxygenated and deoxygenated blood to mix. Pulmonic obstruction is common.

Symptoms	Treatment
<ul><li>Postnatal cyanosis obvious</li><li>Tachycardia and dyspnea</li><li>Increasing hypoxemia and clubbing in older children</li><li>Increased risk for bacterial endocarditis, brain abscess, and stroke</li></ul>	<ul><li>Prostaglandin (alprostadil) is administered, to keep the ductus arteriosus and foramen ovale open if there are no septal defects.</li><li>Numerous surgical procedures may be required, including pulmonary artery banding, shunting from the aorta to the pulmonary arteries, Glenn procedure (connecting superior vena cava to pulmonary artery to allow deoxygenated blood to flow to the lungs), atrial septostomy to enlarge the opening between the atria, and the Fontan corrective procedure (usually done at 2-4 years after previous stabilizing procedures).</li></ul>

TRANSPOSITION OF THE GREAT VESSELS

Transposition of great arteries occurs when the aorta and pulmonary artery arise from the wrong ventricle (aorta from the right ventricle and pulmonary artery from the left). This means there is no connection between pulmonary and systemic circulation, with deoxygenated blood being pumped back to the body, and the oxygenated blood from the lungs is pumped back to the lungs. Septal defects may also occur, allowing some mixing of blood, and the ductus arteriosus allows mixing until it closes. Symptoms vary depending upon whether mixing of blood occurs.

Symptoms	Treatment
• Mild to severe cyanosis • Symptoms of congestive heart failure • Cardiomegaly develops in the weeks after birth • Heart sounds vary depending upon the severity of the defects	• Prostaglandin is administered to keep the ductus arteriosus and foramen ovale open. • Balloon atrial septostomy to increase size of foramen ovale. • Surgical repair with cardiopulmonary bypass and aortic cross-clamping to transpose arteries to the normal position ("arterial switch") as well as repair septal defects and other abnormalities.

TETRALOGY OF FALLOT (TOF)

Tetralogy of Fallot (TOF) is a combination of four different defects:

- Ventricular septal defect (usually with a large opening)
- Pulmonic stenosis with decreased blood flow to lungs
- Overriding aorta (displacement to the right so that it appears to come from both ventricles, usually overriding the ventricular septal defect), resulting in mixing of oxygenated and deoxygenated blood
- Right ventricular hypertrophy

Infants are often acutely cyanotic immediately after birth while others with less severe defects may have increasing cyanosis over the first year.

Symptoms	Treatment
• Intolerance to feeding or crying, resulting in increased cyanotic "blue spells" or "tet spells" • Failure to thrive with poor growth • Clubbing of fingers may occur over time • Intolerance to activity as child grows • Increased risk for emboli, brain attacks, brain abscess, seizures, fainting or sudden death	Total surgical repair at the age of one year or younger is now the preferred treatment rather than palliative procedures formerly used.

HYPOPLASTIC LEFT HEART SYNDROME

Hypoplastic left heart syndrome (HLHS) is underdevelopment of the left ventricle and ascending aortic atresia, causing inability of the heart to pump blood. Because of this, most blood flows from the left atrium through the foramen ovale to the right atrium and to the lungs, with the descending aorta receiving blood through the ductus arteriosus. There may be valvular abnormalities as well. Mortality rates are 100% without surgical correction and 25% with correction.

Symptoms may be mild until the ductus arteriosus closes at about 2 weeks, causing a marked increase in cyanosis and decreased cardiac output leading to cardiovascular collapse.

Treatment is through surgical procedures. These include a series of three staged operations:

1. The **Norwood procedure** connects the main pulmonary artery to the aorta, a shunt for pulmonary blood flow, and creates a large atrial septal defect.
2. The **Glenn procedure** then detaches the superior vena cava from the heart and to the pulmonary artery.
3. Finally, the **Fontan repair procedure** is used to detach the inferior vena cava from the heart and to the pulmonary artery.

Heart transplantation in infancy is preferred in many cases, but the shortage of hearts limits this option.

TRUNCUS ARTERIOSUS

Truncus arteriosus is the blood from both ventricles flowing into one large artery with one valve, with more blood flowing to the lower pressure pulmonary arteries than to the body, resulting in low oxygen saturation and hypoxemia. Usually, there is a ventricular septal defect so the blood in the ventricles mixes.

Symptoms	Treatment
• Congestive heart failure with pulmonary edema because of increased blood flow to lungs • Typical symptoms of congestive heart failure • Cyanosis, especially about the face (mouth and nose) • Dyspnea, increasing on feeding or exertion • Poor feeding and failure to thrive • Heart murmur • Increased risk for brain abscess and bacterial endocarditis	• Palliative banding of the pulmonary arteries to decrease the flow of blood to the lungs. • Surgical repair with cardiopulmonary bypass includes closing the ventricular defect, utilizing the existing single artery as the aorta by separating the pulmonary arteries from it and creating a conduit between the pulmonary arteries and the right ventricle.

EBSTEIN'S ANOMALY

Ebstein's anomaly is an abnormality of the tricuspid valve separating the right atrium from the right ventricle with some valve leaflets displaced downward and one adhering to the wall so that there is backflow into the atrium when the ventricle contracts. This usually results in enlargement of the right atrium and congestive heart failure. As pressure increases in the right atrium, it usually forces the foramen ovale to stay open so that the blood is shunted to the left atrium, mixing the deoxygenated blood with oxygenated blood that then leaves through the aorta. Symptoms vary widely depending upon the degree of defect and range from asymptomatic to life threatening. Ebstein's anomaly may occur with other cardiac defects. Many children are not diagnosed until their teens.

Symptoms	Treatment
• Cyanosis with low oxygen saturation • Congestive heart failure • Palpitations, arrhythmias • Dyspnea on exertion • Increased risk for bacterial endocarditis	• ACE inhibitors, diuretics, and digoxin • Surgical repair of abnormalities with valve repair or replacement

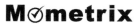

TOTAL ANOMALOUS PULMONARY VENOUS RETURN

Total anomalous pulmonary venous return is a defect in which the four pulmonary veins connect to the right atrium by an anomalous connection rather than the left atrium, so there is no direct blood flow to the left side of the heart. This condition commonly occurs with an atrial septal defect, which allows for the mixed oxygenated and deoxygenated blood to shunt to the left and enter the aorta. There are four different types of anomalies, and in some cases pulmonary vein obstruction. If the pulmonary veins are not obstructed, children may be asymptomatic initially.

Symptoms	Treatment
<ul><li>Heart murmur</li><li>Severe post-natal cyanosis or mild cyanosis</li><li>Dyspnea with grunting and sternal retraction or dyspnea on exertion</li><li>Low oxygen saturation (in the 80s if there is no pulmonary obstruction)</li><li>Cardiomegaly (right-sided hypertrophy)</li></ul>	Surgical repair to attach the pulmonary veins to the left atrium and correct any other defects may be done immediately after birth or delayed for 1-2 months.

CONGESTIVE HEART FAILURE IN CHILDREN

Congestive heart failure is a symptom rather than a disease. It results from the inability of the heart to adequately pump the blood that is needed for the body. In children (primarily infants) it most often occurs secondary to cardiac abnormalities with resultant increased blood volume and blood pressure:

- **Right-sided failure** occurs if the right ventricle cannot effectively contract to pump blood into the pulmonary artery, causing pressure to build in the right atrium and the venous circulation. This venous hypertension can result in peripheral edema or ascites and hepatosplenomegaly.
- **Left-sided failure** occurs if the left ventricle cannot effectively pump blood into the aorta and systemic circulation, increasing pressure in the left atrium and the pulmonary veins, with resultant pulmonary edema and increased pulmonary pressure.

Children often have some combination of both right and left-sided failure, depending on their cardiac defect.

SYMPTOMS IN INFANTS AND CHILDREN

Congestive heart failure symptoms vary widely depending upon the type and degree, the primary cause, and the child's age. Because of increased pressure in the lungs after birth, symptoms may be delayed in infants for the first week or two:

- **Infants** with left failure typically suffer respiratory distress with tachypnea, grunting respirations, sternal retraction, and rales, but the most common symptom is failure to thrive and difficulty eating, often leaving the child exhausted and sweaty. Those with right-sided failure may have more generalized edema of lower extremities, distended abdomen from ascites, hepatomegaly, and jugular venous distension. Tachycardia and low cardiac output occur with both types of heart failure, resulting in sweating, pallor, and hypotension.
- **Older children** typically suffer from inability to tolerate activity or exercise, becoming short of breath on exertion. Appetite is often poor with weight loss.
- In **adolescents**, CHF may be caused by the use of illicit drugs if there is no structural or acquired heart disease.

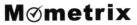

MANAGEMENT IN INFANTS AND CHILDREN

Management of congestive heart failure (CHF) in infants and children can be difficult. It is extremely important to establish the etiology and to treat the underlying cause. For infants with structural cardiac abnormalities, surgical repair may be needed to resolve the CHF. There are some medical treatments that can relieve symptoms:

- **Diuretics**, such as furosemide (Lasix), metolazone, or hydrochlorothiazide, can reduce pulmonary and peripheral edema.
- **Antihypertensives**, such as Captopril or Propranolol, can decrease heart workload.
- **Cardiac glycosides**, such as Lanoxin, may relieve symptoms if above medicines are not successful.
- **High caloric feedings**, either by bottle or nasogastric feeding, provide sufficient nutrients.
- **Oxygen** may be useful for some children with weak hearts.
- **Restriction of activities** reduces stress on the heart.
- **Dopamine or dobutamine** may be given to increase the contractibility of the heart.

CARDIAC HYPERTROPHY

Cardiac hypertrophy occurs when the heart responds to stresses, such as an increase in blood pressure or structural abnormality that interferes with normal functioning, by adapting its size and shape according to the increased effort required to function. As the heart adapts, the heart muscle enlarges, but this change is not the result of proliferation of cells but an increase in the size of existing myocytes (muscles cells). Thus, the cells are not dividing and providing more cells but simply getting bigger, and sometimes crowding out and killing other cells, further increasing the stress on the heart and again causing the cells to enlarge in a cycle that progressively weakens the musculature or the heart. Recent studies show 12% of children with HIV demonstrate cardiac hypertrophy, and 55% of children with renal transplants showed left ventricular hypertrophy, suggesting that many of these children are at risk for congestive heart failure. Treating the cause of hypertrophy does not always reduce the hypertrophic changes.

ACUTE CORONARY SYNDROMES

Acute coronary syndrome (ACS) is the impairment of blood flow through the coronary arteries, leading to ischemia of the cardiac muscle. Angina frequently occurs in ACS, manifesting as crushing pain substernally, radiating down the left arm or both arms. However, in females, elderly, and diabetics, symptoms may appear less acute and include nausea, shortness of breath, fatigue, pain/weakness/numbness in arms, or no pain at all (*silent ischemia*). There are multiple **classifications of angina**:

- **Stable angina**: Exercise-induced, short lived, relieved by rest or nitroglycerin. Other precipitating events include decrease in environmental temperature, heavy eating, strong emotions (such as fright or anger), or exertion, including coitus.
- **Unstable angina** (preinfarction or crescendo angina): A change in the pattern of stable angina, characterized by an increase in pain, not responding to a single nitroglycerin or rest, and persisting for >5 minutes. May cause a change in EKG, or indicate rupture of an atherosclerotic plaque or the beginning of thrombus formation. Treat as a medical emergency, indicates impending MI.
- **Variant angina** (Prinzmetal's angina): Results from spasms of the coronary arteries. Associated with or without atherosclerotic plaques and is often related to smoking, alcohol, or illicit stimulants, but can occur cyclically and at rest. Elevation of ST segments usually occurs with variant angina. Treatment is nitroglycerin or calcium channel blockers.

> **Review Video: Coronary Artery Disease**
> Visit mometrix.com/academy and enter code: 950720

156

MYOCARDIAL INFARCTIONS
NSTEMI AND STEMI

Non–ST-segment elevation MI (NSTEMI): ST elevation on the electrocardiogram (ECG) occurs in response to myocardial damage resulting from infarction or severe ischemia. The absence of ST elevation may be diagnosed as unstable angina or NSTEMI, but cardiac enzyme levels increase with NSTEMI, indicating partial blockage of coronary arteries with some damage. Symptoms are consistent with unstable angina, with chest pain or tightness, pain radiating to the neck or arm, dyspnea, anxiety, weakness, dizziness, nausea, vomiting, and heartburn. Initial treatment may include nitroglycerin, β-blockers, antiplatelet agents, or antithrombotic agents. Ongoing treatment may include β-blockers, aspirin, statins, angiotensin-converting enzyme inhibitors, angiotensin-receptor blockers, and clopidogrel. Percutaneous coronary intervention is not recommended.

ST-segment elevation MI (STEMI): This more severe type of MI involves complete blockage of one or more coronary arteries with myocardial damage, resulting in ST elevation. Symptoms are those of acute MI. As necrosis occurs, Q waves often develop, indicating irreversible myocardial damage, which may result in death, so treatment involves immediate reperfusion before necrosis can occur.

> **Review Video: Myocardial Infarction**
> Visit mometrix.com/academy and enter code: 148923

Q-WAVE AND NON-Q-WAVE MYOCARDIAL INFARCTIONS

Formerly classified as transmural or non-transmural, myocardial infarctions are now classified as Q-wave or non-Q-wave:

- **Q-Wave**
  - Characterized by a series of abnormal Q waves (wider and deeper) on ECG, especially in the early morning (related to adrenergic activity).
  - Infarction is usually prolonged and results in necrosis.
  - Coronary occlusion is complete in 80-90% of cases.
  - Q-wave MI is often, but not always, transmural.
  - Peak CK levels occur in about 27 hours.
- **Non-Q-Wave**
  - Characterized by changes in ST-T wave with ST depression (usually reversible within a few days).
  - Usually reperfusion occurs spontaneously, so infarct size is smaller. Contraction necrosis related to reperfusion is common.
  - Non-Q-wave MI is usually non-transmural.
  - Coronary occlusion is complete in only 20-30%.
  - Peak CK levels occur in 12-13 hours.
  - Reinfarction is common.

LOCATIONS AND TYPES

Myocardial infarctions are also classified according to their location and the extent of injury. Q-wave infarctions involve the full thickness of the heart muscle, often producing a series of Q waves on ECG. While an MI most frequently damages the left ventricle and the septum, the right ventricle may be damaged as well, depending upon the area of the occlusion:

- **Anterior** (V_2 to V_4): Occlusion in the proximal left anterior descending (LAD) or left coronary artery. Reciprocal changes found in leads II, III, aV_F.
- **Lateral** (I, aV_L, V_5, V_6): Occlusion of the circumflex coronary artery or branch of left coronary artery. Often causes damage to anterior wall as well. Reciprocal changes found in leads II, III, aV_F.
- **Inferior/diaphragmatic** (II, III, aV_F): Occlusion of the right coronary artery and causes conduction malfunctions. Reciprocal changes found in leads I and aV_L.

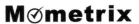

- **Right ventricular** (V_{4R}, V_{5R}, V_{6R}): Occlusion of the proximal section of the right coronary artery and damages in the right ventricle and the inferior wall. No reciprocal changes should be noted on an ECG.
- **Posterior** (V_8, V_9): Occlusion in the right coronary artery or circumflex artery and may be difficult to diagnose. Reciprocal changes found in V_1-V_4.

CLINICAL MANIFESTATIONS AND DIAGNOSIS

Clinical manifestations of myocardial infarction may vary considerably. More than half of all patients present with acute MIs with no prior history of cardiovascular disease.

Signs/symptoms: Angina with pain in chest that may radiate to neck or arms, palpitations, hypertension or hypotension, dyspnea, pulmonary edema, dependent edema, nausea/vomiting, pallor, skin cold and clammy, diaphoresis, decreased urinary output, neurological/psychological disturbances: anxiety, light-headedness, headache, visual abnormalities, slurred speech, and fear.

Diagnosis is based on the following:

- ECG obtained immediately to monitor heart changes over time. Typical changes include T-wave inversion, elevation of ST segment, abnormal Q waves, tachycardia, bradycardia, and dysrhythmias.
- Echocardiogram: decreased ventricular function is possible, especially for transmural MI.
- Labs:
  - **Troponin**: Increases within 3–6 hours, peaks 14–20; elevated for up to 1-2 weeks.
  - **Creatinine kinase (CK-MB)**: Increases 4–8 hours and peaks at about 24 hours (earlier with thrombolytic therapy or PTCA).
  - **Ischemia Modified Albumin (IMA)**: Increase within minutes, peak 6 hours and return to baseline; verify with other labs.
  - **Myoglobin**: Increases in 0.5–4.0 hours, peaks 6–7 hours. While an increase is not specific to an MI, a failure to increase can be used to rule out an MI.

PAPILLARY MUSCLE RUPTURE

Papillary muscle rupture is a rare but often deadly complication of myocardial ischemia/infarct. It most commonly occurs with inferior infarcts. The papillary muscles are part of the cardiac wall structure. Attached to the lower portion of the ventricles, they are responsible for the opening and closing of the tricuspid and mitral valve and preventing prolapse during systole. Rupture of the papillary muscle can occur with myocardial infarct or ischemia in the area of the heart surrounding the papillary muscle. Since the papillary muscles support the mitral valve, rupture will cause severe mitral regurgitation that may result in cardiogenic shock and subsequent death. Rupture of the papillary muscle may be partial or complete and is considered a life-threatening emergency.

Signs and symptoms: Acute heart failure, pulmonary edema, and cardiogenic shock (tachycardia, diaphoresis, loss of consciousness, pallor, tachypnea, mental status changes, weak or thready pulse, and decreased urinary output).

Diagnosis: Transesophageal echocardiography (TEE) to visualize the papillary muscles, color flow Doppler, echocardiogram, and physical assessment. In patients with papillary muscle rupture, a holosystolic murmur starting at the apex and radiating to the axilla may be present.

Treatment: Emergent surgical intervention to repair the mitral valve.

In the cases of complete rupture, patients often experience the rapid development of cardiogenic shock and subsequent death.

CARDIOMYOPATHY
DILATED CARDIOMYOPATHY

Dilated cardiomyopathy (DCM) occurs when some precipitating factor leads to decreased cardiac perfusion. The resulting ischemic cardiac tissue is replaced with scar tissue, and the healthy cells are forced to over-compensate, causing hypertrophy and over stretching. Eventually, the muscle cells become stretched beyond compensation, and dilated and weak chamber results, unable to properly contract. This causes a decrease in stroke volume and cardiac output, with the end result being enlargement of the mitral and tricuspid valves and severe valve regurgitation. While DCM is the most common form of cardiomyopathy, causes include:

- **Vascular**: Cardiac ischemia, hypertension, atherosclerosis
- **Metabolic**: Diabetes, uremia, thyrotoxicosis, and acromegaly, muscular dystrophy
- **Genetics** (familial DCM), and childbirth (peripartum DCM)
- **Viral infections**, particularly adenovirus, Varicella zoster, HIV, and Hepatitis C may cause DCM
- **Alcohol poisoning or cocaine addiction**
- **Radiation or heavy metal poisoning**, specifically cobalt

Signs/Symptoms: Dyspnea, SOB, tachycardia, S3/S4 heart sounds, holosystolic murmur, wheezes/crackles, pleural effusions, edema, JVD, ascites

Diagnosis: EKG (tachycardia/T wave changes), chest x-ray (cardiomegaly), 2D Echocardiogram (valve regurgitation/EF).

Treatment includes:

- Treat underlying cause if possible; supportive care
- Heart transplant if patient is a candidate and damage is permanent

HYPERTROPHIC CARDIOMYOPATHY

Hypertrophic cardiomyopathy (HCM) is a genetic disorder that causes idiopathic thickening of the heart muscle, primarily involving the ventricular septum and portions of the left ventricle. Patients with HCM produce abnormal sarcomeres and misalignment of muscle cells (myocardial disarray). Basically, HCM is characterized by ventricular hypertrophy, an asymmetrical septum, forceful systole, cardiac dysrhythmias, and myocardial disarray. Because the abnormal cells develop over time, it is common for HCM to remain undiagnosed until middle or late adulthood.

Signs/Symptoms: Exertional or atypical chest pain, dyspnea at rest, syncope, frequent palpitations (common due to reoccurring dysrhythmias).

Diagnosis: 2D echo (structure and EF), EKG (pathological Q waves and dysrhythmias), x-ray (cardiomegaly), Family history (especially cardiac death, reoccurring dysrhythmias, or myocardial hypertrophy).

Treatment includes:

- **Surgery**: Septal myectomy is gold standard: high mortality (3-10%), but increases cardiac output and quality of life.
- **Alcohol-based septal ablation**: Ethanol 100% injected into a branch of the LAD, creating a controlled area of infarction and consequently thinning the septum.

RESTRICTIVE CARDIOMYOPATHY

Restrictive cardiomyopathy (RCM) occurs when the ventricles become stiff and noncompliant, resulting in decreased end-diastolic cardiac refill volume. The ventricular stiffening is caused by the infiltration of fibroelastic tissue into the cardiac muscle (such as in amyloidosis or sarcoidosis). Atrial enlargement can be seen in most cases of RCM as a result of the increased effort required to push blood from the atria into the ventricles. It is not uncommon for a patient to be in atrial fibrillation secondary to atrial enlargement. In advanced cases, ventricular dysrhythmias may also be seen.

Signs/Symptoms: Exercise intolerance/fatigue, edema, crackles, elevated CVP, S3/S4, murmur, SOB at rest

Diagnosis: 2D echo (enlarged atria, decreased compliance of ventricle), hemodynamic monitoring (increased right atrial pressure and pulmonary wedge pressure, and SVR), x-ray (cardiomegaly), EKG (atrial fibrillation), endomyocardial biopsy (to differentiate from constrictive pericarditis).

Treatment includes:

- **Medications**: β-blockers increase ventricular filling; antiarrhythmics may be ordered
- **Surgical**: Heart transplant, if patient is a candidate

DYSRHYTHMIAS
SINUS BRADYCARDIA
There are 3 primary types of **sinus node dysrhythmias**: sinus bradycardia, sinus tachycardia, and sinus arrhythmia. **Sinus bradycardia (SB)** is caused by a decreased rate of impulse from sinus node. The pulse and ECG usually appear normal except for a slower rate.

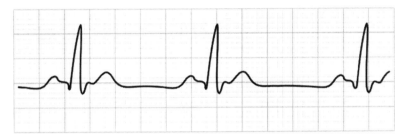

SB is characterized by a regular pulse <50-60 bpm with P waves in front of QRS, which are usually normal in shape and duration. PR interval is 0.12-0.20 seconds, QRS interval is 0.04-0.11 seconds, and P:QRS ratio of 1:1. SB may be caused by several factors:

- May be normal in athletes and older adults; generally not treated unless symptomatic
- Conditions that lower the body's metabolic needs, such as hypothermia or sleep
- Hypotension and decrease in oxygenation
- Medications such as calcium channel blockers and β-blockers
- Vagal stimulation that may result from vomiting, suctioning, defecating, or certain medical procedures (carotid stent placement, etc.)
- Increased intracranial pressure
- Myocardial infarction

Treatment: involves eliminating cause if possible, such as changing medications. Atropine 0.5-1.0 mg may be given IV to block vagal stimulation or increase rate if symptomatic.

SINUS TACHYCARDIA

Sinus tachycardia (ST) occurs when the sinus node impulse increases in frequency. ST is characterized by a regular pulse >100 with P waves before QRS but sometimes part of the preceding T wave. QRS is usually of normal shape and duration (0.04-0.11 seconds) but may have consistent irregularity. PR interval is 0.12-0.20 seconds and P:QRS ratio of 1:1.

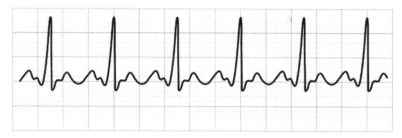

The rapid pulse decreases diastolic filling time and causes reduced cardiac output with resultant hypotension. Acute pulmonary edema may result from the decreased ventricular filling if untreated. ST may be **caused** by a number of factors:

- Acute blood loss, shock, hypovolemia, anemia
- Sinus arrhythmia, hypovolemic heart failure
- Hypermetabolic conditions, fever, infection
- Exertion/exercise, anxiety, stress
- Medications, such as sympathomimetic drugs

Treatment: eliminating precipitating factors, calcium channel blockers and β-blockers to reduce heart rate.

SUPRAVENTRICULAR TACHYCARDIA

Supraventricular tachycardia (SVT) (>100 BPM) may have a sudden onset and result in congestive heart failure. Rate may increase to 200–300 BMP, which will significantly decrease cardiac output due to decreased filling time. SVT originates in the atria rather than the ventricles but is controlled by the tissue in the area of the AV node rather than the SA node. Rhythm is usually rapid but regular. The P wave is present but may not be clearly defined as it may be obscured by the preceding T wave, and the QRS complex appears normal. The PR interval is 0.12-0.20 seconds and the QRS interval is 0.04-0.11 seconds with a P:QRS ratio of 1:1.

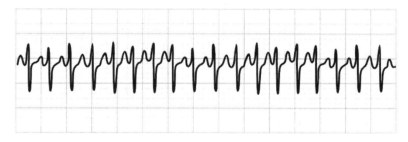

SVT may be episodic with periods of normal heart rate and rhythm between episodes of SVT, so it is often referred to as paroxysmal SVT (PSVT).

Treatment: Adenosine, digoxin (Lanoxin), Verapamil (Calan, Verelan), vagal maneuvers, cardioversion.

SINUS ARRHYTHMIA

Sinus arrhythmia (SA) results from irregular impulses from the sinus node, often paradoxical (increasing with inspiration and decreasing with expiration) because of stimulation of the vagal nerve during inspiration and rarely causes a negative hemodynamic effect. These cyclic changes in the pulse during respiration are quite common in both children and young adults and often lesson with age but may persist in some adults. Sinus arrhythmia can, in some cases, relate to heart or valvular disease and may be increased with vagal stimulation for suctioning, vomiting, or defecating. Characteristics of SA include a regular pulse 50-100 BPM, P waves in front of QRS with duration (0.04-0.11 seconds) and shape of QRS usually normal, PR interval of 0.12-0.20 seconds, and P:QRS ratio of 1:1.

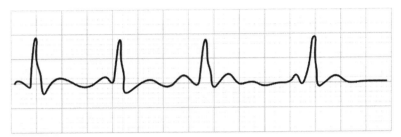

Treatment is usually not necessary unless it is associated with bradycardia.

PREMATURE ATRIAL CONTRACTION

There are 3 primary types of **atrial dysrhythmias**: premature atrial contraction, atrial flutter, and atrial fibrillation. Premature atrial contraction (PAC) is essentially an extra beat precipitated by an electrical impulse to the atrium before the sinus node impulse. The extra beat may be caused by alcohol, caffeine, nicotine, hypervolemia, hypokalemia, hypermetabolic conditions, atrial ischemia, or infarction. Characteristics include an irregular pulse because of extra P waves, the shape and duration of QRS is usually normal (0.04-0.11 seconds) but may be abnormal, PR interval remains between 0.12-0.20, and P:QRS ratio is 1:1. Rhythm is irregular with varying P-P and R-R intervals.

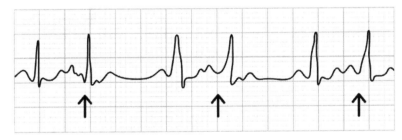

PACs can occur in an essentially healthy heart and are not usually cause for concern unless they are frequent (>6 per hr) and cause severe palpitations. In that case, atrial fibrillation should be suspected.

ATRIAL FLUTTER

Atrial flutter (AF) occurs when the atrial rate is faster, usually 250-400 beats per minute, than the AV node conduction rate so not all of the beats are conducted into the ventricles. The beats are effectively blocked at the AV node, preventing ventricular fibrillation although some extra ventricular impulses may pass though. AF is caused by the same conditions that cause A-fib: coronary artery disease, valvular disease, pulmonary disease, heavy alcohol ingestion, and cardiac surgery. AF is characterized by atrial rates of 250-400 with ventricular rates of 75-150, with ventricular rate usually being regular. P waves are saw-toothed (referred to as F waves), QRS shape and duration (0.04-0.11 seconds) are usually normal, PR interval may be hard to calculate because of F waves, and the P:QRS ratio is 2:1 to 4:1. Symptoms include chest pain, dyspnea, and hypotension.

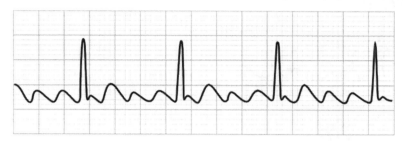

Treatment includes:

- Emergent cardioversion if condition is unstable
- Medications to slow ventricular rate and conduction through AV node: non-dihydropyridine calcium channel blockers (Cardizem, Calan) and beta blockers
- Medications to convert to sinus rhythm: Corvert, Tikosyn, Amiodarone; also used in practice: Cardioquin, Norpace, Cordarone

ATRIAL FIBRILLATION

Atrial fibrillation (A-fib) is rapid, disorganized atrial beats that are ineffective in emptying the atria, so that blood pools in the chambers. This can lead to thrombus formation and emboli. The ventricular rate increases with a decreased stroke volume, and cardiac output decreases with increased myocardial ischemia, resulting in palpitations and fatigue. A-fib is caused by coronary artery disease, valvular disease, pulmonary disease, heavy alcohol ingestion, infection, and cardiac surgery; however, it can also be idiopathic. A-fib is characterized by a very irregular pulse with atrial rate of 300-600 and ventricular rate of 120-200, shape and duration (0.04-0.11 seconds) of QRS is usually normal. Fibrillatory (F) waves are seen instead of P waves. The PR interval cannot be measured and the P:QRS ratio is highly variable.

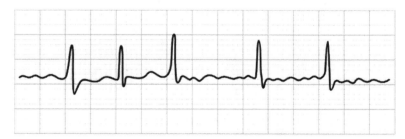

Treatment is the same as atrial flutter.

Review Video: EKG Interpretation: Afib and Aflutter
Visit mometrix.com/academy and enter code: 263842

PREMATURE JUNCTIONAL CONTRACTION

The area around the AV node is the junction, and dysrhythmias that arise from that area are called junctional dysrhythmias. Premature junctional contraction (PJC) occurs when a premature impulse starts at the AV node before the next normal sinus impulse reaches the AV node. PJC is similar to premature atrial contraction (PAC) and generally requires no treatment although it may be an indication of digoxin toxicity. The ECG may appear basically normal with an early QRS complex that is normal in shape and duration (0.04-0.11 seconds). The P wave may be absent or it may precede, be part of, or follow the QRS with a PR interval of 0.12 seconds. The P:QRS ratio may vary from <1:1 to 1:1 (with inverted P wave). The underlying rhythm is usually regular at a heart rate of 60-100. Significant symptoms related to PJC are rare.

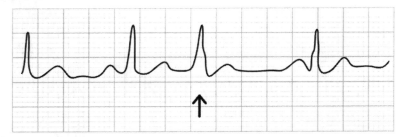

JUNCTIONAL RHYTHMS

Junctional rhythms occur when the AV node becomes the pacemaker of the heart. This can happen because the sinus node is depressed from increased vagal tone or a block at the AV node prevents sinus node impulses from being transmitted. While the sinus node normally sends impulses 60-100 beats per minute, the AV node junction usually sends impulses at 40-60 beats per minute. The QRS complex is of usual shape and duration (0.04-0.11 seconds). The P wave may be inverted and may be absent, hidden or after the QRS. If the P wave precedes the QRS, the PR interval is <0.12 seconds. The P:QRS ratio is <1:1 or 1:1. The junctional escape rhythm is a protective mechanism preventing asystole with failure of the sinus node. An **accelerated junctional rhythm** is similar, but the heart rate is 60-100. **Junctional tachycardia** occurs with heart rate of >100.

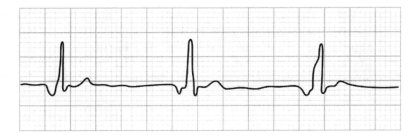

AV NODAL REENTRY TACHYCARDIA

AV nodal reentry tachycardia occurs when an impulse conducts to the area of the AV node and is then sent in a rapidly repeating cycle back to the same area and to the ventricles, resulting in a fast ventricular rate. The onset and cessation are usually rapid. AV nodal reentry tachycardia (also known as paroxysmal atrial tachycardia or supraventricular tachycardia if there are no P waves) is characterized by atrial rate of 150-250 with ventricular rate of 75-250, P wave that is difficult to see or absent, QRS complex that is usually normal and a PR interval of <0.12 if a P wave is present. The P:QRS ratio is 1-2:1. Precipitating factors include nicotine, caffeine, hypoxemia, anxiety, underlying coronary artery disease and cardiomyopathy. Cardiac output may be decreased with a rapid heart rate, causing dyspnea, chest pain, and hypotension.

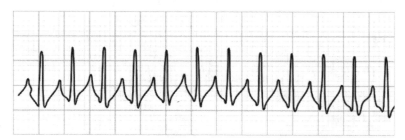

Treatment includes:

- Vagal maneuvers (carotid sinus massage, gag reflex, holding breath/bearing down)
- Medications (adenosine, verapamil, or diltiazem)
- Cardioversion if other methods unsuccessful

PREMATURE VENTRICULAR CONTRACTIONS

Premature ventricular contractions (PVCs) are those in which the impulse begins in the ventricles and conducts through them prior to the next sinus impulse. The ectopic QRS complexes may vary in shape, depending upon whether there is one site (unifocal) or more (multifocal) that stimulates the ectopic beats. PVCs usually cause no morbidity unless there is underlying cardiac disease or an acute MI. PVCs are characterized by an irregular heartbeat, QRS that is ≥0.12 seconds and oddly shaped. PVCs are often not treated in otherwise healthy people. PVCs may be precipitated by electrolyte imbalances, caffeine, nicotine, or alcohol. Because PVCs may occur with any supraventricular dysrhythmia, the underlying rhythm must be noted as well as the PVCs. If there are more than six PVCs in an hour, that is a risk factor for developing ventricular tachycardia.

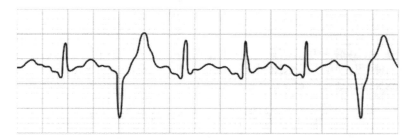

Bigeminy is a rhythm where every other beat is a PVC. **Trigeminy** is a rhythm where every third beat is a PVC.

Ventricular bigeminy is a rhythm where every other beat is a PVC. **Ventricular trigeminy** is a rhythm where every third beat is a PVC.

Treatment: Lidocaine (affects the ventricles, may cause CNS toxicity with nausea and vomiting), Procainamide (affects the atria and ventricles and may cause decreased BP and widening of QRS and QT); treat underlying cause.

VENTRICULAR TACHYCARDIA

Ventricular tachycardia (VT) is greater than 3 PVCs in a row with a ventricular rate of 100-200 beats per minute. Ventricular tachycardia may be triggered by the same factors as PVCs and often is related to underlying coronary artery disease. The rapid rate of contractions makes VT dangerous as the ineffective beats may render the person unconscious with no palpable pulse. A detectable rate is usually regular and the QRS complex is ≥0.12 seconds and is usually abnormally shaped. The P wave may be undetectable with an irregular PR interval if P wave is present. The P:QRS ratio is often difficult to ascertain because of the absence of P waves.

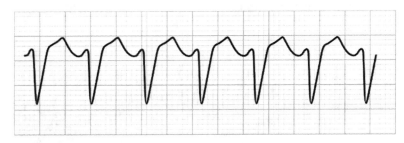

Treatment is as follows:

- With pulse: Synchronized cardioversion, adenosine
- No pulse: Same as ventricular fibrillation

NARROW COMPLEX AND WIDE COMPLEX TACHYCARDIAS

Tachycardias are classified as narrow complex or wide complex. Wide and narrow refer to the configuration of the QRS complex.

- **Wide complex tachycardia (WCT)**: About 80% of cases of WCT are caused by ventricular tachycardia. WCT originates at some point below the AV node and may be associated with palpitations, dyspnea, anxiety, diaphoresis, and cardiac arrest. Wide complex tachycardia is diagnosed with more than 3 consecutive beats at a heart rate >100 BPM and QRS duration ≥0.12 seconds.

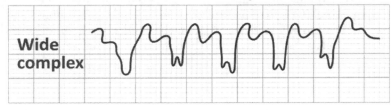

- **Narrow complex tachycardia (NCT)**: NCT is associated with palpitations, dyspnea, and peripheral edema. NCT is generally supraventricular in origin. Narrow complex tachycardia is diagnosed with ≥3 consecutive beats at heart rate of >100 BPM and QRS duration of <0.12 seconds.

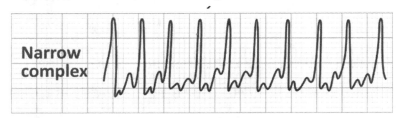

VENTRICULAR FIBRILLATION

Ventricular fibrillation (VF) is a rapid, very irregular ventricular rate >300 beats per minute with no atrial activity observable on the ECG, caused by disorganized electrical activity in the ventricles. The QRS complex is not recognizable as ECG shows irregular undulations. The causes are the same as for ventricular tachycardia and asystole. VF is accompanied by lack of palpable pulse, audible pulse, and respirations and is immediately life threatening without defibrillation.

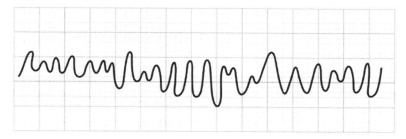

Treatment includes:

- Emergency defibrillation, the cause should be identified and treated
- Epinephrine 1 mg q 3-5minutes then amiodarone 300mg (2nd dose: 150mg) IV push

> **Review Video: EKG Interpretation: Ventricular Arrythmias**
> Visit mometrix.com/academy and enter code: 933152

IDIOVENTRICULAR RHYTHM

Ventricular escape rhythm (idioventricular) occurs when the Purkinje fibers below the AV node create an impulse. This may occur if the sinus node fails to fire or if there is blockage at the AV node so that the impulse does not go through. Idioventricular rhythm is characterized by a regular ventricular rate of 20-40 BPM. Rates >40 BPM are called accelerated idioventricular rhythm. The P wave is missing and the QRS complex has a very bizarre and abnormal shape with duration of ≥0.12 seconds. The low ventricular rate may cause a decrease in cardiac output, often making the patient lose consciousness. In other patients, the idioventricular rhythm may not be associated with reduced cardiac output.

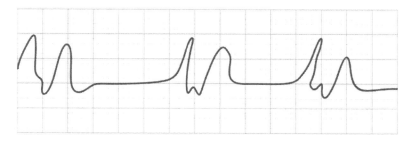

VENTRICULAR ASYSTOLE

Ventricular asystole is the absence of audible heartbeat, palpable pulse, and respirations, a condition often referred to as "cardiac arrest." While the ECG may show some P waves initially, the QRS complex is absent although there may be an occasional QRS "escape beat" (agonal rhythm). Cardiopulmonary resuscitation is required with intubation for ventilation and establishment of an intravenous line for fluids. Without immediate treatment, the patient will suffer from severe hypoxia and brain death within minutes. Identifying the cause is critical for the patient's survival. Consider the "Hs & Ts": hypovolemia, hypoxia, hydrogen ions (acidosis), hypo/hyperkalemia, hypothermia, tension pneumothorax, tamponade (cardiac), toxins, and thrombosis (pulmonary or coronary). Even with immediate treatment, the prognosis is poor and ventricular asystole is often a sign of impending death.

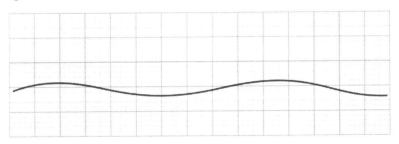

Treatment includes:

- CPR only; Asystole is not a shockable rhythm therefore defibrillation is not indicated
- Epinephrine 1 mg q 3-5 minutes

SINUS PAUSE

Sinus pause occurs when the sinus node fails to function properly to stimulate heart contractions, so there is a pause on the ECG recording that may persist for a few seconds to minutes, depending on the severity of the dysfunction. A prolonged pause may be difficult to differentiate from cardiac arrest. During the sinus pause, the P wave, QRS complex and PR and QRS intervals are all absent. P:QRS ratio is 1:1 and the rhythm is irregular. The pulse rate may vary widely, usually 60-100 BPM. Patients with frequent pauses may complain of dizziness or syncope. The patient may need to undergo an electrophysiology study and medication reconciliation to determine the cause. If measures such as decreasing medication are not effective, a pacemaker is usually indicated (if symptomatic).

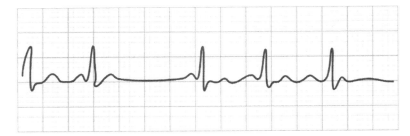

FIRST-DEGREE AV BLOCK

First-degree AV block occurs when the atrial impulses are conducted through the AV node to the ventricles at a rate that is slower than normal. While the P and QRS are usually normal, the PR interval is >0.20 seconds, and the P:QRS ratio is 1:1. A narrow QRS complex indicates a conduction abnormality only in the AV node, but a widened QRS indicates associated damage to the bundle branches as well. *Chronic* first-degree block may be caused by fibrosis/sclerosis of the conduction system related to coronary artery disease, valvular disease, cardiac myopathies and carries little morbidity, thus is often left untreated. *Acute* first-degree block, on the other hand, is of much more concern and may be related to digoxin toxicity, β-blockers, amiodarone, myocardial infarction, hyperkalemia, or edema related to valvular surgery.

Treatment: involves eliminating cause if possible, such as changing medications. Atropine 0.5-1.0 mg may be given IV if rate falls.

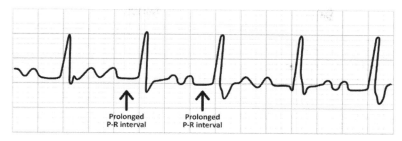

Prolonged P-R interval

Prolonged P-R interval

SECOND-DEGREE AV BLOCK

Second-degree AV block occurs when some of the atrial beats are blocked. Second-degree AV block is further subdivided according to the patterns of block.

TYPE I

Mobitz type I block (Wenckebach) occurs when each atrial impulse in a group of beats is conducted at a lengthened interval until one fails to conduct (the PR interval progressively increases), so there are more P waves than QRS complexes, but the QRS complex is usually of normal shape and duration. The sinus node functions at a regular rate, so the P-P interval is regular, but the R-R interval usually shortens with each impulse. The P:QRS ratio varies, such as 3:2, 4:3, 5:4. This type of block by itself usually does not cause significant morbidity unless associated with an inferior wall myocardial infarction.

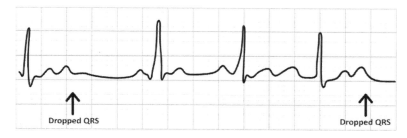

Dropped QRS

Dropped QRS

TYPE II

In Mobitz type II, only some of the atrial impulses are conducted unpredictably through the AV node to the ventricles, and the block always occurs below the AV node in the bundle of His, the bundle branches, or the Purkinje fibers. The PR intervals are the same if impulses are conducted, and the QRS complex is usually widened. The P:QRS ratio varies 2:1, 3:1, and 4:1. Type II block is more dangerous than Type I because it may progress to complete AV block and may produce Stokes-Adams syncope. Additionally, if the block is at the Purkinje fibers, there is no escape impulse. Usually, a transcutaneous cardiac pacemaker and defibrillator should be at the patient's bedside. **Symptoms** may include chest pain if the heart block is precipitated by myocarditis or myocardial ischemia.

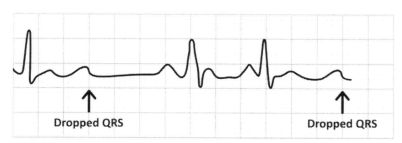

Dropped QRS

Dropped QRS

THIRD-DEGREE

With third-degree AV block, there are more P waves than QRS complexes, with no clear relationship between them. The atrial rate is 2-3 times the pulse rate, so the PR interval is irregular. If the SA node malfunctions, the AV node fires at a lower rate, and if the AV node malfunctions, the pacemaker site in the ventricles takes over at a bradycardic rate; thus, with complete AV block, the heart still contracts, but often ineffectually. With this type of block, the atrial P (sinus rhythm or atrial fibrillation) and the ventricular QRS (ventricular escape rhythm) are stimulated by different impulses, so there is AV dissociation.

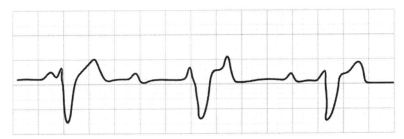

The heart may compensate at rest but can't keep pace with exertion. The resultant bradycardia may cause congestive heart failure, fainting, or even sudden death, and usually conduction abnormalities slowly worsen. **Symptoms** include dyspnea, chest pain, and hypotension, which are treated with IV atropine. Transcutaneous pacing may be needed. Complete persistent AV block normally requires implanted pacemakers, usually dual chamber.

> **Review Video: AV Heart Blocks**
> Visit mometrix.com/academy and enter code: 487004

BUNDLE BRANCH BLOCKS

A **right bundle branch block (RBBB)** occurs when conduction is blocked in the right bundle branch that carries impulses from the Bundle of His to the right ventricle. The impulse travels through the left ventricle instead, and then reaches the right ventricle, but this causes a slight delay in contraction of the right ventricle. A RBBB is characterized by normal P waves (as the right atrium still contracts appropriately), but the QRS complex is widened and notched (referred to as an "RSR pattern" that resembles the letter "M") in lead V1, which is a reflection of the asynchronous ventricular contraction. The PR interval is normal or prolonged, and the QRS interval is > 0.12 seconds. P:QRS ratio remains 1:1 with regular rhythms.

A **left bundle branch block (LBBB)** occurs when there is a delay in conduction between the left atrium and left ventricle. It is also characterized by normal or inverted P waves, but the QRS complex may be widened with a deep S wave and an interval of >0.12 seconds (in lead V1) that resembles a "W." The PR interval may be normal or prolonged. The P:QRS ratio is 1:1 and the rhythm is regular.

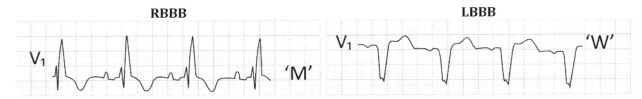

MITRAL STENOSIS

Mitral stenosis is a narrowing of the mitral valve that allows blood to flow from the left atrium to the left ventricle. Pressure in the left atrium increases to overcome resistance, resulting in enlargement of the left atrium and increased pressure in the pulmonary veins and capillaries of the lung (pulmonary hypertension). Mitral stenosis can be caused by infective endocarditis, calcifications, or tumors in the left atrium.

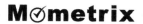

Signs/Symptoms: Exertional dyspnea, orthopnea/nocturnal dyspnea, right-sided heart failure, loud S_1 and S_2, and mid-diastolic murmur.

Diagnosis: Cardiac catheterization, chest x-ray, echocardiogram, ECG.

Treatment includes:

- **Medications**: Antiarrhythmic, anticoagulant, and antihypertensive medications
- **Surgical**: Open/closed commissurotomy, balloon valvuloplasty, and mitral valve replacement

MITRAL VALVE INSUFFICIENCY

Mitral valve insufficiency occurs when the mitral valve fails to close completely so that there is backflow into the left atrium from the left ventricle during systole, decreasing cardiac output. It may occur with mitral stenosis or independently. Mitral valve insufficiency can result from damage caused by rheumatic fever, myxomatous degeneration, infective endocarditis, collagen vascular disease (Marfan's syndrome), or cardiomyopathy/left heart failure. There are **three phases** of the disease:

- **Acute**: May occur with rupture of a chordae tendineae or papillary muscle causing sudden left ventricular flooding and overload.
- **Chronic compensated**: Enlargement of the left atrium to decrease filling pressure, and hypertrophy of the left ventricle.
- **Chronic decompensated**: Left ventricle fails to compensate for the volume overload; decreased stroke volume and increased cardiac output.

Symptoms: Orthopnea/dyspnea, split S_2/S_3/S_4 heart sounds, systolic murmur, palpitations, right-sided heart failure, fatigue, angina (rare).

Diagnosis: Cardiac catheterization, chest x-ray, echocardiogram, ECG.

Treatment includes:

- **Medications**: Antiarrhythmic, anticoagulant, and antihypertensive medications.
- **Surgical**: Annuloplasty or valvuloplasty, and mitral valve replacement.

AORTIC STENOSIS

Aortic stenosis is a stricture (narrowing) of the aortic valve that controls the flow of blood from the left ventricle. This causes the left ventricular wall to thicken as it increases pressure to overcome the valvular resistance, increasing afterload and increasing the need for blood supply from the coronary arteries. This condition may result from a birth defect or childhood rheumatic fever, and tends to worsen over the years as the heart grows.

Symptoms: Angina, exercise intolerance, dyspnea, split S_1 and S_2, systolic murmur at base of carotids, hypotension on exertion, syncope, left-sided heart failure; sudden death can occur.

Diagnosis: Cardiac catheterization, chest x-ray, echocardiogram, ECG.

Treatment includes:

- **Medications**: Antiarrhythmic, anticoagulant, and antihypertensive medications
- **Surgical**: Balloon valvuloplasty, and aortic valve replacement

PULMONIC STENOSIS

Pulmonic stenosis is a stricture of the pulmonary blood that controls the flow of blood from the right ventricle to the lungs, resulting in right ventricular hypertrophy as the pressure increases in the right ventricle and decreased pulmonary blood flow. The condition may be asymptomatic or symptoms may not be evident until adulthood, depending upon the severity of the defect. Pulmonic stenosis may be associated with a number of other heart defects.

Symptoms: May be asymptomatic; dyspnea on exertion, systolic heart murmur, right-sided heart failure.

Diagnosis: Cardiac catheterization, chest x-ray, echocardiogram, ECG.

Treatment includes:

- **Medications**: Antiarrhythmic, anticoagulant, and antihypertensive medications
- **Surgical**: Balloon valvuloplasty, valvotomy, valvectomy with or without transannular patch, and pulmonary valve replacement

PERIPHERAL ARTERIAL AND VENOUS INSUFFICIENCY

Characteristics of peripheral arterial and venous insufficiency are listed below:

- **Arterial insufficiency**
  - **Pain**: Ranging from intermittent claudication to severe and constant shooting pain
  - **Pulses**: Weak or absent
  - **Skin**: Rubor on dependency, but pallor of foot on elevation; pale, shiny, and cool skin with loss of hair on toes and foot; nails thick and ridged
  - **Ulcers**: Painful, deep, circular, often necrotic ulcers on toe tips, toe webs, heels, or other pressure areas
  - **Edema**: Minimal
- **Venous insufficiency**
  - **Pain**: Aching/cramping
  - **Pulses**: Strong/present
  - **Skin**: Brownish discoloration around ankles and anterior tibial area
  - **Ulcers**: Varying degrees of pain in superficial, irregular ulcers on medial or lateral malleolus and sometimes the anterior tibial area
  - **Edema**: Moderate to severe

ACUTE PERIPHERAL VASCULAR INSUFFICIENCY

Acute peripheral arterial insufficiency can occur when sudden occlusion of a blood vessel causes tissue ischemia, ultimately leading to cellular death and necrosis. This can occur as a result of traumatic injury or non-traumatic events such as arterial thrombus or embolism, vasospasm, or severe swelling (compartment syndrome). Risk factors for acute peripheral arterial insufficiency include age, tobacco use, diabetes mellitus, hyperlipidemia, and hypertension.

- **Signs and symptoms**: Classic 6 P's: Pain (extreme, unrelieved by narcotics), pallor, pulselessness, poikilothermia (the inability to regulate body temperature; extremity is room temperature), paresthesias, and paralysis (late).
- **Diagnosis**: Ultrasound, angiography, and physical exam; labs—coagulation studies, CBC, BMP, creatinine phosphokinase
- **Treatment**: Re-establishment of blood flow to the affected area
- **Arterial thrombus or embolism**: Mechanical thrombolysis may be performed to remove the clot occluding the vessel.
  - **Trauma**: Surgical repair of the severed/injured vessels. Fasciotomy may be performed in the event of compartment syndrome to relieve pressure.
  - **Other treatment options**: Hyperbaric oxygen therapy, anti-platelet therapy for the prevention of arterial thrombosis and anti-coagulant therapy for the prevention of venous thrombosis

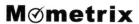

ACUTE VENOUS THROMBOEMBOLISM

Acute venous thromboembolism (VTE) is a condition that includes both deep vein thrombosis (DVT) and pulmonary emboli (PE). VTE may be precipitated by invasive procedures, lack of mobility, and inflammation, so it is a common complication in critical care units. **Virchow's triad** comprises common risk factors: blood stasis, injury to endothelium, and hypercoagulability. Some patients may be initially asymptomatic, but **symptoms** may include:

- Aching or throbbing pain
- Positive Homan's sign (pain in calf when foot is dorsiflexed)
- Unilateral erythema and edema
- Dilation of vessels
- Cyanosis

Diagnosis: ultrasound and/or D-dimer test, which tests the serum for cross-linked fibrin derivatives. A CT scan, pulmonary angiogram, and ventilation-perfusion lung scan may be used to diagnose pulmonary emboli.

Treatment includes:

- Medications: IV heparin, tPA, or other anticoagulation; analgesia for pain
- Surgical: May have to surgically remove clot if large
- Bed rest, elevation of affected limb; stockings on ambulation

Prevention: Use of sequential compression devices (SCDs) or foot pumps, routine anticoagulant use for those at highest risk (Heparin SQ), early and frequent ambulation

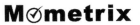

Neurological Pathophysiology

INCREASED INTRACRANIAL PRESSURE

Increased intracranial pressure is a pressure build up inside the cranium that results in altered neurological function. Causes can include intracranial bleeding, tumors, cerebrospinal fluid (CSF) build up, or edema. These alterations can be caused by head trauma, hydrocephalus, meningitis, encephalitis, brain tumors, intracerebral hemorrhage, or Guillain-Barre syndrome. The brain has mechanisms to deal with rising intracranial volume; when the rising volume is too much for these mechanisms, less blood will be able to get to the brain, leading to increased edema which further raises the ICP. This cycle will continue until no blood reaches the brain and the brain dies. If the brain stem is pushed downwards and herniates, the body's vital functions cease to operate.

MONITORING OF INTRACRANIAL PRESSURE

Monitoring of intracranial pressure in pediatric patients is of special importance because of the danger of herniation with increased pressure. Studies indicate that intracranial pressure requires treatment if ≥20 mmHg, although some authorities believe that infants and young children may need treatment at lower pressures. **Monitoring** of intracranial pressure can be done in a number of ways:

- Intraventricular catheter attached to a transducer to record pressure (most accurate)
- Subarachnoid bolt
- Epidural or subdural catheter
- Fiber-optic transducer-tipped catheter placed in the ventricular or subdural space
- External anterior fontanel monitor

CSF may be drained continuously or intermittently and must be monitored hourly for amount, color, and character. For ICP measurement, the patient's head must be elevated to 30-45° and the transducer leveled to the outer canthus of the eye. Normal ICP values (manometer):

- Infant: 1.5-6.0 mmHg
- Young child: 3-7 mmHg
- Older child: 2-7 mmHg
- 18 years: 0-15 mmHg

MONRO-KELLIE HYPOTHESIS AND SYMPTOMS OF INCREASED ICP

The Monro-Kellie hypothesis states that to maintain a normal intracranial pressure (ICP), a change in volume in one compartment must be compensated by a reciprocal change in volume in another compartment. The three brain compartments are brain tissue, CSF, and blood. The CSF and blood can change more easily to accommodate changes in pressure than tissue, so medical intervention focuses on cerebral blood flow and drainage. **Symptoms** include:

- **Infants**: Bulging fontanels without normal pulsations, distention of scalp veins, and increased head circumference. Infants may be irritable with high-pitched cries and poor feeding.
- **Children**: Headache, vomiting without associated nausea, double and blurred vision, and seizures. Behavioral and personality changes may occur, increased lethargy, memory loss, and inability to follow directions.
- **Late signs**: Decreased level of consciousness, motor response, and response to painful stimuli. Pupil size and reactivity change, decerebrate or decorticate posturing, respiratory depression with Cheyne-Stokes and papilledema. Cushing's triad:
  - Increased systolic pressure with widened pulse pressure
  - Bradycardia in response to increased pressure
  - Decreased respirations

As the pressure becomes severe, the child will become lethargic which may progress to coma, be unable to move on command, react more violently to pain stimuli, have decreased pupil size and reactivity, display decerebrate (the arms and legs will extend and turn inward) or decorticate (the arms are flexed toward the body, hands clenched on chest, with legs extended) posturing, have swelling of the optic nerve at the back of the eye, and/or have abnormal respirations.

DIAGNOSIS AND CARE

ICP is measured by various means. CT or MRI is used to find the cause of the increased ICP. The child should be monitored for changes in vital signs, LOC, activity, behavior, and pupils. Various tools to measure ICP can be used: intraventricular catheter, subarachnoid screw, fiber-optic sensor, or fiber-optic transducer-tipped catheter. Medications include diuretics and corticosteroids. The head and neck should be kept in a neutral, well-aligned position to prevent compression. Suctioning and respiratory PT may increase ICP and should be avoided. Maintain good respiratory status and O_2 saturation. Keep fluids balanced. Monitor I&Os. Prevent constipation and straining by using laxatives and diet control. Provide a nutritious diet to prevent weight loss. Watch for skin breakdown. Watch for signs of diabetes insipidus (low BP, high HR, weight loss, thirst, apathy or depression, excess urination, constipation, dilute urine, low blood volume and high blood sodium) and syndrome of inappropriate antidiuretic hormone (weight gain, high BP, seizures, coma, vomiting, concentrated low volume urine output, increased blood volume, and low blood sodium).

HYDROCEPHALUS IN PEDIATRIC PATIENTS

Symptoms of hydrocephalus depend on the age of onset. In early infancy, before closure of cranial sutures, head enlargement is the most common presentation, but in older children with less elasticity in the skull, neurological symptoms usually relate to increasing pressure on structures of the brain:

- **Early infancy**: Bulging, non-pulsating fontanels (usually anterior) usually with increasing head circumference, dilated scalp veins, separating sutures, and positive Macewen sign (resonance on tapping near the frontal-temporal-parietal juncture)
- **Later signs**: Enlargement of frontal area with depressed eyes, setting sun sign (sclera evident above iris), and pupils sluggish and unequally reactive
- **Throughout infancy**: Increased irritability, lethargy, high-pitched crying, delayed responses, change in level of consciousness, opisthotonos, spasticity, difficulty feeding, and cardiopulmonary compromise
- **Childhood** (related to increased intracranial pressure): Headache relieved by vomiting, papilledema, strabismus, ataxia, irritability, lethargy, confusion, and difficulty communicating

TREATMENT

Hydrocephalus is diagnosed through CT and MRI, which help to determine the cause. Treatment may vary somewhat depending upon the underlying disorder, which may require treatment. For example, if obstruction is caused by a tumor, surgical excision to directly remove the obstruction is required. Generally, however, most hydrocephalus is **treated** with shunts:

- **Ventricular-peritoneal shunt**: This procedure is the most common and consists of placement of a ventricular catheter directly into the ventricles (usually lateral) at one end with the other end in the peritoneal area to drain away excess CSF. There is a one-way valve near the proximal end that prevents backflow but opens when pressure rises to drain fluid. In some cases, the distal end drains into the right atrium.
- **Third ventriculostomy**: A small opening is made in the base of the third ventricle so CSF can bypass an obstruction. This procedure is not common and is done with a small endoscope.

ENCEPHALOCELE

Encephalocele is a neural defect that involves a bony defect and herniation of the brain and cerebrospinal fluid through part of the skull in a skin-covered sac. In the United States, most commonly the mass is midline in the occipital and occasionally the frontal area. The encephalocele may be as large as the skull or may look like a small nasal polyp. In many cases, other abnormalities may exist, so thorough examination, including angiography and MRI are usually required. Often, the part of the brain that herniates is disorganized, so the condition may be associated with cognitive impairment although in mild cases the child has normal mentation. Surgical repair to place the herniated mass inside the skull and to repair the bony defect is the standard treatment. If the sac is left in place, the skin can erode, resulting in meningitis.

ARTERIOVENOUS MALFORMATION

Arteriovenous malformation (AVM) is a congenital abnormality within the brain consisting of a tangle of dilated arteries and veins without a capillary bed. AVMs can occur anywhere in the brain and may cause no significant problems. Usually the AVM is "fed" by one or more cerebral arteries, which enlarge over time, shunting more blood through the AVM. The veins also enlarge in response to increased arterial blood flow because of the lack of a capillary bridge between the veins and arteries. Because vein walls are thinner and lack the muscle layer of an artery, the veins tend to rupture as the AVM becomes larger, causing a subarachnoid hemorrhage. Chronic ischemia that may be related to the AVM can result in cerebral atrophy. Sometimes small leaks, usually accompanied by headache and nausea and vomiting, may occur before rupture. AVMs may cause a wide range of neurological **symptoms**, including changes in mentation, dizziness, sensory abnormalities, confusion, increasing ICP, and dementia. **Treatment** includes:

- Supportive management of symptoms
- Surgical repair or focused irradiation (definitive treatments)

SURGICAL EXCISION

Surgical excision of AVM is the **definitive treatment** for AVMs as both embolization and radiotherapy treatment pose the risk that the abnormal vessels will recur. Sometimes, 2-3 different surgeries may be required for large AVMs. Usually, nonfunctioning brain tissue surrounds the AVM, so it is possible to remove this AVM without damaging brain tissue. However, reperfusion bleeding may occur, as blood is diverted to surrounding arterials that had dilated because of chronic ischemia. The sudden increase in blood flow and pressure may cause leakage of blood from the vessels. There may be extensive blood loss during surgery, so constant monitoring of arterial pressure and multiple IV cannulas are important. Embolization may be done prior to surgery to reduce bleeding. Hyperventilation and mannitol are often used and β-blockers may be used to prevent hypertension and cerebral edema. Postoperatively, blood pressure is kept low to prevent reperfusion bleeding.

NEUROLOGICAL INFECTIOUS DISEASES

BACTERIAL MENINGITIS IN CHILDREN

Bacterial meningitis may be caused by a wide range of pathogenic organisms, with the predominant agents varying with the child's age:

- ≤1 month: *E. coli*, Group B *streptococci*, *Listeria monocytogenes*, and *Neisseria meningitidis*
- 1-2 months: Group B *streptococci*
- >2 months: *Streptococcus pneumoniae*, *Neisseria meningitidis*. Unvaccinated (Hib vaccine) children are at risk for *Haemophilus influenzae*

Bacterial infections usually arise from the spread of distant infections although they can enter the CNS from surgical wounds, invasive devices, nasal colonization, or penetrating trauma. The infective process includes inflammation, exudates, white blood cell accumulation, and tissue damage with the brain showing evidence of hyperemia and edema. Purulent exudate covers the brain and invades and blocks the ventricles, obstructing CSF and leading to increased intracranial pressure. Since antibodies specific to bacteria do not cross the blood-brain barrier, the body's ability to fight the infection is very poor. Diagnosis is usually based on lumbar puncture examination of cerebrospinal fluid and symptoms.

AGE-RELATED SYMPTOMS

Bacterial meningitis may **manifest** differently, depending upon the age of the child:

- **Neonates:** Signs may be very non-specific, such as weight loss, hypo- or hyperthermia, jaundice, irritability, lethargy, and irregular respirations with periods of apnea. More specific signs may include increasing signs of illness, difficulty feeding with loss of suck reflex, hypotonia, weak cry, seizures, and bulging fontanels (may be a late sign). Nuchal rigidity does not usually occur with neonates.
- **Infants and young children:** Classic symptoms usually do not appear until ≥2 years. Signs may include fever, poor feeding, vomiting, irritability, and bulging fontanel. Nuchal rigidity in some children.
- **Older children and adolescents:** Abrupt onset, including fever, chills, headache, and alterations of consciousness with seizures, agitation, and irritability. May have photophobia, hallucinations, and aggressive behavior or become stuporous and lapse into coma. Nuchal rigidity progressing to opisthotonos. Reflexes are variable but positive Kernig and Brudzinski signs. Signs may relate to particular bacteria, such as rashes, sore joints, or draining ear.

SIGNS

Patients with bacterial meningitis may exhibit signs to help support the diagnosis. While the following are not universally present, they are specific to meningitis and are rarely positive with other disorders:

- **Kernig's sign:** Flex each hip and then try to straighten the knee while the hip is flexed. Spasm of the hamstrings makes this painful and difficult with meningitis.
- **Brudzinski's sign:** With the child lying supine, flex the neck by pulling head toward chest. The neck stiffness causes the hips and knees to pull up into a flexed position with meningitis.
- **Jolt accentuation maneuver:** (Used if nuchal rigidity is not present.) Ask child to rapidly move his/her head from side to side horizontally. Increase in headache is positive for meningitis.

INFECTIOUS ENCEPHALOPATHY

Infectious encephalopathy is an encompassing term describing encephalopathies caused by a wide range of bacteria, viruses, or prions. Common to all infections are altered brain function that results in alterations in consciousness and personality, cognitive impairment, and lethargy. A wide range of neurological symptoms may occur, including myoclonus, seizures, dysphagia, dysphonia, neuromuscular impairment with muscle atrophy, and tremors or spasticity. **Treatment** depends on the underlying cause and response to treatment. Prior infections are not treatable, but bacterial infections may respond to antibiotic therapy and viral infections may be self-limiting. HIV-related encephalopathy results from opportunistic infections as immune responses decrease, usually indicated by CD4 counts <50. Aggressive antiretroviral treatment and treatment of the infection may reverse symptoms if permanent damage has not occurred for HIV-related encephalopathy. Treatment for other infectious encephalopathies varies according to the type of infection and underlying causes.

VARICELLA ZOSTER VIRUS (CHICKEN POX)

Chicken pox, caused by the varicella zoster virus, during the first 20 weeks of pregnancy can result in an infant with congenital varicella syndrome, which can cause a number of abnormalities of the skin, extremities, eyes, and central nervous system. Children are often unusually small, with distinctive cicatrix scarring on the skin and chorioretinitis. Brain abnormalities may include microcephaly, hydrocephalus, cortical atrophy, enlargement of the ventricles, and damage to the sympathetic nervous system. The child may suffer intellectual disability and developmental delays as well as lack of psychomotor coordination. If the mother is infected at the end of pregnancy and develops a rash from 5 days before to 2 days after delivery, the child may develop neonatal varicella, which poses a high risk to the child, with mortality rates of about 30%. Vaccination prior to pregnancy is the best preventive. Premature neonates exposed after birth with ≤28 weeks gestation or ≥28 weeks if the mother has no immunity should receive varicella zoster immunoglobulin (VZIG).

TOXOPLASMA GONDII

Toxoplasma gondii is a single-celled parasite that is transmitted from cat feces and poorly-cooked or raw meat, and if a pregnant woman is infected with toxoplasmosis, the infant can develop congenital toxoplasmosis, with transmission rates estimated at 20-50%. Symptoms in the neonate are most severe if the mother developed the infection in the first trimester. Congenital abnormalities include hydrocephalus, cerebral calcifications, and chorioretinitis (classic triad of disorders). Additionally, the child may suffer from seizure disorders, microcephaly, and encephalitis. There may be other abnormalities as well, including hepatomegaly, splenomegaly, anemia, jaundice, and deafness. **Treatment** of the infected mother to prevent transmission to the fetus includes initially spiramycin (Rovamycin), which reduces risk. Pyrimethamine (Daraprim) and sulfonamide are usually given after the 18th week. Some studies have indicated that treatment does not reduce the rate of mother-infant transmission but does reduce the severity of abnormalities the child manifests.

RUBELLA AND CYTOMEGALOVIRUS

Rubella virus is an RNA virus that causes rubella (German measles), but infection in a pregnant woman during the first or second trimester can transmit to the infant congenital rubella syndrome (CRS). CRS can result in eye defects, congenital heart defects, hearing loss, hepatomegaly, hyperbilirubinemia, and a number of defects of the central nervous system: microencephaly, seizures, intellectual disability, delay in development, and meningoencephalitis. With vaccinations, this condition is now extremely rare in the United States.

Cytomegalovirus (CMV) infection during pregnancy can transmit to the infant cytomegalic inclusion disease, which can cause respiratory infections, bleeding, anemia, hepatic disorders, and vision impairment. Central nervous system defects include microcephaly, cerebral calcifications, seizure disorders, and intellectual disability. CMV is the virus most frequently transmitted congenitally and most infants suffer no ill effects, but some develop severe disabilities. Infants of mothers with their first infection during pregnancy are at highest risk for developing abnormalities.

WEST NILE VIRUS

West Nile virus is an RNA virus, spread by infected mosquitoes. Infection has been traced to donor organs, blood transfusions, and breast milk although the blood supply has been monitored for WNV since 2003. While WNV is more common in adults, especially the elderly, it can affect infants and children. Infected children show symptoms more readily than adults. The incubation period ranges from 2-14 days. There are three **types** of infection:

- **Viremia**: 80%, infection but no symptoms.
- **Mild**: 20% (West Nile fever), characterized by fever, malaise, lymphadenopathy, headache, rash, nausea, and vomiting. The acute stage is usually self-limiting within a few days, but symptoms can persist for weeks, including muscular weakness, fatigue, concentration problems, fever, and headache. About 30% require hospitalization.
- **Severe**: <1%, severe neurological symptoms, with meningitis and associated symptoms being the most common in children and young adults.

Treatment is supportive during illness and preventive (insect repellant).

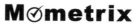

ARBOVIRUSES

There are a number of arboviruses in addition to West Nile virus that can cause flu-like symptoms that progress to viral encephalitis, and incidence is increasing across the United States, often spread by mosquitoes. Because many people are unaware of emerging causes for diseases, the cause of the ensuing encephalitis is frequently misdiagnosed. Encephalitis is an infection of the brain tissue and usually lasts for 2-3 weeks. **Symptoms** vary somewhat from one type of infection to another, but they have similar characteristics.

- Onset usually involves flu-like symptoms with sore throat, headaches, muscle aches, fever and chills, and myalgia. In some cases, a rash may appear.
- Progressive symptoms include photophobia, vomiting, and increased weakness.
- Advanced symptoms may include altered mental status, seizures, memory loss, coma, and death.

Encephalitis may also result from complications of Lyme disease, spread by infected ticks. One of the most common causes of encephalitis is the herpes simplex virus.

ARBOVIRAL ENCEPHALITIDES FOUND IN THE US

Arboviral encephalitides include:

- **Eastern equine encephalitis virus (EEEV)** (Togaviridae) has a high mortality rate and is most common in the eastern and gulf coast areas of the US. Sporadic outbreaks occur. Half of survivors have residual neurological damage, especially children.
- **Western equine encephalitis (WEE)** (Togaviridae) is similar to EEE but found on the west coast and the Midwest.
- **Venezuelan equine encephalitis** (Togaviridae) occurs primarily in Florida and southwestern US.
- **St. Louis encephalitis** (Flaviviridae) occurs throughout the US, but most infections are sub-clinical; however, if symptoms are present, about 50% of those under age 20 develop encephalitis and 5-15% die.
- **La Crosse encephalitis** (Bunyaviridae) is scattered and rare and usually results in mild disease with mortality rate <1%.
- **Cache Valley virus** (Bunyaviridae) has occurred in the southeastern US and Wisconsin and is believed to be under-reported. It occurs primarily in children <16. Mortality rates are <1%, but neurological damage may persist.

MIGRAINE AND TENSION HEADACHES

Headaches are common in children and usually benign. About 3% of children develop migraine headaches before age 7 and up to 23% by age 11 or older, and many experience tension headaches. Sudden onset of headache or persistent or severe headache may indicate a pathological condition, such as increased intracranial pressure or tumor, so headaches should be evaluated carefully.

Type	Symptoms	Treatment
Migraine	Unilateral or bilateral, moderate to severe throbbing pain persisting ≤72 hours and sometimes preceded by visual or motor aura. Co-morbidities include nausea, vomiting, photophobia, or phonophobia. Young children may exhibit head banging, irritability, general malaise, and head holding.	NSAIDs, acetaminophen Relaxation techniques Biofeedback Adolescents: Sumatriptan nasal spray Identifying and eliminating triggers, such as caffeine, foods, or additives

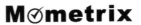
Type	Symptoms	Treatment
Tension	Dull, aching, mild to moderate bilateral constricting pain about head, neck, and sometimes shoulders persisting hours or days. Pain unrelated to physical activity.	NSAIDs, acetaminophen Ice pack Rest Relaxation techniques

REBOUND AND SINUS- OR DENTAL-RELATED HEADACHES

Type	Symptoms	Treatment
Rebound (from excess medication use)	Vary but may be bilateral or unilateral in frontal area with frequency increasing with increased medication use. Tend to occur at least 5 times weekly or 15 times per month.	Withdrawal of medications (NSAIDs, acetaminophen, other drugs). Substitution with other drugs if headaches persist. Clonidine for withdrawal symptoms if necessary.
Sinus- or dental-related	Dull constant pain and pressure over affected areas of sinus or dental abscess. Fever. Changing head position may vary pain.	NSAIDs, acetaminophen. Antibiotics. Application of cold or heat. Surgical drainage of sinus may be indicated for severe infection. Dental treatment as needed.

SPINA BIFIDA AND MYELOMENINGOCELE

The terms spina bifida and myelomeningocele are often used interchangeably, but there is a distinction. Spina bifida is a neural tube defect with an incomplete spinal cord and often missing vertebrae that allow the meninges and spinal cord to protrude through the opening. There are five basic types:

- **Spina bifida**: Defect in which the vertebral column is not closed, with varying degrees of herniation through the opening
- **Spina bifida occulta**: Failure of the vertebral column to close, but no herniation through the opening so the defect may not be obvious
- **Spina bifida cystica**: Defect in closure with external sac-like protrusion with varying degrees of nerve involvement
- **Meningocele**: Spina bifida cystica with meningeal sac filled with spinal fluid
- **Myelomeningocele**: Spina bifida cystica with meningeal sac containing spinal fluid and part of the spinal cord and nerves

PHYSICAL MANIFESTATIONS AND MANAGEMENT RELATED TO MYELOMENINGOCELE

Myelomeningocele, which involves spina bifida cystica with a meningeal sac containing spinal fluid and part of the spinal cord and nerves, comprises about 75% of the total cases of spina bifida. There are numerous physical manifestations:

- **Exposed sac** poses the danger of infection and cerebrospinal fluid leakage; so surgical repair is usually done within the first 48 hours although it may be delayed for a few days, especially if the sac is intact.
- **Chiari type II malformation** comprises hypoplasia of the cerebellum and displacement of the lower brainstem into the upper cervical area, which impairs circulation of spinal fluid. It may result in symptoms of cranial nerve dysfunction (dysphonia, dysphagia) and weakness and lack of coordination of upper extremities.
- **Neurogenic bladder** is common and may require credé massage for infants and later intermittent clean catheterization.
- **Fecal incontinence** is common and may be controlled, as the child gets older, with diet and bowel training.

- **Musculoskeletal abnormalities** depend upon the level of the myelomeningocele and the degree of impairment but often involve the muscle and joints of the lower extremities and sometimes the upper. Dysfunction often increases with the number of shunts. Scoliosis and lumbar lordosis are common. Hip contractures may cause dislocations.
- **Paralysis/paresis** may vary considerably and be spastic or flaccid. Many children require wheelchairs for mobility although some are fitted with braces for assisted ambulation.
- **Seizures** occur in about a quarter of those affected, sometimes related to shunt malfunction.
- **Hydrocephalus** is present in about 25-35% of infants at birth and 60-70% after surgical repair with ventriculoperitoneal shunt. Untreated, the ventricles will dilate and brain damage can occur.
- **Tethered spinal cord** occurs when the distal end of the spinal cord becomes attached to the bone or site of surgical repair and does not move superiorly with growth, causing increased pain, spasticity, and disability and requiring surgical repair.

NEUROMUSCULAR DISORDERS

MULTIPLE SCLEROSIS

Multiple sclerosis is an autoimmune disorder of the CNS in which the myelin sheath around the nerves is damaged and replaced by scar tissue that prevents conduction of nerve impulses.

Symptoms vary widely and can include problems with balance and coordination, tremors, slurring of speech, cognitive impairment, vision impairment, nystagmus, pain, and bladder and bowel dysfunction. Symptoms may be relapsing-remitting, progressive, or a combination. Onset is usually at 20-30 years of age, with incidence higher in females. Patient may initially present with problems walking or falling or optic neuritis (30%) causing loss of central vision. Males may complain of sexual dysfunction as an early symptom. Others have dysuria with urinary retention.

Diagnosis is based on clinical and neurological examination and MRI. **Treatment** is symptomatic and includes treatment to shorten duration of episodes and slow progress.

- **Glucocorticoids**: Methylprednisolone
- **Immunomodulator**: Interferon beta, glatiramer acetate, natalizumab
- **Immunosuppressant**: Mitoxantrone
- **Hormone**: Estriol (for females)

> **Review Video: Multiple Sclerosis**
> Visit mometrix.com/academy and enter code: 417355

ALS

Amyotrophic lateral sclerosis (ALS) is a progressive degenerative disease of the upper and lower motor neurons, resulting in progressively severe symptoms such as spasticity, hyperreflexia, muscle weakness, and paralysis that can cause dysphagia, cramping, muscular atrophy, and respiratory dysfunction. ALS may be sporadic or familial (rare). Speech may become monotone; however, cognitive functioning usually remains intact. Eventually, patients become immobile and cannot breathe independently.

Diagnosis is based on history, electromyography, nerve conduction studies, and MRI. Treatment includes riluzole to delay progression of the disease. Patients in the ED usually have been diagnosed and have developed an acute complication, such as acute respiratory failure, aspiration pneumonia, or other trauma.

Treatment includes:

- Nebulizer treatments with bronchodilators and steroids
- Antibiotics for infection
- Mechanical ventilation

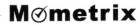

If **ventilatory assistance** is needed, it is important to determine if the patient has a living will expressing the wish to be ventilated or not or has assigned power of attorney for health matters to someone to make this decision.

PARKINSON'S DISEASE

Parkinson's disease (PD) is an extrapyramidal movement motor system disorder caused by loss of brain cells that produce dopamine. Typical symptoms include tremor of face and extremities, rigidity, bradykinesia, akinesia, poor posture, and a lack of balance and coordination causing increasing problems with mobility, talking, and swallowing. Some may suffer depression and mood changes. Tremors usually present unilaterally in an upper extremity.

Diagnosis includes:

- **Cogwheel rigidity test**: The extremity is put through passive range of motion, which causes increased muscle tone and ratchet-like movements.
- **Physical and neurological exam**
- **Complete history** to rule out drug-induced Parkinson akinesia

Treatment includes:

- Symptomatic support
- Dopaminergic therapy: Levodopa, amantadine, and carbidopa
- Anticholinergics: Trihexyphenidyl, benztropine
- For drug-induced Parkinson's, terminate drugs

Drug therapy tends to decrease in effectiveness over time, and patients may present with a marked increase in symptoms. Discontinuing the drugs for 1 week may exacerbate symptoms initially, but functioning may improve when drugs are reintroduced.

GUILLAIN-BARRÉ SYNDROME

Guillain-Barré syndrome (GBS) is an autoimmune disorder of the myelinated motor peripheral nervous system, causing ascending and descending paralysis. GBS is often triggered by a viral infection, but may be idiopathic in origin. Diagnosis is by history, clinical symptoms, and lumbar puncture, which often show increased protein with normal glucose and cell count although protein may not increase for a week or more.

> **Review Video: Guillain-Barre Syndrome**
> Visit mometrix.com/academy and enter code: 742900

Symptoms include:

- Numbness and tingling with increasing weakness of lower extremities that may become generalized, sometimes resulting in complete paralysis and inability to breathe without ventilatory support.
- Deep tendon reflexes are typically absent and some people experience facial weakness and ophthalmoplegia (paralysis of muscles controlling movement of eyes).

Treatment includes:

- Supportive: Fluids, physical therapy, and antibiotics for infections
- Patients should be hospitalized for observation and placed on ventilator support if forced vital capacity is reduced.
- While there is no definitive treatment, plasma exchange or IV immunoglobulin may shorten the duration of symptoms.

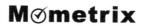

MUSCULAR DYSTROPHY

Muscular dystrophies are genetic disorders with gradual degeneration of muscle fibers and progressive weakness and atrophy of skeletal muscles and loss of mobility. **Pseudohypertrophic (Duchenne) muscular dystrophy** is the most common form and the most severe. It is an X-linked disorder in about 50% of the cases with the rest sporadic mutations, affecting males almost exclusively. Children typically have some delay in motor development with difficulty walking and have evidence of muscle weakness by about age 3. Pseudohypertrophic refers to enlargement of muscles by fatty infiltration associated with muscular atrophy, which causes contractures and deformities of joints. Abnormal bone development results in spinal and other skeletal deformities. The disease progresses rapidly, and most children are wheelchair bound by about 12 years of age. As the disease progresses, it involves the muscles of the diaphragm and other muscles needed for respiration. Mild to frank mental deficiency is common. Facial, oropharyngeal, and respiratory muscles weaken late in the disease. Cardiomegaly commonly occurs. Death most often relates to respiratory infection or cardiac failure by age 25. Treatment is supportive.

CEREBRAL PALSY

Cerebral palsy (CP) is a non-progressive motor dysfunction related to CNS damage associated with congenital, hypoxic, or traumatic injury before, during, or ≤2 years after birth. It may include visual defects, speech impairment, seizures, and intellectual disability. There are four **types of motor dysfunction:**

- **Spastic**: Damage to the cerebral cortex or pyramidal tract. Constant hypertonia and rigidity lead to contractures and curvature of the spine.
- **Dyskinetic**: Damage to the extrapyramidal, basal ganglia. Tremors and twisting with exaggerated posturing and impairment of voluntary muscle control.
- **Ataxic**: Damage to the extrapyramidal cerebellum. Atonic muscles in infancy with lack of balance, instability of muscles, and poor gait.
- **Mixed**: Combinations of all three types with multiple areas of damage.

Characteristics of CP include:

- Hypotonia or hypertonia with rigidity and spasticity
- Athetosis (constant writhing motions)
- Ataxia
- Hemiplegia (one-sided involvement, more severe in upper extremities)
- Diplegia (all extremities involved, but more severe in lower extremities)
- Quadriplegia (all extremities involved with arms flexed and legs extended)

MYASTHENIA GRAVIS

Myasthenia gravis is an autoimmune disorder that results in sporadic, progressive weakness of striated (skeletal) muscles because of impaired transmission of nerve impulses. Myasthenia gravis usually affects muscles controlled by the cranial nerves although any muscle group may be affected. Many patients also have thymomas.

Signs and symptoms include weakness and fatigue that worsens throughout the day. Patients often exhibit ptosis and diplopia. They may have trouble chewing and swallowing and often appear to have masklike facies. If respiratory muscles are involved, patients may exhibit signs of respiratory failure. Myasthenic crisis occurs when patients can no longer breathe independently.

Diagnosis includes electromyography and the Tensilon test (an IV injection of edrophonium or neostigmine, which improves function if the patient has myasthenia gravis, but does not improve function if the symptoms are from a different cause). CT or MRI to diagnose thymoma.

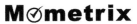

Treatment includes anticholinesterase drugs (neostigmine, pyridostigmine) to relieve some muscle weakness, but these drugs lose effectiveness as the disease progresses. Corticosteroids may be used. Thymectomy is performed if thymoma is present. Tracheotomy and mechanical ventilation may be needed for myasthenic crisis.

> **Review Video: <u>Myasthenia Gravis</u>**
> Visit mometrix.com/academy and enter code: 162510

SEIZURE DISORDERS
PARTIAL SEIZURES

Partial seizures are caused by electrical discharges to a localized area of the cerebral cortex, such as the frontals, temporal, or parietal lobes with seizure characteristics related to the area of involvement. They may begin in a focal area and become generalized, often preceded by an aura.

- **Simple partial:** Unilateral motor symptoms including somatosensory, psychic, and autonomic
  - Aversive: Eyes and head turned away from focal side
  - Sylvan (usually during sleep): Tonic-clonic movements of the face, salivation, and arrested speech
- **Special sensory:** Various sensations (numbness, tingling, prickling, or pain) spreading from one area. May include visual sensations, posturing or hypertonia.
- **Complex (psychomotor):** No loss of consciousness, but altered consciousness and non-responsive with amnesia. May involve complex sensorium with bad tastes, auditory or visual hallucinations, feeling of déjà vu, strong fear. May carry out repetitive activities, such as walking, running, smacking lips, chewing, or drawling. Rarely aggressive. Seizure usually followed by prolonged drowsiness and confusion. Most common ages 3 through adolescence.

> **Review Video: <u>Seizures</u>**
> Visit mometrix.com/academy and enter code: 977061

GENERALIZED SEIZURES

Generalized seizures lack a focal onset and appear to involve both hemispheres, usually presenting with loss of consciousness and no preceding aura.

- **Tonic-clonic (Grand Mal)**: Occurs without warning
  - Tonic period (10-30 seconds): Eyes roll upward with loss of consciousness, arms flexed; stiffen in symmetric tonic contraction of body, apneic with cyanosis and salivating
  - Clonic period (10 seconds to 30 minutes, but usually 30 seconds). Violent rhythmic jerking with contraction and relaxation. May be incontinent of urine and feces. Contractions slow and then stop.

Following seizures, there may be confusion, disorientation, and impairment of motor activity, speech, and vision for several hours. Headache, nausea, and vomiting may occur. Person often falls asleep and awakens more lucid.

- **Absence (Petit Mal):** Onset is at ages 4-12 and usually ends in puberty. Onset is abrupt with brief loss of consciousness for 5-10 seconds and slight loss of muscle tone but often appears to be daydreaming. Lip smacking or eye twitching may occur.

EPILEPSY

Epilepsy is diagnosed based on a history of seizure activity as well as supporting EEG findings. Treatment is individualized. First line treatments include antiepileptic medications for partial and generalized tonic-clonic seizures. Usually, treatment is started with one medication, but this may need to be changed, adjusted, or an additional medication added until the seizures are under control or to avoid adverse effects, which include allergic reactions, especially skin irritations and acute or chronic toxicity. Milder reactions often subside with time or adjustment in doses. Toxic reactions may vary considerably, depending upon the medication and duration of use, so close monitoring is essential. Severe rash and hepatotoxicity are common toxic reactions that occur with many of the antiepileptic drugs. Dosages of drugs may need to be adjusted to avoid breakthrough seizures during times of stress, such as during illness or surgery. Alcohol/drug abuse and sleep deprivation may also cause breakthrough seizures. Most anticonvulsant drugs are teratogenic.

STATUS EPILEPTICUS

Status epilepticus (SE) is usually generalized tonic-clonic seizures that are characterized by a series of seizures with intervening time too short for regaining of consciousness. The constant assault and periods of apnea can lead to exhaustion, respiratory failure with hypoxemia and hypercapnia, cardiac failure, and death.

Causes: Uncontrolled epilepsy or non-compliance with anticonvulsants, infections such as encephalitis, encephalopathy or stroke, drug toxicity (isoniazid), brain trauma, neoplasms, and metabolic disorders.

Treatment includes:

- Anticonvulsants usually beginning with a fast-acting benzodiazepine (lorazepam), often in steps, with administration of medication every 5 minutes until seizures subside.
- If cause is undetermined, acyclovir and ceftriaxone may be administered.
- If there is no response to the first 2 doses of anticonvulsants (refractory SE), rapid sequence intubation (RSI), which involves sedation and paralytic anesthesia, may be done while therapy continues. Combining phenobarbital and benzodiazepine can cause apnea, so intubation may be necessary.
- Antiepileptic medications are added.

BRAIN TUMORS

Any type of brain tumor can occur in adults. Brain tumors may be primary, arising within the brain, or secondary as a result of metastasis:

- **Astrocytoma**: This arises from astrocytes, which are glial cells. It is the most common type of tumor, occurring throughout the brain. There are many types of astrocytomas, and most are slow growing. Some are operable while others are not. Radiation may be given after removal. Astrocytomas include glioblastomas, aggressively malignant tumors occurring most often in adults 45-70.
- **Glioblastoma**: This is the most common and most malignant adult brain tumor/astrocytoma. Treatment includes surgery, radiation, and chemotherapy, but survival rates are very low.
- **Brain stem glioma**: This may be fast or slow growing but is generally not operable because of location, although it may be treated with radiation or chemotherapy.
- **Craniopharyngioma**: This is a congenital, slow-growing, recurrent (especially if >5 cm) and benign cystic tumor that is difficult to resect and is treated with surgery and radiation.
- **Meningioma**: Slow growing recurrent tumors are usually benign and most often occur in women, ages 40-70; however, they can cause severe impairment/death, depending on size and location. Meningiomas are surgically removed if causing symptoms.
- **Ganglioglioma**: This can occur anywhere in the brain and is usually slow growing and benign.
- **Medulloblastoma**: There are many types of medulloblastoma, most arising in the cerebellum, malignant, and fast growing. Surgical excision is often followed by radiation and chemotherapy although recent studies show using just chemotherapy controls recurrence with less neurological damage.
- **Oligodendroglioma**: This tumor most often occurs in the cerebrum, primarily the frontal or temporal lobes, involving the myelin sheath of the neurons. It is slow growing and most common in those age 40-60.

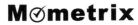

- **Optical nerve glioma**: This slow growing tumor of the optic nerve is usually a form of astrocytoma. Optic nerve glioma is often associated with neurofibromatosis type I (NF1), occurring in 15-40% of patients with NF1. Despite surgical, chemotherapy, or radiotherapy treatment, it is usually fatal.

STROKES
HEMORRHAGIC STROKES

Hemorrhagic strokes account for about 20% of all strokes and result from a ruptured cerebral artery, causing not only a lack of oxygen and nutrients but also edema that causes widespread pressure and damage:

- **Intracerebral** is bleeding into the substance of the brain from an artery in the central lobes, basal ganglia, pons, or cerebellum. Intracerebral hemorrhage usually results from atherosclerotic degenerative changes, hypertension, brain tumors, anticoagulation therapy, or use of illicit drugs, such as cocaine.
- **Intracranial aneurysm** occurs with ballooning cerebral artery ruptures, most commonly at the Circle of Willis.
- **Arteriovenous malformation**. Rupture of AVMs can cause brain attack in young adults.
- **Subarachnoid hemorrhage** is bleeding in the space between the meninges and brain, resulting from aneurysm, AVM, or trauma. This type of hemorrhage compresses brain tissue.

Treatment includes: The patient may need airway protection/artificial ventilation if neurologic compromise is severe. Blood pressure is lowered to control rate of bleeding but with caution to avoid hypotension and resulting cerebral ischemia (Goal – CPP >70). Sedation can lower ICP and blood pressure, and seizure prophylaxis will be indicated as blood irritates the cerebral cells. An intraventricular catheter may be used in ICP management; correct any clotting disorders if identified.

> **Review Video: Overview of Strokes**
> Visit mometrix.com/academy and enter code: 310572

ISCHEMIA STROKES

Strokes (brain attacks, cerebrovascular accidents) result when there is interruption of the blood flow to an area of the brain. The two basic types are ischemic and hemorrhagic. About 80% are **ischemic**, resulting from blockage of an artery supplying the brain:

- **Thrombosis** in a large artery, usually resulting from atherosclerosis, may block circulation to a large area of the brain. It is most common in the elderly and may occur suddenly or after episodes of transient ischemic attacks.
- **Lacunar infarct** (a penetrating thrombosis in a small artery) is most common in those with diabetes mellitus and/or hypertension.
- **Embolism** travels through the arterial system and lodges in the brain, most commonly in the left middle cerebral artery. An embolism may be cardiogenic, resulting from cardiac arrhythmia or surgery. An embolism usually occurs rapidly with no warning signs.
- **Cryptogenic** has no identifiable cause.

Medical management of ischemic strokes with tissue plasminogen activator (tPA) (Activase), the primary treatment, should be initiated within 3 hours (or up to 4.5 hours if inclusion criteria are met):

- **Thrombolytic,** such as tPA, which is produced by recombinant DNA and is used to dissolve fibrin clots. It is given intravenously (0.9 mg/kg up to 90 mg) with 10% injected as an initial bolus and the rest over the next hour.
- **Antihypertensives** if MAP >130 mmHg or systolic BP >220
- **Cooling** to reduce hyperthermia

- **Osmotic diuretics** (mannitol), hypertonic saline, loop diuretics (Lasix), and/or corticosteroids (dexamethasone) to decrease cerebral edema and intracranial pressure
- **Aspirin/anticoagulation** may be used with embolism
- Monitor and treat hyperglycemia
- **Surgical Intervention:** Used when other treatment fails, may go in through artery and manually remove the clot

SYMPTOMS OF BRAIN ATTACKS IN RELATION TO AREA OF BRAIN AFFECTED

Brain attacks most commonly occur in the right or left hemisphere, but the exact location and the extent of brain damage from a brain attack affects the type of presenting symptoms. If the frontal area of either side is involved, there tends to be memory and learning deficits. Some symptoms are common to specific areas and help to identify the area involved:

- **Right hemisphere**: This results in left paralysis or paresis and a left visual field deficit that may cause spatial and perceptual disturbances, so people may have difficulty judging distance. Fine motor skills may be impacted, resulting in trouble dressing or handling tools. People may become impulsive and exhibit poor judgment, often denying impairment. Left-sided neglect (lack of perception of things on the left side) may occur. Difficulty following directions, short-term memory loss, and depression are also common. Language skills usually remain intact.
- **Left hemisphere**: Results in right paralysis or paresis and a right visual field defect. Depression is common and people often exhibit slow, cautious behavior, requiring repeated instruction and reinforcement for simple tasks. Short-term memory loss and difficulty learning new material or understanding generalizations is common. Difficulty with mathematics, reading, writing, and reasoning may occur. Aphasia (expressive, receptive, or global) is common.
- **Brain stem**: Because the brain stem controls respiration and cardiac function, a brain attack in the brain stem frequently causes death, but those who survive may have a number of problems, including respiratory and cardiac abnormalities. Strokes may involve motor or sensory impairment or both.
- **Cerebellum**: This area controls balance and coordination. Brain attacks in the cerebellum are rare but may result in ataxia, nausea and vomiting, and headaches and dizziness or vertigo.

TIA

Transient ischemic attacks (TIAs) from small clots cause similar but short-lived (minutes to hours) symptoms. Emergent treatment includes placing patient in semi-Fowlers or Fowler's position and administering oxygen. The patient may require oral suctioning if secretions pool. The patient's circulation, airway, and breathing should be assessed and IV access line placed. Thrombolytic therapy to dissolve blood clots should be administered within 1 to 3 hours. While a patient can recover fully from a TIA, they should be educated, because having a TIA increases an individual's risk for a stroke.

Gastrointestinal Pathophysiology

ACUTE GASTROINTESTINAL BLEEDING

Gastrointestinal bleeding is unusual in children, but the age of the child and the symptoms present can indicate the area that is bleeding:

- **Neonates**: Apparent bleeding may occur from the infant swallowing maternal blood during delivery or from allergy to milk protein, but actual bleeding may result from mucosal erosion from increased gastric acid or from maternal medications (aspirin, phenobarbital) that cause problems with coagulation, or medications to the infant, such as indomethacin and dexamethasone. Bleeding indicates necrotizing enterocolitis, Hirschsprung's disease, volvulus, or coagulopathies.
- **Older infants**: Intussusception and mucosal lesions cause most bleeding.
- **Children/adolescents**: Wide range of disorders may cause bleeding, including ulcers, inflammatory bowel disease, infectious diarrhea. Stress ulcers may relate to system disease.

Symptoms	Treatment
Vomiting blood	Fluid replacement with transfusions is necessary
Bloody or tarry stools	Identification and treatment of underlying problem
Abdominal distension	Endoscopy or push enteroscopy for upper GI bleeding
Hypotension with tachycardia	Colonoscopy for lower GI bleeding

STRESS-RELATED EROSIVE SYNDROME

Stress-related erosive syndrome (SRES) (stress ulcers) occurs most frequently in children who are critically ill, such as those with severe or multi-organ trauma, mechanical ventilation, sepsis, severe burns, and head injury with increased intracranial pressure. Stress induces changes in the gastric mucosal lining and decreased perfusion of the mucosa, causing ischemia. SRES involves hemorrhage in ≥30% with mortality rates of 30-80% so prompt identification and treatment is critical. The lesions tend to be diffuse, so they are more difficult to treat than peptic ulcers.

Symptoms:

- Coffee ground emesis
- Hematemesis
- Abdominal discomfort

Treatment is both prophylactic and active.

Prophylaxis in those at risk:

- Sucralfate (Carafate) protects mucosa against pepsin
- Famotidine (Pepcid), nizatidine (Axid), or cimetidine reduces gastric secretions

Treatment for active bleeding includes:

- Intraarterial infusion of vasopressin
- Intraarterial embolization
- Over-sewing of ulcers or total gastrectomy if bleeding persists

MOmetrix

ACUTE ABDOMEN

Acute abdomen is a nonspecific term referring to a child presenting with acute abdominal distress, which could be caused by a number of different disorders. Typical symptoms include abdominal pain, Abdominal distension, guarding, rigidity, and fever. Diagnostic procedures usually include a history of medications and treatment, physical exam, complete blood count, and abdominal ultrasound, CT, or MRI, depending on the severity of symptoms. Other lab tests such as renal and liver function tests may be indicated. Infants and children may cry and pull legs to chest. Differential diagnoses for infants include intussusception, volvulus, and congenital defects. Older children and adolescents may have a strangulated hernia, appendicitis, ulcerative colitis, or irritable bowel syndrome. Children with sickle cell disease may be experiencing a crisis. Ketoacidosis may also cause symptoms consistent with an acute abdomen. The primary focus of care is to eliminate possible differential diagnoses.

HYPERTROPHIC PYLORIC STENOSIS

Hypertrophic pyloric stenosis (PS) is obstruction of the pyloric sphincter between the gastric pylorus and small intestine, caused by hypertrophy and hyperplasia of the circular muscle of the pylorus so the enlarged tissue obstructs the sphincter. PS is more common in boys than girls and has a genetic predisposition. Onset of **symptoms** is usually >3 weeks:

- Projectile vomiting (1-4 feet) usually shortly after eating but may be delayed for a few hours. Emesis may be blood-tinged but non-bilious.
- Child is hungry and eats readily, but shows weight loss and sings of dehydration.
- Upper Abdominal distension with palpable mass in epigastrium (to right of umbilicus).
- Visible left to right peristaltic waves.

Diagnosis is based on ultrasound. Decreased sodium and potassium levels may not be evident with dehydration.

Treatment includes:

- Intravenous fluids to restore hydration and electrolyte balance
- Surgical pyloromyotomy: Longitudinal incisions through the circular muscle fibers down to the submucosa to release the restriction and allow the muscle to expand

MALROTATION/VOLVULUS

Malrotation is a congenital defect in which the intestines are attached to the back of the abdominal wall by one single attachment rather than a broad band of attachments across the abdomen, essentially suspending the bowels so that they can easily twist, resulting in a **volvulus** (twisted bowel), cutting off blood supply. It may untwist but can lead to bowel infarction. Some children with malrotation have no symptoms, but most develop **symptoms** by 1 year:

- Cycles of cramping pain about every 15-30 minutes that cause the child to cry and pull knees to chest
- Distended painful abdomen
- Diarrhea, bloody stools, or no stools
- Vomiting (occurring soon after crying begins usually indicates small intestine obstruction; later vomiting usually indicated large intestine blockage)
- Tachycardia and tachypnea
- Decreased urinary output
- Fever

189

Treatment:

- Surgical repair (Ladd procedure) is indicated immediately if there is volvulus. Most malrotations require surgical repair even with less severe symptoms.

INTUSSUSCEPTION

Intussusception is a telescoping of one portion of the intestine into another, usually at the ileocecal valve, causing an obstruction. As the walls of the intestine come in contact, inflammation and edema cause decreased perfusion, which can result in infarction with peritonitis and death. Fecal material cannot move past the obstruction. It is most common between 3-12 months but can occur until 6 years and may relate to viral infections.

Symptoms	Treatment
<ul><li>"Currant jelly stool" composed of blood and mucous (occurs with 60%)</li><li>Sudden acute episodes of severe abdominal pain during which child pulls knees to chest</li><li>Vomiting</li><li>Lethargy and weakness</li><li>Distended abdomen, painful to palpation</li><li>Sausage-shaped mass in RUQ of abdomen</li><li>Progressive fever and prostration if peritonitis occurs</li></ul>	<ul><li>Barium or air enema to diagnose and apply pressure that may resolve the intussusception</li><li>Surgical repair if there is shock, peritonitis, intestinal perforation, or failure to resolve with barium/air enema</li></ul>

MESENTERIC ISCHEMIA

Mesenteric ischemia occurs when intestinal circulation decreases because of thrombus formation (arterial or venous), arterial embolus, or systemic shock or drugs (such as cocaine, digoxin, and α-adrenergic agonists) resulting in intestinal vasoconstriction. Mesenteric ischemia is most common in the elderly but can occur in children. Mortality rates are very high if diagnosis and treatment is delayed for >12 hours or after onset of peritonitis. Abdominal examination may be fairly normal initially, except for pain, but progresses to indications of peritonitis and shock, with fever, pain, and Abdominal distension.

Symptoms (vary)	Treatment (cause-dependent)
<ul><li>Pain: Severe with sudden onset (embolism) or increasing in intensity with history of pain after meals, not usually localized</li><li>Nausea, vomiting, and diarrhea</li><li>Melena, hematochezia, occult blood</li><li>Pneumatosis intestinalis (gas in intestinal wall) on radiograph</li></ul>	<ul><li>IV fluids</li><li>Intubation with ventilation if necessary</li><li>Broad-spectrum antibiotics</li><li>Analgesics (opioids)</li><li>Thrombolytics (tPA)</li><li>Papaverine infusion (if non-occlusive)</li></ul>

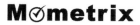

ADHESIONS

Adhesions are fibrous bands that cause intestinal loops to adhere to areas within the abdomen that heal slowly or scar after surgery. These bands can loop around the intestines and cause them to kink or bind them to other internal organs, sometimes resulting in partial or complete intestinal obstruction. Adhesions can occur in children who have had abdominal surgery or abdominal radiation treatments or may be congenital. Adhesions may increase in size over time and become more constrictive. Long-term sequelae include infertility in adulthood (females). **Symptoms**, usually general abdominal discomfort, may be minimal unless obstruction occurs, at which time pain and distention becomes acute. **Diagnosis** is often made through exploratory surgery, as adhesions are not evident on x-ray or ultrasound. Partial obstructions may be treated with dietary modifications (liquid/low residue), although severe or complete obstructions require surgical repair.

OMPHALOCELE

Omphalocele is a congenital herniation of intestines or other organs through the base of the umbilicus with a protecting amniotic membrane but no skin. The sac may contain only a loop or most of the bowel and the internal abdominal organs. This sac differentiates gastroschisis from omphalocele. **Diagnosis** is usually with fetal ultrasound. **Symptoms** vary widely. Maintaining integrity of tissues by keeping exposed sac or viscera moist and providing intravenous fluids is important. Small omphaloceles are repaired immediately, but more extensive repair is usually delayed until the infant is stable if the sac is intact. Silvadene cream toughens the sac, which is usually covered with a silastic (plastic) pouch to protect the tissue. The abdomen may be unusually small, making correction difficult, so surgeons may wait 6-12 months while the abdominal cavity grows. Surgical repair may be done in stages over 8-10 days.

GASTROSCHISIS

Gastroschisis is extrusion of the non-rotated midgut through the abdominal wall to the right of the umbilicus with no protective membrane covering matted, thickened loops of intestine. The abnormality is usually small, but the stomach and almost all of the small and large intestines can protrude. Because the intestines float without protection in amniotic fluid, there may be severe damage to the intestines with bowel atresia and ischemia. Gastroschisis is usually diagnosed with fetal ultrasound and is obvious at birth. These infants lose body temperature, fluids, and electrolytes and receive intravenous fluids. The exposed organs are covered with sterile plastic film for protection and to prevent fluid loss, and a naso-gastric feeding tube is inserted. Primary closure is done when infant stabilizes for small abnormalities. Larger abnormalities may require staged surgeries with only part of organs returned to cavity and the remaining covered with a Silastic pouch until the abdominal cavity grows and surgical repair can be completed.

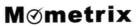

NEC

Necrotizing enterocolitis is an inflammatory bowel disease affecting primarily preterm/premature infants, characterized by an immature bowel that has suffered a hypoxic episode with resultant inflammation and necrosis of the intestinal wall, allowing gas into tissues of the wall, the portal venous system, and/or the peritoneal cavity. It may result in infarction and/or perforation. The distal ileum and proximal colon are the most commonly affected. The cause is not clearly understood, but appears related to an ischemic episode, colonization by bacteria, and excess/rapid enteral feedings. Mortality rates are about 30%.

Symptoms	Treatment
• Gastric retention/Abdominal distension • Periods of apnea • Vomiting (bilious) • Occult or frank blood (25%) in stool • Pneumatosis intestinalis (gas in intestinal wall) (75%) • Portal venous gas (10-30%) • Decrease in urinary output • Jaundice • Unstable temperature	• Cessation of oral feeding • NG decompression • Systemic antibiotics • Correcting fluid and electrolyte imbalance • Surgical repair with bowel resection may be necessary

HIRSCHSPRUNG'S DISEASE

Hirschsprung's disease (congenital aganglionic megacolon) is failure of ganglion nerve cells to migrate to part of the bowel (usually the distal colon), so that part of the bowel lacks enervation and peristalsis, causing stool to accumulate and leading to distention and megacolon. There is a genetic predisposition to the disease that affects more males than females and is associated with trisomy 21 (Down syndrome). **Symptoms** include:

- Failure to pass meconium in 24-48 hours
- Poor feeding
- Bilious vomitus
- Abdominal distension

Delayed diagnosis:

- Chronic constipation
- Failure to thrive
- Periods of diarrhea and vomiting
- (With infection) Severe prostration with watery diarrhea, fever, and hypotension

Childhood symptoms:

- Chronic constipation with ribbon-like stools.
- Abdominal distension with visible peristalsis and palpable fecal mass. Poorly-nourished, anemic, child.

Treatment:

- Resection of aganglionic section and colorectal anastomosis. There are a number of procedures (Swenson, Duhamel, and Soave) but recently laparoscopic or trans-anal minimally-invasive approaches have proven successful.

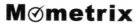

ABDOMINAL WALL MALROTATION DEFECT

INCARCERATED HERNIA

Hernias are protrusions into or through the abdominal wall and may occur in children and adults. Hernias may contain fat, tissue, or bowel. There are a number of types that are common in children. Hernias are evident on clinical examination. Incarceration (strangulation of an organ in the hole of the hernia) is a life-threatening condition that requires immediate surgical repair.

- **Indirect inguinal hernias** related to congenital defect are most common on the right in males and can incarcerate, especially during the first year and in females.
- **Umbilical hernias** occur in children, especially African American children, and rarely incarcerate.
- **Incisional hernias** occur, usually related to obesity or wound infections, and may incarcerate.

Symptoms	Treatment
<ul><li>Severe abdominal pain</li><li>Nausea and vomiting</li><li>Soft mass at hernia site</li><li>Tachycardia</li><li>Fever</li></ul>	<ul><li>Intravenous fluids</li><li>Immediate surgical excision and fixation</li><li>Broad-spectrum antibiotics</li></ul>

UMBILICAL HERNIA

Umbilical hernia is a skin-covered herniation of intestine and omentum through an abdominal wall defect near the umbilicus caused by an incomplete closure of the umbilical ring. The herniation may range from 1-5 cm in size and may be obvious on physical examination or felt on palpation. It may appear flat when the child is supine but protrude when the child is upright or crying. Approximately 1 in 6 infants are born with umbilical hernias. **Symptoms** are usually absent unless strangulation of the hernia occurs, and then the infant may cry with pain, feed poorly, vomit, and have an increase in temperature. The abdomen may become distended. In this case, emergency surgical repair must be done. **Treatment** usually involves just observing the hernia for complications as, in most cases, it will reduce on its own. If the hernia is still present at 3-4 years, a simple surgical repair of the hernia may be done.

CONGENITAL DIAPHRAGMATIC HERNIA

Congenital diaphragmatic hernia is herniation of abdominal contents into chest cavity. During fetal development, a hole in the diaphragm that should close at about 3 months stays open, allowing loops of the intestine or the stomach to herniate into the chest and preventing adequate development of the lungs (pulmonary hypoplasia) and/or heart. The infants are usually very dyspneic at birth and may need to be ventilated. They may need temporary heart/bypass as well. The kidneys are often enlarged. Radiographic studies are done to show the extent of the abnormality, usually showing a high gastrointestinal obstruction, often at the duodenum. A nasogastric feeding tube is inserted, and an intravenous line is inserted as well. Supportive treatment is given for dyspnea as well as correction of acidosis. Surgical repair may be done after birth or delayed for weeks until the child stabilizes. Surgical repair may be done in one stage or more, depending upon the degree of abnormality.

ENCOPRESIS AND FECAL INCONTINENCE

Encopresis is the voluntary or involuntary passage of stool in places or manners that are inappropriate for a child. 80% of children with encopresis are male, 4 years or older. There are two types: retentive encopresis, which accounts for about 80% of those affected, and non-retentive, which accounts for the other 20%. Retentive encopresis is characterized by a history of long term, painful constipation and the development of overflow diarrhea. The chronic constipation causes distention of the rectum and stretching of both the internal and external anal sphincters. As a result, the child may no longer feel the urge to defecate, so stool eventually leaks from the rectum, causing **chronic fecal incontinence**. Non-retentive encopresis, usually involving passage of normally formed stools on a daily basis, does not involve constipation or bowel abnormalities,

193

except in a small subset that may have irritable bowel syndrome. It is generally a behavioral/psychological problem.

DIARRHEA

Diarrhea is common in infants and children and can be caused by a variety of different infections and conditions. Diarrhea accounts for about 20% of hospitalizations of children <2 and causes about 500 deaths in children <4 in the United States each year. Because of the potential for loss of fluids, electrolytes, and nutrition, and the danger of ulceration and bleeding, diarrhea should be monitored carefully to determine the **cause**:

- **Osmotic**: Increased fluid in the stool and may be related to lactose intolerance and overfeeding.
- **Secretory**: Inhibited electrolyte (ion) absorption or increased electrolyte secretion related to bacterial endotoxins.
- **Motility disorders**: Interfere with absorption of fluids, including bile salt or pancreatic enzyme deficiencies.
- **Inflammatory**: Related to Crohn's disease or ulcerative colitis.
- **Viral/bacterial**: The most common cause of diarrhea in children. A wide range of viral and bacterial pathogens can cause mild to severe life-threatening diarrhea.

BACTERIAL CAUSES

A wide range of bacterial and viral pathogens can cause mild to severe life-threatening diarrhea:

- ***Campylobacter jejuni*** transmitted from pets to children <7 through contaminated food and water, usually in the summer. Diarrhea with fever, vomiting, and abdominal pain persists for 7-12 days. **Treatment**: Erythromycin (40 mg/kg/day) in 3 doses daily for 5-7 days.
- ***Clostridioides difficile*** occurs secondary to antibiotic use. Some children are asymptomatic carriers, but severe illness is life threatening with bloody diarrhea and abdominal pain leading to megacolon. **Treatment**: Metronidazole 30 mg/kg/day in 4 doses or Vancomycin 40 mg/kg/day in 4 doses for 7-10 days.
- ***Yersinia enterocolitica*** found in uncooked pork or unpasteurized milk causes secretory diarrhea in all ages with fever, foul, green and bloody stool, and pain in right lower abdomen. Usually resolves in 3-4 days.
- ***Shigella*** is transmitted by the fecal-oral route from contaminated food and water and occurs from 6-36 months. Characterized by bloody diarrhea, abdominal pain, and fever. **Treatment**: TMP-SMZ 8 mg TMP/kg/day in 2 doses for 7-10 days.

SALMONELLA

Salmonella causes up to 4 million infections in the United States, resulting in 500 deaths, primarily of young children. *Salmonella* is spread by the fecal-oral route through ingestion of contaminated food or water, including all meats, milk, eggs, and vegetables. Raw or undercooked meat, unpasteurized milk, and unwashed produce are high-risk. *Salmonella* may be found in the feces of pets, particularly reptiles such as snakes and turtles. Small children should not have reptiles as pets. **Symptoms** appear 12-72 hours after infection and include bloody diarrhea with abdominal pain, fever, and vomiting. Most cases resolve within 7-10 days, but in some cases, life-threatening sepsis may occur, requiring **treatment** with antibiotics. Amoxicillin 40 g/kg/day in 3 doses for 7-10 days is the antibiotic of choice. Antibiotic prophylaxis is usually contraindicated except in children <1 year that are at risk for bacteremia or those who are immunocompromised.

ESCHERICHIA COLI

Escherichia coli is part of the normal flora of the intestines and serves to inhibit other bacteria, but 5 serotypes can cause intestinal disease and severe diarrhea. Some types are more common in developing countries and may occur in children who are traveling in areas where feces have contaminated food supplies and water. Severe outbreaks of *E. coli* infection have occurred in the United States with a toxic strain, O157:H7, which produces a toxin that can cause damage to the intestinal lining, including blood vessels, resulting in

194

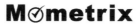

hemorrhage and watery diarrhea that becomes bloody. This hemorrhagic colitis usually clears with supportive treatment after 10 days. However, about 15% of children develop sepsis and hemolytic uremic syndrome with kidney failure, hemolytic anemia, and thrombocytopenia. Death rates are 3-5%, but residual renal and neurological damage may result. **Treatment** is supportive with intravenous therapy, blood transfusions, and kidney dialysis. Antibiotics and antidiarrheals are contraindicated as they may worsen *E. coli* infections.

SHORT GUT SYNDROME

Short gut (bowel) syndrome occurs when removal of part of the small intestine results in a malabsorptive condition. **Symptoms** relate to the amount of bowel removed and the area of resection:

- Resection of the terminal ileum interferes with absorption of bile salts and vitamin B_{12}. If <100 cm removed, malabsorption of bile salts causes watery diarrhea. Treatment includes salt binding resins (cholestyramine 2-4 g three times daily). If >100 cm removed, steatorrhea with resultant malabsorption of fat-soluble vitamins occurs. Additional treatment includes a low-fat diet, vitamins, and calcium supplements to prevent oxalate kidney stone.
- Resection of >40-50% of small bowel results in weight loss, diarrhea, and electrolyte imbalance. If colon and 100 cm of proximal jejunum are retained, a low fat, high complex carbohydrate diet, and electrolytes may maintain nutrition, but if the colon is removed, 200 cm of jejunum is required for adequate nutrition. Otherwise, parenteral nutrition is required, and this can lead to liver failure and death or liver/intestine transplantation.

CELIAC DISEASE, LACTOSE INTOLERANCE AND PARASITIC DISEASES

	Pathology	Symptoms	Treatment
Celiac Disease	Autoimmune disorder with intolerance to gluten, which causes destruction of surface epithelium of the small intestine	Loss of weight, diarrhea, bloating, steatorrhea (fatty stools), azotorrhea (nitrogenous wastes in stool-urine), anemia, vitamin/iron deficiency	Gluten-free diet
Lactose Intolerance	Deficiency of intestinal lactase causes increased lactose in intestine	Diarrhea, cramping.	Oral lactase (Lactaid) or a dairy-free diet
Parasitic Diseases (Giardiasis, Strongyloidiasis, Coccidiosis)	Parasites live and multiply within the intestines, causing damage to the intestinal mucosa	(Varies with parasitic agent). Loss of weight, diarrhea, steatorrhea	Antiparasitic drugs as indicated for the specific parasite

> **Review Video: Lactose Intolerance**
> Visit mometrix.com/academy and enter code: 672651

CROHN'S DISEASE

Crohn's disease manifests with inflammation of the GI system. Inflammation is transmural (often leading to intestinal stenosis and fistulas), focal, and discontinuous with aphthous ulcerations progressing to linear and irregular shaped ulcerations. Granulomas may be present. Common sites of inflammation are the terminal ileum and cecum. This condition is usually chronic, but an acute flare-up may mimic appendicitis. Children may have delayed development and stunted growth. There is a genetic component to the disease.

Copyright © Mometrix Media. You have been licensed one copy of this document for personal use only. Any other reproduction or redistribution is strictly prohibited. All rights reserved. This content is provided for test preparation purposes only and does not imply an endorsement by Mometrix of any particular political, scientific, or religious point of view.

Symptoms:

- Perirectal abscess/fistula may be present in advanced disease.
- Diarrhea is usually present with colonic disease. May have nocturnal bowel movements, watery stools, and rectal hemorrhage.
- Anemia may develop with chronic bleeding.
- Abdominal pain is most common in the lower right quadrant, usually indicating transmural inflammation; this may include post-prandial pain and cramping.
- Nausea and vomiting (usually related to strictures of small intestine)
- Weight loss (with small intestine involvement)
- Fever
- Night sweats

Treatment:

- Corticosteroids and antibiotics for acute exacerbations
- Immunomodulatory agents (cyclosporine, methotrexate)
- Antidiarrheals
- Aminosalicylates

ULCERATIVE COLITIS

Ulcerative colitis is superficial inflammation of mucosa of colon and rectum, causing ulcerations in the areas where inflammation has destroyed cells. These ulcerations, ranging from pinpoint to extensive, may bleed and produce purulent material. The mucosa of the bowel becomes swollen, erythematous, and granular. Onset is usually between ages 15 and 30, and there is a genetic component. Ulcerative colitis may affect only the rectum (ulcerative proctitis), the entire colon (pancolitis), or only the left colon (limited or distal colitis).

Symptoms	Treatment
<ul><li>Abdominal pain may be absent or mild unless there is severe disease.</li><li>Bloody diarrhea/rectal bleeding in absence of infection may result in anemia and fluid and electrolyte depletion. Diarrhea is more frequent as colonic involvement increases.</li><li>Fecal urgency and tenesmus may occur.</li><li>Anorexia may occur, resulting in weight loss, fatigue.</li><li>Systemic disorders with eye inflammation, arthritis, liver disease, and osteoporosis occur as the immune system triggers generalized inflammation.</li></ul>	<ul><li>Aminosalicylates</li><li>Steroids</li><li>Immunomodulatory agents</li><li>Antispasmodics</li><li>Iron supplementation</li><li>High-protein diet with decreased fiber</li></ul>

> **Review Video: Ulcerative Colitis**
> Visit mometrix.com/academy and enter code: 584881

PERITONITIS

Peritonitis (inflammation of the peritoneum) may be primary (from infection of blood or lymph) or, more commonly, secondary, related to perforation or trauma of the gastrointestinal tract. Common causes include perforated bowel, ruptured appendix, abdominal trauma, abdominal surgery, peritoneal dialysis or chemotherapy, or leakage of sterile fluids, such as blood, into the peritoneum.

Symptoms: Diffuse abdominal pain with rebound tenderness (Blumberg's sign), abdominal rigidity, paralytic ileus, fever (with infection), nausea and vomiting, and sinus tachycardia.

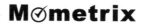

Diagnosis: Increased WBC (>15,000), abdominal x-ray/CT, paracentesis, blood and peritoneal fluid culture.

Treatment includes:

- Intravenous fluids and electrolytes
- Broad-spectrum antibiotics
- Laparoscopy as indicated to determine cause of peritonitis and effect repair

APPENDICITIS

Appendicitis is inflammation of the appendix often caused by luminal obstruction and pressure within the lumen; secretions build up and can eventually perforate the appendix. Diagnosis can be made difficult by the fact that there is some variation in the exact location of the appendix in some patients. Appendicitis can occur in all ages, but children younger than 2 years usually present with peritonitis or sepsis because of difficulty in early diagnosis. **Symptoms** include:

- Acute abdominal pain, which may be epigastric, periumbilical, right lower quadrant, or right flank with rebound tenderness
- Anorexia
- Nausea and vomiting
- Positive psoas and obturator signs
- Fever may develop after 24 hours
- Malaise
- Bowel irregularity and flatulence

Diagnosis is based on clinical presentation, CBC (although leukocytosis may not be present), urinalysis, and imaging studies (usually an abdominal CT with contrast).

CHOLECYSTITIS

Cholecystitis can result in obstruction of the bile duct related to calculi as well as pancreatitis from obstruction of the pancreatic duct. In acute cholecystitis, there is fever, leukocytosis, right upper quadrant abdominal pain, and inflammation of the gallbladder. The disease is most common in overweight women 20-40 years of age, but can occur in pregnant women and people of all ages, especially those who are diabetic or elderly. Cholecystitis may develop secondary to cystic fibrosis, obesity, or total parenteral nutrition. Many times, cholecystitis may resolve in about 7-10 days on its own, but acute cholecystitis may need surgical intervention to prevent complications such as gangrene in the gallbladder or perforation. Diagnosis is confirmed by ultrasound of gallbladder showing thickening of gallbladder walls or positive Murphy's sign, or a HIDA scan showing failure to fill.

Symptoms:

- Severe right upper quadrant or epigastric pain (ranging from 2-6 hours per episode)
- Nausea and vomiting
- Jaundice
- Altered mental status
- Positive Murphy's sign

Treatment:

- Antibiotics for sepsis/ascending cholangitis
- Antispasmodic agents (glycopyrrolate) for biliary colic and vomiting
- Analgesics (note that opioids result in increased sphincter of Oddi pressure)

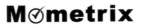

- Antiemetics
- Surgical consultation for possible laparoscopic or open cholecystectomy

EROSIVE VS. NONEROSIVE GASTRITIS

Gastritis is inflammation of the epithelium or endothelium of the stomach. Types include:

- **Erosive**: Typically caused by alcohol, NSAIDs, illness, portal hypertension, and/or stress. Risk factors include severe illness, mechanical ventilation, trauma, sepsis, organ failure, and burns. Patients may be essentially asymptomatic but may have hematemesis or "coffee ground" emesis. Treatment depends on cause and severity but often includes a proton pump inhibitor (such as omeprazole 20-40 mg per day). Some may receive an H2-rceptor (such as famotidine). Those with portal hypertension may respond to propranolol or nadolol or portal decompression.
- **Nonerosive**: Typically caused by Helicobacter pylori infection or pernicious anemia. H. pylori infection can lead to gastric and duodenal ulcers. Treatment for H. pylori is per antibiotics and proton pump inhibitors with standard triple or standard quadruple therapy. Pernicious anemia is treated with vitamin B-12. Gastritis may also be caused by a wide range of pathogens, including parasites, so treatment depends on the causative agent.

GASTROENTERITIS

VIRAL GASTROENTERITIS

Viral gastroenteritis (commonly referred to as stomach flu) is characterized by nausea, vomiting, abdominal cramping, watery (may become bloody) diarrhea, headache, muscle aches, and fever. Viral gastroenteritis is spread through the fecal-oral route. Common **causes** include:

- **Norovirus**: Symptoms generally include diarrhea and vomiting with symptoms persisting for 1-3 days. Most people do not require treatment, but if diarrhea or vomiting is severe, an antiemetic or antidiarrheal may be prescribed if the patient is younger than 65. If severe dehydration occurs, the patient may require intravenous fluids until she is able to resume adequate oral intake.
- **Rotavirus**: Symptoms include watery diarrhea, nausea, vomiting, abdominal pain and cramping, lack of appetite and fever. Patients may become easily dehydrated and require rehydration with Pedialyte or Rice-Lyte or IV fluids. Medications are usually not needed but the rotavirus vaccine prevents severe rotavirus-related diarrhea and is given in 3 doses (2 months, 4 months, and 6 months).

BACTERIAL GASTROENTERITIS

Bacterial gastroenteritis generally results in cramping, nausea, and severe diarrhea. Some bacteria cause gastroenteritis because of enterotoxins that adhere to the mucosa of the intestines and others because of exotoxins that remain in contaminated food. Some bacteria directly invade the intestinal mucosa. Bacterial gastroenteritis is commonly **caused** by:

- *Salmonella*: Sudden onset of bloody diarrhea, abdominal cramping, nausea, and vomiting, leading to dehydration. Infection may become systemic and life-threatening. Treatment is supportive although antibiotics may be administered to those at risk.
- *Campylobacter*: Bloody diarrhea, cramping, fever, for up to 7 days that usually resolves but may become systemic in those who are immunocompromised. Treatment is primarily supportive with antibiotics only for those at risk.
- *Shigella* spp.: Most common in children <5 and presents with fever, abdominal cramping, and bloody diarrhea, persisting 5-7 days. Treatment is primarily supportive (rehydration) although those at risk (very young, old, immunocompromised) may receive antibiotics because the disease may become systemic.
- *Escherichia coli*: Different strains are associated with traveler's diarrhea and food-borne illnesses, and severity varies. Most result in diarrhea, nausea, vomiting, and cramping, but some strains (O157) may develop into life-threatening hemolytic uremic syndrome (HUS). Treatment is supportive. Antibiotics increase risk of developing HUS.

PARASITIC GASTROENTERITIS

Parasitic gastroenteritis is generally caused by infection with protozoa (one-celled pathogens):

- *Giardia intestinalis*: Common cause of waterborne (drinking and recreational) disease and non-bacterial diarrhea, resulting from fecal contamination. Symptoms include diarrhea, abdominal cramping, flatulence, greasy floating stools, nausea and vomiting as well as weight loss. Symptoms usually persist for up to 3 weeks although some develop chronic disease. Metronidazole is the drug of choice: Adults, 250 mg TID for 5-7 days. Pediatrics, 15 mg/kg/day in 3 doses for 5-7 days.
- *Cryptosporidium parvum*: About 10,000 cases occur in the US each year, usually from contact with fecal-contaminated water. Symptoms include watery diarrhea, abdominal pain, nausea, vomiting, weight loss, and fever and persist for up to 2 weeks although a severe chronic infection may occur in those who are immunocompromised. Treatment for non-HIV-infected patients (medications ineffective for HIV patients): Adults and children >11, Nitazoxanide 500 mg BID for 3 days. Pediatrics, 1-3 years 100 mg BID for 3 days; 4-11 years 200 mg BID for 3 days.

CONSTIPATION AND IMPACTION

Constipation is a condition with bowel movements less frequent than normal for a person, or hard, small stool that is evacuated fewer than 3 times weekly. Food moves through the GI from the small intestine to the colon in semi-liquid form. Constipation results from the colon, where fluid is absorbed. If too much fluid is absorbed, the stool can become too dry. People may have Abdominal distension and cramps and need to strain for defecation.

Fecal impaction occurs when the hard stool moves into the rectum and becomes a large, dense, immovable mass that cannot be evacuated even with straining, usually as a result of chronic constipation. In addition to abdominal cramps and distention, the person may feel intense rectal pressure and pain accompanied by a sense of urgency to defecate. Nausea and vomiting may also occur. Hemorrhoids will often become engorged. Fecal incontinence, with liquid stool leaking about the impaction, is common.

MEDICAL PROCEDURES TO EVALUATE CAUSES OF CONSTIPATION

Medical procedures to evaluate causes of constipation should be preceded by a careful history as this may help to define the type and guide the choice of diagnostic procedures. Most tests are necessary only for severe constipation that does not respond to treatment. Medical **diagnostic procedures** may include the following:

- **Physical exam** should include rectal exam and abdominal palpation to assess for obvious hard stool or impaction.
- **Blood tests** can identify hypothyroidism and excess parathyroid hormone.
- **Abdominal x-ray** may show large amounts of stool in the colon.
- **Barium enema** can indicate tumors or strictures causing obstruction.
- **Colonic transit studies** can show defects of the neuromuscular system.
- **Defecography** shows the defecation process and abnormalities of anatomy.
- **Anorectal manometry studies** show malfunction of anorectal muscles.
- **Colonic motility studies** measure the pattern of colonic pressure.
- **Colonoscope** allows direct visualization of the lumen of the rectum and colon.

BOWEL OBSTRUCTIONS

Bowel obstruction occurs when there is a mechanical obstruction of the passage of intestinal contents because of constriction of the lumen, occlusion of the lumen, adhesion formation, or lack of muscular contractions (paralytic ileus). **Symptoms** include abdominal pain, rigidity, and distention, n/v, dehydration, constipation, respiratory distress from the diaphragm pushing against the pleural cavity, sepsis, and shock. **Treatment** includes strict NPO, insertion of naso/orogastric tube, IV fluids and careful monitoring; may correct spontaneously, severe obstruction requires surgery.

BOWEL INFARCTIONS

Bowel infarction is ischemia of the intestines related to severely restricted blood supply. It can be the result of a number of different conditions, such as strangulated bowel or occlusion of arteries of the mesentery, and may follow untreated bowel obstruction. Patients present with acute abdomen and shock, and mortality rates are very high even with resection of infarcted bowel. **Treatment** includes replacing volume, correcting the underlying issue, improving blood flow to the mesentery, insertion of NGT, and/or surgery.

INTESTINAL PERFORATION

Intestinal perforation is a partial or complete tear in the intestinal wall, leaking intestinal contents into the peritoneum. Causes include trauma, NSAIDs (elderly, patients with diverticulitis), acute appendicitis, PUD, iatrogenic (laparoscopy, endoscopy, colonoscopy, radiotherapy), bacterial infections, IBS, and ingestion of toxic substances (acids) or foreign bodies (toothpicks). The danger posed by infection after perforation varies depending upon the site. The stomach and proximal portions of the small intestine have little bacteria, but the distal portion of the small intestine contains aerobic bacteria, such as *E. coli,* as well as anaerobic bacteria.

Signs/Symptoms: (appear within 24-48 hours): Abdominal pain and distention and rigidity, fever, guarding and rebound tenderness, tachycardia, dyspnea, absent bowel sounds/paralytic ileus with nausea and vomiting; Sepsis and abscess or fistula formation can occur.

Diagnosis: Labs: elevated WBC; lactic acid and pH change as late signs. X-ray and CT will show free air in abdominal cavity.

Treatment includes:

- Prompt antibiotic therapy and surgical repair with peritoneal lavage
- The abdominal wound may be left open to heal by secondary intention and to prevent compartment syndrome

IMPERFORATE ANUS

Imperforate anus (anorectal malfunction) is a congenital abnormality where the rectum is absent, malformed, or displaced from normal position. It may include disorders of the urinary tract. Imperforate anus occurs in 1 in 5000 births, more commonly in males than females. Imperforate anus may include stenosis or atresia of anus. There are three main **categories**, classified according to relationship of rectum to puborectalis musculature:

- **Low anomalies**: No external opening, but rectum is otherwise in normal position through the puborectalis muscle, with normal function, and no connection to the genitourinary tract.
- **Intermediate anomalies**: Rectum is at or below the level of puborectalis muscle and an anal dimple is evident. The external sphincter is in normal position.
- **High anomalies**: Rectum ends above the puborectalis muscles, and internal sphincter is absent. Frequently, there is a rectourethral fistula in males or a rectovaginal fistula in females. There may be fistulas to the bladder or perineum.

Symptoms	Diagnosis	Treatment
Absence of anal opening: There is no meconium in 24-48 hours, Abdominal distension, and vomiting. **Rectovaginal fistula or rectourethral fistula**: Symptoms may not be evident at first because stool passes through the fistula. **Fistula between the rectum and the bladder**: Gas or fecal material may be expelled per the urethra. **Displacement of the anus**: Chronic constipation develops over time.	Physical examination. Digital or endoscopic examination. Contrast radiography with the infant inverted and an opaque marker at the anal dimple will outline the location of a pouch in relation to the normal position of the anus.	Most forms of imperforate anus require treatment by surgery. The type depends on the extent of the abnormality: Simple excision of anal opening may suffice. 2-3 step procedures for higher anomalies in which a colostomy is first performed with later reconstruction of the anus in the proper position, involving anoplasty and pull through procedures. Manual dilation may treat stenosis.

CYSTIC FIBROSIS

Cystic fibrosis (CF) is a genetic disease. It affects the respiratory, gastrointestinal, reproductive and cardiovascular systems. The body produces excess secretions that are thick; these secretions build up in the respiratory system, resulting in obstructions which contribute to respiratory infections, which lead to fibrosis and bronchiectasis.

- **Respiratory symptoms** include shortness of breath, cyanosis, wheezing, cough, atelectasis, emphysema, and chronic infections such as sinusitis, bronchitis, and pneumonia.
- **GI symptoms** include thick meconium trapped in the ileus at birth, rectal prolapse, stools that are fatty, loose, and frothy, big appetite while losing weight, vitamin deficiencies, and intestinal obstruction.
- **Reproductive problems** include delayed puberty and decreased fertility in females, and males are usually not fertile.
- **Cardiovascular issues** include the right side of the heart becoming enlarged and failing, blood sodium levels drop, and sodium and chloride are excreted in the sweat of the child (tastes excessively salty). A sweat test will show chloride levels greater than 60 mEq/L, the stool will have excess fat in it, and a chest x-ray will reveal atelectasis and obstructive emphysema.

BILIARY ATRESIA

Biliary atresia is atresia (absence or closure) of bile ducts outside the liver, related to congenital abnormality, an autoimmune reaction, or viral process. Biliary atresia is progressive with inflammation causing further scarring and obstruction of bile ducts inside the liver. The bile retained in the liver causes distention and scarring. The pathologic process may begin in the fetus or shortly after birth. Surgical repair must be done within the first 2-3 months after birth to prevent irreversible damage to the liver.

Symptoms	Treatment
<ul><li>Jaundice (2-3 weeks after birth)</li><li>Hepatomegaly with Abdominal distension</li><li>Light-colored stools and dark urine</li><li>Failure to thrive related to poor metabolism of fat</li><li>Irritability</li><li>Splenomegaly (late sign)</li></ul>	<ul><li>The Kasai (Roux-en-Y hepatoportojejunostomy) surgical procedure removes exterior ducts, transects the small intestine, and connects the distal segment directly to the liver to provide bile drainage. The proximal segment is attached to the distal segment, below the liver-intestine anastomosis.</li><li>Liver transplant is required in about 20% of children</li></ul>

GASTROESOPHAGEAL REFLUX

Gastroesophageal reflux (GER) occurs when the lower esophageal sphincter fails to remain closed, allowing the contents of the stomach to back into the esophagus. This reflux of the acid containing contents of the stomach may cause irritation of the lining of the esophagus. Over time, damage to the lining of the esophagus can occur. In some patients, this may lead to the formation of Barrett's esophagus. In Barrett's esophagus, the lining of the esophagus begins to resemble the tissue lining the intestine. Patients with Barrett's esophagus have an increased risk of developing esophageal adenocarcinoma.

Signs and symptoms: Heartburn, dysphagia, belching, water brash, sore throat, hoarseness, and chest pain.

Diagnosis: Clinical signs/symptoms, ambulatory esophageal reflux monitoring (this test uses a thin pH probe that is placed in the esophagus). Data is collected on the amount of acid entering the esophagus along with the presence of clinical symptoms. Endoscopy may be used in the diagnosis of GERD in patients with persistent or progressive symptoms.

Treatment: GER is often treated with proton pump inhibitors (inhibit gastric acid secretion). Surgical therapy may be utilized if medical management is unsuccessful. Patients are taught to eliminate foods that trigger symptoms (chocolate, caffeine, alcohol, and highly acidic foods). In addition, patients with GERD should avoid meals 2-3 hours before bed and may find it helpful to sleep with the head of the bed elevated to alleviate symptoms.

PEPTIC ULCER DISEASE

Peptic ulcer disease (PUD) includes both ulcerations of the duodenum and stomach. They may be primary (usually duodenal) or secondary (usually gastric). Gastric ulcers are commonly associated with **H. pylori** infections (80%) but may be caused by aspirin and NSAIDs. *H. pylori* are spread in the fecal-oral route from person to person or contaminated water and cause a chronic inflammation and ulcerations of the gastric mucosa. PUD is 2 to 3 times more common in males and is associated with poor economic status that results in a crowded, unhygienic environment, although it can occur in others. Usually, other family members have a history of ulcers as well.

Symptoms include abdominal pain, nausea, vomiting, and GI bleeding in children younger than 6 years with epigastric and postprandial pain and indigestion in older children and adults.

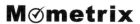

Treatment includes:

- Antibiotics for *H. pylori*: amoxicillin, clarithromycin, metronidazole
- Proton pump inhibitors: lansoprazole or omeprazole
- Bismuth
- Histamine-receptor antagonists: cimetidine or famotidine

Review Video: Peptic Ulcers and GERD
Visit mometrix.com/academy and enter code: 184332

INFLAMMATORY BOWEL DISEASE

ULCERATIVE COLITIS

Ulcerative colitis is superficial inflammation of the mucosa of the colon and rectum, causing ulcerations in the areas where inflammation has destroyed cells. These ulcerations, ranging from pinpoint to extensive, may bleed and produce purulent material. The mucosa of the bowel becomes swollen, erythematous, and granular. Patients may present emergently with **severe ulcerative colitis** (having >6 blood stools a day, fever, tachycardia, anemia) or with **fulminant colitis** (>10 blood stools per day, severe bleeding, and toxic symptoms) These patients are at high risk for megacolon and perforation. For patients with severe and fulminant ulcerative colitis:

Symptoms:

- Abdominal pain
- Anemia
- F&E depletion
- Bloody diarrhea/rectal bleeding
- Diarrhea
- Fecal urgency
- Tenesmus
- Anorexia
- Weight loss
- Fatigue
- Systemic disorders: Eye inflammation, arthritis, liver disease, and osteoporosis as immune system triggers generalized inflammation

Treatment:

- Glucocorticoids
- Aminosalicylates
- Antibiotics if signs/symptoms of toxicity
- D/C anticholinergics, NSAIDS, and antidiarrheals
- If fulminant: Admitted & monitored for deterioration. Kept NPO, and given IV F&E replacement. NGT for decompression if intestinal dilation is present. Knee-elbow position to reposition gas in bowel. Colectomy for those with megacolon or who are unresponsive to therapy.

CROHN'S DISEASE

Crohn's disease manifests with inflammation of the GI system. Inflammation is transmural (often leading to intestinal stenosis and fistulas), focal, and discontinuous with aphthous ulcerations progressing to linear and irregular-shaped ulcerations. Granulomas may be present. Common sites of inflammation are the terminal ileum and cecum. The condition is chronic, but patients with severe or fulminant disease (fevers, persistent vomiting, abscess, obstruction) often present emergently for treatment.

Symptoms:

- Perirectal abscess/fistula in advanced disease
- Diarrhea
- Watery stools
- Rectal hemorrhage
- Anemia
- Abdominal pain (commonly RLQ)
- Cramping
- Weight loss
- Nausea and vomiting
- Fever
- Night sweats

Treatment:

- Triamcinolone for oral lesions, aminosalicylates, glucocorticoids, antidiarrheals, probiotics, avoid lactose, and identify and eliminate food triggers.
- For patients who present with toxic symptoms: hospitalization for careful monitoring, IV glucocorticoids, aminosalicylates, antibiotics, and bowel rest. Parenteral nutrition for the malnourished.
- For repeated relapses (refractory):
  - Immunomodulatory agents (azathioprine, mercaptopurine, methotrexate) or Biologic therapies (infliximab). Bowel resection if unresponsive to all treatment or with ischemic bowel.

DIVERTICULAR DISEASE

Diverticular disease is a condition in which diverticula (saclike pouchings of the bowel lining that extend through a defect in the muscle layer) occur anywhere within the GI tract. About 20% of patients with diverticular disease will develop acute diverticulitis, which occurs as diverticula become inflamed when food or bacteria are retained within the diverticula. This may result in abscess, obstruction, perforation, bleeding, or fistula. Diagnosis is best confirmed by abdominal CT with contrast (showing a localized thickening of the bowel wall, increased density of soft tissue, and diverticula in the colon). Many patients have normal lab studies, but some present with leukocytosis, elevated serum amylase, and pyuria on urinalysis.

Symptoms (similar to appendicitis):

- Steady pain in left lower quadrant
- Change in bowel habits
- Tenesmus
- Dysuria from irritation
- Recurrent urinary infections from fistula
- Paralytic ileus from peritonitis or intra-abdominal irritation
- Toxic reactions: fever, severe pain, leukocytosis

Treatment:

- Rehydration and electrolytes per IV fluids
- Nothing by mouth initially
- Antibiotics, broad spectrum (IV if toxic reactions)
- NG suction if necessary, for obstruction
- Careful observation for signs of perforation or obstruction

Genitourinary Pathophysiology

ACUTE PANCREATITIS

Acute pancreatitis is related to chronic alcoholism or cholelithiasis in 90% of patients, but may have unknown etiology. It may also be triggered by a variety of drugs (tetracycline, thiazides, acetaminophen, and oral contraceptives). Complications may include shock, acute respiratory distress syndrome, and MODs.

Signs/Symptoms: acute pain (mid-epigastric, LUQ, or generalized), nausea and vomiting, Abdominal distension.

Diagnosis: Serum lipase (>2x normal), amylase (less accurate), CT with contrast, abdominal U/S, MRI cholangiopancreatography, ERCP.

Treatment (supportive) includes:

- **Medications**: IV fluids, antiemetics, antibiotics (if necrosis is secondary to infection), and analgesia. NOTE: do not give morphine, can cause spasms in sphincter of Oddi, making pain worse.
- **TPN, NPO, or restricted to clear liquids** may help manage vomiting, ileus, and aspiration.
- **Surgical**: may remove gallbladder and biliary duct obstructions if cause of recurrent pancreatitis.

Prevention: Avoid smoking and alcohol consumption; limit fat intake and increase fresh fruits/vegetables and water.

URINARY TRACT INFECTION

A urinary tract infection (UTI) is an inflammation of the urethra, bladder, ureters and/or kidneys. If it only involves the lower tract, it is considered uncomplicated. A kidney infection (pyelonephritis) or recurrent infections can cause chronic problems. Usually caused by bacteria (mostly E. coli), UTIs occur mostly in girls, primarily between the ages of 2 and 6. The following can contribute to the development of a UTI:

- Obstructed flow of urine
- Reflux of urine
- Poor fluid intake
- Improper perineal cleansing
- Constipation
- Uncircumcised male
- Catheterization (indwelling)
- Antibiotic use
- Tight underwear
- Perineal infection
- Sexual activity
- Bubble baths

Babies may be irritable, have fever (or hypothermia), be jaundiced, have vomiting, diarrhea and a diaper rash, and poor feeding with weight loss. The older child may have urine that smells bad, blood in urine, frequency, urgency, burning with urination, and stomach pain; if involving the kidneys, the symptoms may include flank pain, fever, and chills.

DIAGNOSTIC TOOLS AND NURSING CARE

Diagnosis is assisted by a urinalysis (blood, protein, or pus in urine), visually assessing the urine (foul odor, cloudy, mucus), a urine culture (detect bacteria), ureteral catheterization, bladder washout or renography (determine where the infection is located), and/or renal ultrasound, IVP, and VCU (assess for structural abnormalities). The nurse should assess the urine appearance, color and odor. Take note of any symptoms the

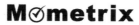

child is having. Give antibiotics as ordered. Use aseptic technique to avoid infection. The child should increase fluid intake, rest, take tub baths to help with burning pain, and take meds as prescribed for pain and fever.

BLADDER EXSTROPHY

Bladder exstrophy is eversion of the posterior wall of the bladder through the anterior wall of the bladder and through the lower abdominal wall with bladder and urethra exposed, a wide pubic arch, anterior displacement of the anus, renal disorders, and abnormalities of reproductive organs in both males and females. Symptoms include urinary and bowel problems related to specific anomalies. **Diagnosis** is by physical examination to assess abnormalities. Renal ultrasound is done to determine the number of kidneys and presence of hydroureteronephrosis.

Treatment is as follows:

First stage:

- **Primary closure of bladder**: No ostomy is necessary if done within 72 hours of birth. Procedures include ureteral stents and suprapubic urinary drainage.
- **Bilateral iliac ostomies**: Necessary after 72 hours because pelvic ring is not malleable.
- **Epispadias repair**: May be done in the first or second stage.

Second stage:

- **Epispadias repair**: Usually done between 6-12 months

Final stage:

- **Bladder neck reconstruction and reimplantation of ureters**
- **Permanent urinary diversion**: Required by 10-15% of individuals with bladder exstrophy

POSTERIOR URETHRAL VALVES

Posterior urethral valves are a urethral abnormality in males where urethral valves have narrow slit-like openings that impede flow and allow reverse flow, damaging urinary organs, which swell and become engorged with urine. 30% will develop long-term kidney failure. **Symptoms** vary, depending upon severity:

- Dysuria: Pain, weak stream, frequency
- Hematuria
- Urinary retention
- Incontinence
- Enlarged bladder palpable as abdominal mass
- Urinary infection (most common after 1 year of age)
- Possible sepsis, metabolic acidosis, and azotemia (increased blood levels of urea and other nitrogenous compounds)

Diagnosis includes the following:

- **Fetal ultrasound**
- **Voiding cystourethrogram (VCUG)**: Evaluate extent of valvular abnormality and other urinary defects
- **Endoscopy**: Examine inside of urinary tract/take tissue samples
- **Blood tests**: Assess kidney function and electrolytes

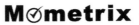

Treatment includes the following:

- **Medical management**: Supportive care, antibiotics, electrolytes, Foley catheter
- **Urinary diversion**: Usually closed after valve repair
- **Endoscopic ablation/resection**: Examine obstruction and remove valve leaflets

ENURESIS

Enuresis is repeated involuntary urinary incontinence in children old enough to have bladder control, usually about 5-6 years old. Diabetes and other disorders should be ruled out although 95% of enuresis cases are not associated with structural or neurological disorders. There are three **types**:

- **Primary**: The child has never been dry at night, and incontinence is associated with delay in maturation and small functional bladder rather than stress or psychiatric disorders.
- **Intermittent**: The child stays dry part of the time with episodes of incontinence at night.
- **Secondary**: The child has had long periods (6-12 months) staying dry and then is incontinent because of infection, stress, or a sleep disorder.

Treatment includes:

- Laboratory assessment and examination to rule out primary causes
- Fluid restriction
- Bladder training and enuresis alarms
- Imipramine (tricyclic antidepressant) is used with many children younger than 6 years of age but requires close monitoring
- Desmopressin nasal spray may be used for short-term control
- Support and acceptance

PRUNE BELLY (EAGLE-BARRETT) SYNDROME

Prune belly (Eagle-Barrett) syndrome is a group of abnormalities involving lack of developed abdominal muscles, undescended testicles, and urinary tract problems. Urinary abnormalities may include large, hypotonic bladder, dilated ureters, and prostatic urethra. Males comprise 96-99% of cases. It may include anomalies of the pulmonary, cardiac, skeletal, and GI tracts. **Symptoms** vary widely, frequently including cardio-pulmonary complications:

- **Prune-like appearance of abdomen** due to fetal Abdominal distension. After birth, abdominal fluid is lost, and the abdomen develops a wrinkled "prune" appearance, noticeable because of undeveloped abdominal muscles.
- **Undescended testicles** bilaterally.
- **Urinary tract abnormalities** such as urinary infections, obstruction, and chronic renal failure.

Diagnosis is by physical examination, chest x-rays to evaluate pulmonary problems, renal ultrasound to evaluate kidneys, and voiding cystourethrogram (VCUG) to evaluate urinary defects.

Treatment: Monitor the condition and provide antibiotics, both therapeutic and prophylactic. Intermittent catheterization is needed.

Surgical repair to correct genitourinary defects varies according to abnormality. Procedures may include a vesicostomy, ureterostomy, or pyelostomy; reduction cystoplasty; urethroplasty; or abdominoplasty.

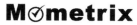

MEGAURETER

Megaureter is dilation of ureters from the normal 3-5 mm to more than 10 mm in diameter with or without obstruction and/or reflux from abnormality of ureters or secondary causes:

- **Primary obstruction**: At point where ureter joins bladder; can cause kidney damage
  o Refluxing: Backward flow of urine from bladder to ureters.
  o Non-obstructing/non-refluxing: Dilated ureters without blockage may resolve over time
  o Obstructed/ refluxing: Ureters continue to dilate with blockage
- **Secondary**: Ureters enlarge because of other conditions, such as neurogenic bladder

Symptoms include urinary tract infection, dysuria, back/flank pain, and fever.

Diagnosis is by:

- Fetal ultrasound: in utero diagnosis
- Ultrasound: To evaluate appearance of the urinary tract
- Voiding cystourethrogram (VCUG): To check for reflux
- Diuretic renal scan: To check for obstruction
- Intravenous pyelogram: To view the urinary system

Treatment includes:

- Antibiotic prophylaxis until surgery
- Ureteral implantation: Trimming the widened portion of the ureter, removing the obstruction, and reattaching

URETEROPELVIC JUNCTION OBSTRUCTION

Ureteropelvic junction obstruction (UPI) is congenital obstruction at the point where the ureter connects to the renal pelvis, unilaterally or bilaterally, causing inadequate urinary flow and hydronephrosis. Some children improve markedly within first 18 months, but others require surgery.

Symptoms include:

- Urinary tract infections
- Abdominal or flank pain
- Palpable mass from hydronephrosis
- Vomiting

Diagnosis is by:

- Fetal ultrasound: For in utero diagnosis
- Renal ultrasound: To show dilation of renal pelvis
- Intravenous pyelogram (IVP): To identify obstruction
- Renal isotope scan: To evaluate and measure kidney function

Treatment includes:

- Fetal urinary diversion: Remains controversial
- Pyeloplasty: Open surgical procedure where ureteropelvic junction is excised and the ureter is reattached to the renal pelvis with wide junction, allowing adequate drainage

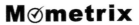

- Laparoscopic pyeloplasty: Through the abdominal wall and abdominal cavity with internal excision of ureteropelvic junction
- Insertion of wire through ureter: To cut the ureteropelvic junction from inside with a ureteral drain left in place for a few weeks

NEUROGENIC BLADDER

Neurogenic bladder is bladder dysfunction from lesions in the peripheral or central nervous system that are related to traumatic or congenital etiologies or that developed from cerebrovascular accident or diabetic neuropathy. Nerve damage can cause an under-active bladder that is unable to contract to effectively empty or an overactive bladder that contracts frequently and ineffectually.

Symptoms include:

- Underactive: Incontinence, dribbling, straining or inability to urinate, retention
- Overactive: Frequency, urgency, dysuria, urinary tract infection, fever

Diagnosis is by:

- Neurological testing (x-rays, MRI, and EEGs): To determine etiology
- 24-hour urine collection: To determine volume and urine patterns
- Bladder stress test: To determine reaction to full bladder while bending over, coughing, walking, or doing other activities

Treatment includes:

- Antibiotics: To control infections
- Clean intermittent catheterization (CIC): To empty bladder
- Endoscopy: Combined with cutting of external sphincter or injecting sphincter with paralytic agents to allow urination
- Surgical repair: Placing of permanent stents at bladder neck, bladder augmentation to increase bladder size, repair of vesicoureteral reflux, or urinary diversion

VESICOURETERAL REFLUX

Vesicoureteral reflux is an abnormality where urine flows from the bladder back up the ureters. Reflux is graded on the international scale of 1 to 5, depending upon degree of dilation of the ureters and renal pelvis.

- **Primary**: Congenital defect with impaired valve where ureter opens to bladder. The ureter may be too short so the valve doesn't close properly.
- **Secondary**: Caused by infection or other cause of obstruction

Symptoms include:

- Neonates: Fever, irritability, lethargy, emesis
- Older infants, children: Abdominal pain, emesis, diarrhea, fever, dysuria with enuresis, frequency, urgency, cloudy/foul urine
- Late symptoms: Hypertension, dysuria with difficulty urinating, proteinuria, chronic renal insufficiency

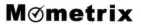

Diagnosis is by:

- Ultrasound: Evaluate appearance of urinary system
- Voiding cystourethrogram (VCUG): Identify reflux (after infection has cleared)
- Intravenous pyelogram: Reveal obstructions
- Nuclear scans: Show urinary functioning
- Cystoscopy: View bladder interior

Treatment includes:

- Antibiotics: For infection
- Surgical repair or reconstruction: Usually involves severing ureter from bladder and reattaching at a different angle to prevent reflux

RENAL TRAUMA

Most renal trauma in children is the result of blunt trauma associated with motor vehicle accidents, falls, sports injuries, and child abuse, although gunshot wounds and stabbings also occur with increasing frequency. Various staging systems are used, but overall injuries are **graded by severity**:

- Grade A: Contusion of cortex with fracture (tear) of small confined area
- Grade B: Major fracture with peri-renal hematoma and/or extravasation of urine
- Grade C: Multiple fractures with extensive bleeding
- Grade D: Severe vascular disruption decreasing perfusion of kidney

Kidney injuries are often accompanied by other trauma (75%) so **symptoms** may be complex:

- Pain in abdominal or flank area
- Hematuria
- Abrasions or contusions in flank or abdominal area
- Shock
- Delayed symptoms include hypertension, hydronephrosis

Treatment includes:

- Treatment is usually non-operative if the child is hemodynamically stable, based on evaluation by CT, especially for blunt trauma.
- Bed rest is required.

POLYCYSTIC KIDNEY DISEASE

Polycystic kidney disease (PK) is caused by renal cysts (fluid-filled sacs in renal tissue), which may be genetic or acquired. The cysts develop from nephrons and can cause gross enlargement of kidneys. Cysts may be single or multiple (polycystic) and may involve one or both kidneys. PK is often associated with cystic disease in other organs as well.

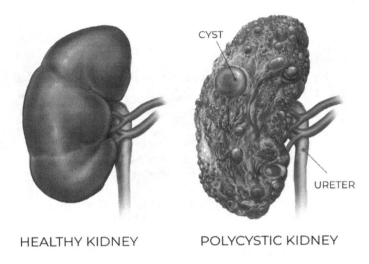

HEALTHY KIDNEY   POLYCYSTIC KIDNEY

There are three **types** of PK:

- **Autosomal dominant** is the most common (90%), but symptoms are usually delayed until adulthood although they can occur in childhood. However, it may progress to ESRD over time. Symptoms include urinary and cyst infections, rupture of cysts with hematuria, hypertension, and renal calculi.
- **Autosomal recessive** is rarer and symptoms arise much earlier, sometimes in the fetus.
- **Acquired** usually does not affect children because it develops from long-term kidney disease or dialysis.

Treatment cannot cure but can delay effects:

- Antihypertensives
- Antibiotics for infections
- Analgesia
- Growth hormone (autosomal recessive)
- Long-term: dialysis and transplantation

OBSTRUCTIVE UROPATHY WITH NEPHROSIS

Obstructive uropathy with nephrosis may present with a variety of **symptoms** depending upon the underlying cause, but most include:

- Pain in flank area
- Recurrent urinary infections with associated pain and fever
- Dysuria decreased urinary output, foul urine, and/or hematuria
- Edema
- Renal failure

Sometimes obstructions will resolve over time and may not constitute medical emergencies, especially if only one side is involved. However, if blockage is causing severe symptoms or does not resolve, various **treatments** may be used:

- Prenatal shunts may be done if the condition is identified through ultrasound. The procedure carries risk, so it is done primarily if the life of the fetus is threatened.
- A ureteral/urethral stent may be inserted to maintain patency of ureter.
- Urinary diversions, such as ileal conduit or cutaneous ureterostomy may be indicated in cases of severe obstruction, especially those associated with congenital abnormalities.
- Antibiotics are given for infections.

ACUTE TUBULAR NECROSIS

Acute tubular necrosis (ATN) occurs when a hypoxic condition causes renal ischemia that damages tubular cells of the glomeruli so they are unable to adequately filter the urine, leading to acute renal failure. Causes include hypotension, hyperbilirubinemia, sepsis, surgery (especially cardiac or vascular), and birth complications. ATN may result from nephrotoxic injury related to obstruction or drugs, such as chemotherapy, acyclovir, and antibiotics, such as sulfonamides and streptomycin. Symptoms may be non-specific initially and can include life-threatening complications.

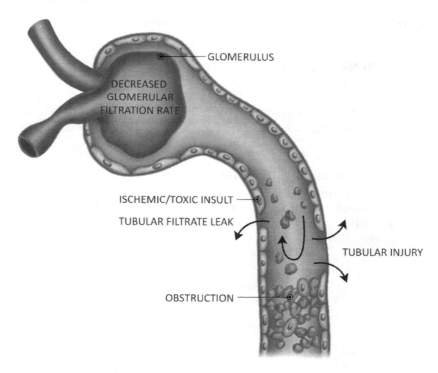

Symptoms include:

- Lethargy
- Nausea and vomiting
- Hypovolemia with low cardiac output and generalized vasodilation
- Fluid and electrolyte imbalance leading to hypertension, CNS abnormalities, metabolic acidosis, arrhythmias, edema, and congestive heart failure
- Uremia leading to destruction of platelets and bleeding, neurological deficits, and disseminated intravascular coagulopathy (DIC)
- Infections, including pericarditis and sepsis

Treatment includes:

- Identifying and treating underlying cause, discontinuing nephrotoxic agents
- Supportive care
- Loop diuretics (in some cases), such as Lasix
- Antibiotics for infection (can include pericarditis and sepsis)
- Kidney dialysis

ACUTE KIDNEY INJURY

Acute kidney injury (AKI), previously known as acute renal failure, is an acute disruption of kidney function that results in decreased renal perfusion, a decrease in glomerular filtration rate and a buildup of metabolic waste products (azotemia). Azotemia is the accumulation of urea, creatinine and other nitrogen containing end products into the bloodstream. The regulation of fluid volume, electrolyte balance and acid base balance is also affected. The causes of acute kidney injury are divided into pre-renal (caused by a decrease in perfusion), intrarenal or intrinsic (occurring within the kidney) and post-renal (caused by the inadequate drainage of urine). Acute kidney injury is common in hospitalized patients and even more common in critically ill patients, carrying a mortality rate of 50-80%. Risk factors for acute kidney injury include advanced age, the presence of co-morbid conditions, pre-existing kidney disease and a diagnosis of sepsis.

Signs and symptoms: Malaise, fatigue, lethargy, confusion, weakness, change in urine color, change in urine volume, and flank pain.

Diagnosis: Urinalysis, serum BUN and creatinine levels, renal ultrasound, CT or MRI and renal biopsy.

Treatment: The treatment of acute kidney injury is based on the underlying cause. Treatment options may include fluid and electrolyte replacement, diuretic therapy, fluid restriction, renal diet, and low dose dopamine to increase renal perfusion. Hemodialysis may also be necessary in patients with acute kidney injury.

PYELONEPHRITIS

Pyelonephritis is a potentially organ-damaging bacterial infection of the parenchyma of the kidney. Pyelonephritis can result in abscess formation, sepsis, and kidney failure. Pyelonephritis is especially dangerous for those who are immunocompromised, pregnant, or diabetic. Most infections are caused by *Escherichia coli*. **Diagnostic studies** include urinalysis, blood and urine cultures. Patients may require hospitalization or careful follow-up.

Symptoms vary widely but can include:

- Dysuria and frequency, hematuria, flank and/or low back pain
- Fever and chills
- Costovertebral angle tenderness
- Change in feeding habits (infants)
- Change in mental status (geriatric)
- Young women often exhibit symptoms more associated with lower urinary infection, so the condition may be overlooked.

Treatment includes:

- Analgesia
- Antipyretics
- Intravenous fluids
- Antibiotics: started but may be changed based on cultures

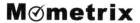

- IV ceftriaxone with fluoroquinolone orally for 14 days
- Monitor BUN. Normal 7-8 mg/dL (8-20 mg/dL >age 60). Increase indicates impaired renal function, as urea is end product of protein metabolism.

CYSTITIS

Cystitis is a common and often-chronic low-grade kidney infection that develops over time, so observing for symptoms of urinary infections and treating promptly are very important.

Changes in **character of urine**:

- **Appearance**: The urine may become cloudy from mucus or purulent material. Hematuria may be present.
- **Color**: Urine usually becomes concentrated and may be dark yellow/orange or brownish in color.
- **Odor**: Urine may have a very strong or foul odor.
- **Output**: Urinary output may decrease markedly.

Pain: There may be lower back or flank pain from inflammation of the kidneys.

Systemic: Fever, chills, headache, and general malaise often accompany urine infections. Some people suffer a lack of appetite as well as nausea and vomiting. Fever usually indicates that the infection has affected the kidneys. Children may develop incontinence or loose stools and cry excessively.

Treatment:

- Increased fluid intake
- Antibiotics

NEPHROTOXIC AGENTS

Medications are a common cause of renal damage, especially among older patients. The **nephrotoxic effects** may be reversible if the drug is discontinued before permanent damage occurs. Those at increased risk include patients who are older than 60, have a history of renal insufficiency, suffer from volume depletion, or have diabetes mellitus, sepsis, or heart failure. Initial signs may be quite subtle. Preventive measures include baseline renal function tests and monitoring of renal function and vital signs during treatment. The following are some common effects, and the drugs that may cause them:

- **Chronic interstitial nephritis**: Acetaminophen, lithium, carmustine, cisplatin, cyclosporine.
- **Acute interstitial nephritis**: NSAIDs, acyclovir, beta-lactams, rifampin, quinolones, sulfonamides, vancomycin, indinavir, loop/thiazide diuretics, lansoprazole, allopurinol, phenytoin.
- **Rhabdomyolysis**: Amitriptyline, diphenhydramine, doxylamine, benzodiazepines, haloperidol, lithium, ketamine, methadone, methamphetamine, statins.
- **Crystal nephropathy**: Acyclovir, foscarnet, ganciclovir, quinolones, sulfonamides, indinavir, methotrexate, triamterene.
- **Tubular cell toxicity**: Aminoglycosides, amphotericin B, pentamidine, adefovir, tenofovir, contrast dye, zoledronate.
- **Thrombotic microangiopathy**: Cyclosporine, clopidogrel, mitomycin-C, quinine.
- **Impaired intraglomerular hemodynamics**: NSAIDs, cyclosporine, tacrolimus, ACE inhibitors.
- **Glomerulonephritis**: NSAIDs, lithium, beta-lactams, interferon-alpha, gold therapy, pamidronate.

Fluid Balance in Infants and Children

Body fluid is primarily **intracellular fluid (ICF)** or **extracellular space (ECF)**. Infants and children have proportionately more extracellular fluid (ECF) than adults. At birth, more than half of the child's weight is ECF, but by 3 years of age, the child's balance is more like adults:

- ECF: 20-30% (interstitial fluid, plasma, transcellular fluid)
- ICF: 40-50% (fluid within the cells)

The fluid compartments are separated by semipermeable membranes that allow fluid and solutes (electrolytes and other substances) to move by osmosis. Fluid also moves through diffusion, filtration, and active transport. In fluid volume deficit, fluid is out of balance and ECF is depleted; an overload occurs with increased concentration of sodium and retention of fluid. Signs of **fluid deficit** include:

- Thirsty, restless to lethargic
- Increasing pulse rate, tachycardia
- Fontanels depressed (infants)
- Decreased urinary output
- Normal BP progressing to hypotension
- Dry mucous membranes
- 3-10% decrease in body weight

Normal Values for Electrolytes in the Pediatric Population

Electrolyte	Normal Range(s)
Potassium	Infant: 4.1-5.3 mEq/L Child: 3.4-4.7 mEq/L
Calcium	11 days to 2 years: 9-11 mg/dL 3-12 years: 8.8-10.8 mg/dL 13-18 years: 8.4-10.2 mg/dL
Phosphate	1-3 years: 3.9-6.5 mg/dL 4-6 years: 4.0-5.4 mg/dL 7-11 years: 3.7-5.6 mg/dL 12-13 years: 3.3-5.4 mg/dL 14-15 years: 2.9-5.4 mg/dL 16-19 years: 2.8-4.6 mg/dL
Magnesium	1.7-2.1 mEq/L

Persistent Cloaca

Persistent cloaca is a condition in females with an imperforate anus and the rectum, vagina, and urethra forming a single channel with a rectal fistula attached to the posterior wall of the channel. **Diagnosis** is made with a physical exam showing a single perineal opening. An abdominal mass (hydrocolpos—distended bladder) may occur. A voiding cystourethrogram (VCUG) will show bladder abnormalities if catheterization is possible.

Treatment includes the following:

- **Colostomy**: Fecal diversion in neonate prevents fecal material from entering urinary system and causing infection.
- **Decompression of vagina**: Prevents infection and scarring and relieves obstruction of urinary tract.
- **Posterior sagittal anorectovagino-urethroplasty (PSARVUP)**: (Usually two months after colostomy.) The rectum is separated from the vagina, and the vagina is separated from the urethra. The urethra is reconstructed, the vagina is reconstructed, and the rectum is reconstructed with anoplasty

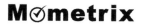

- **Postoperative anal dilation**: Two weeks after surgery until the final size is reached
- **Cystoscopy/vaginoscopy**: Checks for urethrovaginal fistula
- **Colostomy removal**: Anastomosis of colon and rectum and colostomy is removed

ADOLESCENT MENSTRUAL DISORDERS

Menarche occurs between 9-15 years of age in most girls, preceded by development of secondary sexual characteristics. The usual menstrual cycle is every 21-35 days, lasting 2-7 days with blood loss of 35-150 mL per monthly cycle. **Menstrual disorders** may cause considerable discomfort:

- **Dysmenorrhea** is pain associated with menses, usually 6-24 months after menarche. Pain usually lasts about 2 days and is accompanied by mild to severe cramping in the supra-pubic area, lumbar back, and labia. **Treatment** includes:
  - NSAIDs (ibuprofen) 400-900 mg up to 4 times daily
  - Naproxen 250-500 mg every 6-12 hours

- **Endometriosis** occurs when endometrial tissue outside of the pelvic area irritates nerve endings and causes severe pain and uterine cramping during periods, usually preceded by a few days of increasing dysmenorrhea. **Treatment** consists of the following:
  - Referral to gynecologist
  - NSAIDs
  - Oral contraceptives to reduce shedding
  - Gonadotropin-releasing hormone to reduce estrogen and androgen levels
  - Laparoscopy to remove extrauterine endometrial tissue.

- **Dysfunctional uterine bleeding** results from an abnormality in hormones so that shedding of the endometrium is irregular, resulting in excessive bleeding or irregular periods. **Treatment** includes:
  - Hgb >12: NSAIDs with iron supplementation
  - Hgb 10-12 add folic acid supplement
  - Hgb <10 may require hospitalization or referral to gynecologist

- **Mittelschmerz** is pain in the middle of the menstrual cycle, usually dull in the lower abdomen and lasting for minutes to hours, and probably related to enlargement of follicle before rupture. **Treatment** includes the following:
  - Heating pad may relieve discomfort
  - NSAIDs

- **Amenorrhea** may be primary (absence at ≤16 years old) with normal pubertal development (within 3 years) or with no pubertal development. It may also be secondary (no periods for 3 cycles or 6 months), related to excessive exercise or dieting. Primary and secondary amenorrhea requires testing to determine if there are abnormalities in hormones, genetic disorders, obstructive disorders, or other causes. **Treatment** depends on the underlying cause.

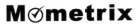

Integumentary Pathophysiology

Tissue Damage Related to Allergic Contact Dermatitis

Contact dermatitis is a localized response to contact with an allergen, resulting in a rash that may blister and itch. Common allergens include poison oak, poison ivy, latex, benzocaine, nickel, and preservatives, but there is a wide range of items, preparations, and products to which people may react.

Treatment includes:

- Identifying the causative agent through evaluating the area of the body affected, careful history, or skin patch testing to determine allergic responses
- Corticosteroids to control inflammation and itching
- Soothing oatmeal baths
- Pramoxine lotion to relieve itching
- Antihistamines to reduce allergic response
- Lesions should be gently cleansed and observed for signs of secondary infection
- Antibiotics are used only for secondary infections as indicated
- Rash is usually left open to dry
- Avoidance of allergen to prevent recurrence

Pressure Ulcers

Pressure ulcers occur when pressure from the weight of the body causes a decrease in perfusion, affecting arterial and capillary blood flow and resulting in ischemia. Ulcers may then develop from pressure, shearing, and friction. Common pressure points include the occiput, scapula, sacrum, buttocks, ischium, and heels. Patients with a decreased level of consciousness, brain/spinal cord injuries, peripheral neuropathies, malnutrition, dehydration, PVD, or impaired mobility are at a higher risk for pressure ulcers. Critically ill patients are at an increased risk due to prolonged immobility, sedation, and often incontinence of urine and stool. In addition, patients on vasopressors are at a higher risk due to the constriction of the peripheral circulation.

Signs and symptoms: Early stages include redness, tenderness, and firmness at the site of the ulcer. Once the ulcer progresses to severe tissue injury, bone, muscle, or tendons may be exposed, and there may be a yellow or black wound base in addition to pain and drainage at the site.

Diagnostics: Skin and wound assessment, including staging of the ulcer.

Treatment: Wet-to-Dry dressings, Wound VAC therapy, and hyperbaric oxygen may be used; a wound care consult is often advised.

Prevention: Begins with a risk assessment; the Braden scale is a commonly used scale. A score of 16 or below indicates that the patient is at risk. At-risk patients or patients with active ulcers should be placed on a turning and positioning schedule or on a specialty bed to relieve pressure. Moisture barriers and skin protectants may also be utilized.

NATIONAL PRESSURE INJURY ADVISORY PANEL STAGING

Pressure ulcers result from pressure or pressure with shear and/or friction over bony prominences. The **National Pressure Injury Advisory Panel (NPIAP) stages** include:

- **Suspected deep tissue injury**: Skin discolored, intact or blood blister
- **Stage I**: Intact skin with non-blanching reddened area
- **Stage II**: Abrasion or blistered area without slough but with partial-thickness skin loss
- **Stage III**: Deep ulcer with exposed subcutaneous tissue; tunneling or undermining may be evident with or without slough
- **Stage IV**: Deep ulcer, full thickness, with necrosis into muscle, bone, tendons, and/or joints
- **Unstageable**: Eschar and/or slough prevents staging prior to debridement

Patients should be placed on pressure-reducing support surfaces and turned at least every two hours, avoiding the area(s) with a pressure ulcer. Wound care depends on the stage of the wound and the amount of drainage but includes irrigation, debridement when necessary, antibiotics for infection, and appropriate dressing. Patients should be encouraged to have adequate protein and iron in their diets to promote healing and to maintain adequate hydration.

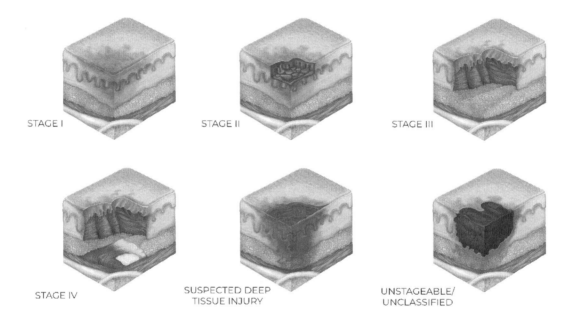

STAGE I   STAGE II   STAGE III

STAGE IV   SUSPECTED DEEP TISSUE INJURY   UNSTAGEABLE/ UNCLASSIFIED

INFECTIOUS WOUNDS

All types of wounds have the potential to become infected. Infectious wounds are commonly health care acquired. Wound infections increase a patient's risk of sepsis, multisystem organ failure and death. Trauma patients are at an increased risk of developing an infected wound due to exposure to various contaminants that they may have encountered during their injury (e.g., dirt from a motor vehicle accident).

Signs and symptoms: Erythema, edema, induration, drainage, increasing pain and tenderness, fever, leukocytosis, and lymphangitis.

Diagnosis: Wound infections are diagnosed by wound cultures (anaerobic and aerobic). Fluid or tissue biopsy may also be performed.

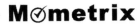

Treatment: Wound infections are treated with antibiotics and a wound care regimen that includes routine cleaning and dressing of the wound. Wound care treatment is based on the type and severity of the wound. Surgical irrigation and debridement may also be indicated. For deep, complex wounds, a wound-care consult is often indicated.

NECROTIZING FASCIITIS

Necrotizing fasciitis is an infection that develops deep within the fascia, causing a rapidly developing tissue necrosis resulting in destruction and death of the soft tissue and nerves. Complications of necrotizing fasciitis may include the loss of the affected limb, sepsis, and death. Group A *Streptococcus*, *Klebsiella*, *Clostridium*, *Escherichia coli*, *Staphylococcus aureus*, and *Aeromonas hydrophila* are organisms that have the potential to cause necrotizing fasciitis.

Signs and symptoms: Edema, erythema, and pain at the affected site. Nausea, vomiting, fatigue, malaise, fever, and chills may also occur.

Diagnosis: Diagnosis is based on physical assessment and patient history. In addition, excisional deep skin biopsy and gram staining may be performed to determine the causative organism. CT/MRI may also be utilized to assess the extent of the infection.

Treatment: Treatment options for necrotizing fasciitis include antibiotics and fasciotomy with radical debridement. Hyperbaric oxygen therapy may also be utilized.

SURGICAL WOUNDS

Surgical wounds or incisions are made during a surgical procedure in a sterile, controlled environment. The American College of Surgeons has defined four classes of surgical wound types. This classification can help to predict how the wound will heal and the risk of infection.

- **Class I** is defined as clean (e.g., laparoscopic surgeries and biopsies).
- **Class II** is defined as clean contaminated (e.g., GI and GU surgeries).
- **Class III** is defined as contaminated (e.g., traumatic wounds such as a gunshot wound).
- **Class IV** is defined as dirty (e.g., traumatic wound from a dirty source).

Surgical wounds should be assessed for signs and symptoms of infection including erythema, edema, fever, increasing pain, and drainage. Surgical drains are commonly placed near the surgical incision to promote drainage—inspect drains for patency, amount, and characteristics of drainage. Patients are often treated with antibiotics prophylactically to help prevent a surgical site infection. Wound vacuum assisted closure devices may also be utilized to remove blood or serous fluid from the surgical wound/incision site.

MANAGEMENT OF INFLAMMATION RESULTING FROM TATTOOS AND PIERCING

Tattoos and piercing have both been implicated in **MRSA infections**. Tattooing uses needles that inject dye, sometimes resulting in local infection with erythema, edema, and purulent discharge. Body piercing for insertion of jewelry carries similar risks. Piercings of concern include the upper ear cartilage, nipples, navel, tongue, lip, penis, and nose. Some people who do piercings use reusable piercing equipment that is difficult to adequately clean and sterilize. Infections resulting from piercing in cartilage are often resistant to antibiotics because of lack of blood supply.

Treatment includes:

- **Cleansing wounds**. Jewelry may need to be removed in some cases.
- **Antibiotics**: Culture should be obtained, but medications for community-acquired MRSA should be started immediately:

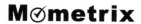

- o **Mupirocin** may be used topically 3 times daily for 7-10 days with or without systemic antimicrobials.
- o **Trimethoprim-sulfamethoxazole DS** (TMP 160 mg/SMX 800 mg), 1-2 tablets twice daily. Children, dose based on TMP: 8-12 mg/kg/day in 2 doses.

TISSUE DAMAGE

Abrasion is damage to superficial layers of skin, such as with road burn or ligature marks.

Contusion occurs when friction or pressure causes damage to underlying vessels, resulting in bruising. Contusions that are bright red/purple with clear margins have occurred within 48 hours and those with receding edges or yellow-brown discoloration are older than 48 hours.

Laceration is a tear in the skin resulting from blunt force, often from falls on protuberances, such as elbows, or other blunt trauma. Lacerations may be partial to full-thickness.

Avulsion is tissue that is separated from its base and lost or without adequate base for attachment.

Treatments include:

- Local anesthetic if needed
- Low pressure, high volume irrigation with 35-50 mL syringe of open wound with normal saline, water, or non-antiseptic nonionic surfactants, and mechanical scrubbing of surrounding tissue with disinfectant
- Topical antibiotics as indicated
- Prophylactic antibiotics or antibiotic irrigation if wound contaminated
- Suturing/debridement as needed
- Hydrocolloids, Steri-Strips, and transparent dressings to stabilize flaps

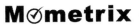

EENT Pathophysiology

INFECTIOUS CONJUNCTIVITIS

Infectious conjunctivitis (**pink eye**) is inflammation of the conjunctiva of the eye from bacteria or viruses. If it occurs less than 30 days after birth, it is referred to as **ophthalmia neonatorum** and is commonly acquired during delivery:

- Pathogenic agents include *Chlamydia trachomatis, Neisseria gonorrhea,* and herpesvirus.
- Antibiotic drops are applied to the newborn's eyes to prevent conjunctivitis. Intravenous acyclovir is given to infants exposed to herpes virus.

Infectious conjunctivitis in older children is usually caused by *Staphylococci, Streptococci, Pneumococci,* or viruses and is extremely contagious, so proper hand hygiene is essential. It is difficult to differentiate between bacterial and viral infections without cultures. The child should be kept from school and other children for 24 hours after starting treatment or until symptoms subside. **Symptoms** include:

- Red, swollen, itchy conjunctiva
- Eye pain
- Purulent discharge
- Scratchy feeling under eyelids
- Mild photophobia

Treatment is usually antibiotic drops or ointment and cool compresses although many cases are caused by viruses and the condition often disappears without treatment in 3-5 days.

STRABISMUS

Strabismus occurs when the muscles of the eyes are not coordinated so that one eye deviates from the axis of the other. Strabismus may be congenital or acquired or associated with other disorders, such as albinism. **Deviations** include:

- **Phoria** is intermittent deviation. The child can still focus eyes and maintain alignment for periods when looking at an object.
- **Tropia** is consistent or intermittent deviation in which the child is unable to maintain alignment of the eyes.
  - Both phorias and tropias may be *hyper* (up), *hypo* (down), *exo* (out), *eso* (in toward nose), or *cyclo* (rotational).

Esotropia is both eyes turning inwards (cross eyes) and **exotropia** is both eyes turning outward (wall eyes). Children often compensate by closing one eye or moving their head. They may have headaches or dizziness. **Treatment** before 24 months reduces **amblyopia** (reduced vision):

- Occlusion therapy: Patching or eye drops to blur vision in óne eye
- Eye exercises
- Corrective lenses and/or prisms
- Surgical repair of rectus muscle

RETINOPATHY OF PREMATURITY

Retinopathy of prematurity (ROP) occurs when small capillaries to the retina constrict, causing necrosis. ROP is associated with infants born ≤28 week and weighing <1600 g (3lb. 8 oz), especially those receiving oxygen therapy. It is also linked to respiratory distress, hypoxia, hypercarbia, acidosis, shock, blood transfusions, and systemic infection. In many cases, revascularization will occur, but ROP may result in myopia, retinal detachment, and blindness. Infants at risk for ROP should have regular evaluations for visual impairment:

- Infants may be unable to follow objects or lights with their eyes and may fail to make eye contact or imitate facial expressions. They may have a vacant stare.
- Toddlers and young children may thrust head forward, hold objects close to eyes, squint or blink frequently, rub or cover their eyes, and bump into objects.

Treatment:

- Corrective lenses
- Cryosurgery or laser surgery to stop disease progression
- Scleral buckle procedure or vitrectomy may be indicated for retinal detachment

GLAUCOMA

Glaucoma is an increase in intraocular pressure caused by abnormal circulation of fluid in the eyes. The ciliary body of the eyes produces aqueous fluid that flows between the iris and lens to the anterior chamber where it collects and increases pressure, which can result in blindness. Glaucoma may affect one eye or both. There are two **types**:

- **Congenital glaucoma** occurs before the age of 3 and includes an abnormality of structures that drain aqueous humor. Treatment is often unsuccessful. Symptoms include:
  - Photophobia
  - Tearing
  - Clouding of cornea
  - Eyelid spasms and enlargement of eyes
- **Secondary/juvenile glaucoma** occurs in children older than 3 and is caused by obstruction related to trauma, infection, tumors, or steroid use. Secondary glaucoma symptoms may be less specific; they include bumping into objects because of loss of visual field and seeing halos about objects.

Treatment:

- Eye drops used for adults are relatively ineffective for children.
- Surgical reduction of pressure is the treatment of choice, and the child may require multiple procedures.

CATARACTS

Cataracts, partial or complete opacity of the lens of one or both eyes preventing refraction of light onto the retina, can be either congenital or acquired and is associated with prenatal infections, (such as rubella and CMV), hypocalcemia, or drug exposure. It can be related to trauma, systemic corticosteroids, genetic defects (albinism, Down syndrome), and prematurity. Clouding of the lens is not always obvious to the naked eye, so careful visual evaluations should be done for those children at risk. **Treatment** depends upon the extent of the cataracts and whether they are unilateral or bilateral. Early diagnosis is important because surgical repair before 2 months is the most successful, with visual acuity in 55% at 20/40. The opaque lens is removed, and the child uses corrective lenses or a lens is implanted. Antibiotic or steroid drops may be used after surgery.

NYSTAGMUS AND BLEPHAROPTOSIS

Nystagmus is involuntary rhythmic movements of one or both eyes, with horizontal, vertical, or circular movements, sometimes accompanied by rhythmic movements of the head. Nystagmus is common in neonates and should resolve in a few weeks but may indicate pathology if it persists. It is often associated with albinism, CNS abnormalities, or diseases of the ear or retina, and sudden onset is cause for concern. There is no specific treatment other than to identify and treat underlying causes.

223

Blepharoptosis is drooping of one or both upper eyelids and may be congenital (autosomal dominant), with defective development of the levator muscles or cranial nerve III, or acquired as the result of trauma or infection. If vision is affected, surgical repair is done early to avoid amblyopia. If vision is unaffected, surgical repair is deferred until the child is 3 or older.

HEARING LOSS

Identifying hearing loss early can facilitate treatment and prevent further deterioration, but most children are not diagnosed until 14-24 months even if hearing loss is profound. Diagnosis is delayed to at most 48 months for less severe hearing loss:

- **Mild hearing loss**: Pure-tone loss of ≥40 decibels at 500, 1000, and 2000 Hz in the better ear
- **Moderate hearing loss**: 40-60 decibel loss
- **Severe hearing loss**: 60-80 decibel loss
- **Profound hearing loss**: ≥80 decibel

There are three **types of hearing loss**:

- **Sensorineural hearing loss (SNHL)**: Damage occurs to the cochlear structure or nerve fibers. Hearing loss is permanent and associated with genetic disorders, birth injury, toxic drugs, head trauma, neoplasms, and viruses. A sub-form is noise-induced hearing loss (NIHL), which is preventable, but also permanent.
- **Conductive hearing loss (CHL)**: Transmission of sound is blocked by infection, foreign object, debris, impacted cerumen, and neoplasms. This type of hearing loss is usually reversible with medication or surgery.
- **Mixed hearing loss (MHL)**: Both conductive and sensorial loss.

COCHLEAR IMPLANTS

While there has been controversy in the deaf community about cochlear implants, by 2012, 38,000 children in the United States had received them. In 2020, the FDA approved lowering the age for cochlear implantation in children from 12 months to 9 months. A **cochlear implant** is an electronic device that provides sound, although not normal hearing, to those who have profound deafness. The person with the implant can often learn to understand speech and environmental sounds. Some use the sounds with lip-reading, but about half are able to understand speech by sound only, depending upon the degree of damage to the auditory nerve. A microphone by the ear picks up sounds that travels to an external speech processor and transmitter, which sends sounds to an implanted receiver where the sound is converted into electrical impulses sent to an internal electrode array implanted in the cochlea. The electrodes send the impulses to the auditory nerve, creating a perception of sound. Some children now receive bilateral cochlear implants. Studies show infants receiving the implant by age 2 acquire normal speech more rapidly than those implanted later.

OCULAR TRAUMA
ORBITAL FRACTURES

Orbital fractures most often occur with blunt force against the globe causing a rupture through the floor of the orbital bone or a direct blow to the orbital rim, often related to an assault. Injuries are most common in adolescents and young adults. **Diagnosis** includes a complete eye (slit lamp) and vision examination, IOP measurement, and CT scan.

Signs and Symptoms	Treatment
• Essentially asymptomatic • Ecchymosis and edema of eyelid • Infraorbital anesthesia from pressure or damage to infraorbital nerve • Decreased sensation of cheek and upper gum on injured side • Diplopia • Enophthalmos (sunken globe)	• Usually supportive • Topical steroids for severe edema • The patient is advised not to blow nose for several weeks. • Surgical repair about 2 weeks after injury when edema has subsided for extensive fracture (≥33% of orbital floor) or enophthalmos >2 mm remaining 10–14 days post-injury.

ZYGOMATIC FRACTURES

Zygomatic fracture involves the arch of bone that forms the lateral border of the eye orbit and the bony cheek prominence, most commonly associated with a blow to the lateral cheek from an altercation or accident. Fracture can result in a tilting of the eye and flattening of the cheek, which may be obscured by initial edema. Fracture may be only of the arch or may be a more extensive tripod fracture of the infraorbital rim, diastasis of the zygomaticofrontal suture, and disruption of the zygomaticotemporal arch junction. **Diagnosis** is by CT scan, which shows the extent of the fracture as well as the amount of displacement. **Treatment** for tripod fracture is referral to a surgeon for open reduction with fixation, exploration, and reconstruction of orbit as needed.

TRAUMATIC HYPHEMA

Traumatic hyphema is characterized by blood coming into the anterior chamber, frequently because of eye injury. Most of the time, the blood will go out of the chamber with no consequences, but sometimes a problem does occur when heightened IOP or blood staining in the cornea results. 71-94% of hyphemas are due to tears in the front of the ciliary body, including disturbance in the primary arterial circle and the branches. It is frequently seen in physically energetic men and boys, and 70% of individuals are less than 20 in age. Ratio of boys to girls is 3:1. The consequences are contingent upon how much blood accumulates in the anterior chamber.

These **forms** of traumatic hyphema may be seen:

- **Microscopic**: Does not have layered blood; flowing red blood cells are seen
- **Grade I**: Affects less than a third of anterior chamber
- **Grade II**: One third to one half of anterior chamber affected
- **Grade III**: More than half of anterior chamber affected
- **Grade IV**: Complete hyphema

Assessments for another problem in the eye should be done, such as iridodialysis, cyclodialysis, lens subluxation, lacerations, detachment of the retina, decreased vision due to commotion in the retina, or fractures in the orbit. When the harm is broad or if there may be something inside the eye, utilize ultrasonography and radiologic imaging. If there may be sickle cell hemoglobinopathy, utilize sickle cell preparation.

CORNEAL ABRASIONS

Corneal abrasion results from direct scratching or scraping trauma to the eye, often involving contact lenses. This causes a defect in the epithelium of the cornea. Infection with corneal ulceration can occur with abrasions.

Symptoms:

- Pain
- Intense photophobia
- Tearing

Determining the **cause and source** of the abrasion is important for treatment, as organic sources pose the danger of fungal infection and soft contact lenses pose the danger of *Pseudomonas* infection.

Diagnosis	Treatment
• Topical anesthetic prior to testing for visual acuity. • Fluorescent staining and examination with cobalt blue light. • Eversion of eyelid to check for foreign body. • Examine cornea and assess anterior chamber with slit lamp.	• Cycloplegic agent to relieve spasm and pain: cyclopentolate 1%. • Erythromycin ophthalmic ointment 4 times daily with or without eye patch if not related to contact lens AND without eye patch if related to organic source. • Tobramycin ophthalmic ointment 4 times daily without eye patch if related to contact lens.

CHEMICAL EYE BURNS

Chemical burns are caused by splashing chemicals (solid, liquid, or fumes) into any part of the eye, often related to facial burns. Chemical burns may damage the cornea and conjunctiva, although other layers of the eye may also be damaged, depending upon the chemical and degree of saturation. Many injuries involve alkali (greater than 7 pH), acid (less than 7 pH; often muriatic acid or sulfuric acid), or other irritants (neutral pH) such as pepper spray. Alkali chemicals (such as ammonia, lime, and lye) usually cause the most serious injuries.

Symptoms	Diagnosis	Treatment
• Pain • Blurring of vision • Tearing • Edema of eyelids	• History of event • Eye exam showing corneal irritation	• Irrigate the eye and other areas of contact with copious amounts of water or normal saline. • Litmus paper exam of the eye to determine residual pH and continue irrigation until pH returns to neutral. • Apply cycloplegic agent to relieve spasm and pain (cyclopentolate 1%). • Apply antibiotic ointment to prevent infection.

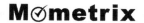

Musculoskeletal Pathophysiology

SLIPPED CAPITAL FEMORAL EPIPHYSIS (SCFE)

A slipped capital femoral epiphysis (SCFE) is an inferior/posterior separation of the ball (proximal femoral epiphysis) of the hip joint from the femur. This separation occurs at the growth plate. A stable SCFE allows ambulation, but an unstable one does not, even with crutches. Unstable SCFE poses an increased risk of avascular necrosis. SCFE is most common in adolescent boys (2.4 times the incidence in girls); especially those who are overweight, have hormonal imbalances, or are experiencing rapid growth. **Symptoms** include limp, knee pain, lateral rotation of the leg, and stiffness in the hip joint. SCFE most frequently involves the left hip. Patients <10 usually have metabolic disorders, such as hypothyroidism and growth hormone disorders. Acute SCFE has duration of <3 weeks and chronic >3 weeks. **Treatment** includes internal fixation with best results found if surgery is done within 24 hours of onset or after 48 hours. Because the condition often occurs in the opposite hip as well, some specialists recommend prophylactic fixation, but this remains controversial in the United States.

SHOULDER DISLOCATION

Shoulder dislocations are common injuries resulting from blunt trauma or hyperextension. Usual **symptoms** include the injured child holding the arm away from the body. (Fractured humerus usually causes the person to hold the arm against the body with the arm across the chest.) There is usually acute severe pain in the shoulder, obvious squaring deformity, and functional loss. There may be numbness or partial paralysis of the arm from compression on nerves or blood vessels. The trainer should not attempt to reduce the dislocation, as this could cause further damage. Initially, the arm should be supported by placing a pillow or another roll (such as a blanket) between the chest wall and the arm. Then, an arm sling with swathing may be applied to prevent pressure on the joint. Pulses and circulation must be monitored. Procedural sedation and analgesia are usually used for reduction with young children, but local intraarticular anesthetic or nerve block may be used in some cases. Radiographs should be taken before and after reduction.

DEVELOPMENTAL DYSPLASIA OF THE HIP

Developmental dysplasia of the hip can be one of several abnormalities, the most common of which is subluxation of the hips. The problems can be associated with other congenital disorders. They can be caused by a breech position or delivery, relaxing of the ligaments (maternal hormones), or genetics. In babies, the practitioner looks for gluteal folds that are not symmetrical, asymmetrical movement of the hips, and several other signs (Ortolani, Barlow, Galeazzi signs, which are manual tests or observations done to determine proper hip movement and placement). Older children may display a limp, odd gait, or Trendelenburg's sign.

LAB FINDINGS, NURSING CARE, AND TREATMENT FOR DDH

X-rays may help with diagnosis after about 6 months of age. An ultrasound, CT scan, or arthrography can also be helpful in diagnosing and treating the disorder. Infants up to six months of age may wear a Pavlik harness, which stabilizes the joint, after which they move into an abduction brace. For older infants, traction following by closed reduction with a cast will stabilize the joint. They may need open reduction followed by a spica cast and abduction splint. Older children usually require surgery. After six years of age, reduction is usually not successful and is not advised. Assess for neurovascular problems while in a cast or brace, and monitor for skin breakdown.

Newborns with this condition are treated with a Pavlik harness that keeps the legs in alignment, which strengthens the ligaments around the joint. Older infants and children are placed into a spica cast for several weeks to maintain proper alignment of the legs for healing.

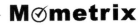

OSTEOGENESIS IMPERFECTA

There are four types of osteogenesis imperfecta (OI) disorders, ranging from mild to severe. This genetic abnormality affects the connective tissue and bones, resulting in loose joints, weak muscles and fractures. The bones become deformed and won't grow correctly. Symptoms include unexplained fractures, loose joints, thin skin, bleeding from the nose, mouth, or throat, bruising, sweating, and blue-tinged sclera. X-rays will show multiple old and new fractures, deformities, and poor bone density. The nurse should handle the child gently at all times and assess for fractures. The family needs the following teaching: make the home safe for the child with OI, enforce a proper diet (low calorie, low fat, high fiber), take special care of teeth, good skin care, and prevention of injuries. The family needs support since this disorder can appear as child abuse to some people. After diagnosis, the parents need to carry a letter explaining the disorder.

GENU VARUM AND GENU VALGUM

Genu varum (bowlegs) and genu valgum (knock-kneed) are normal progressions in straightening of the legs. **Genu varum** (lateral bowing of the tibia) is present in infants until after they begin to walk and strengthen muscles. It is clinically significant if the measured distance between the knees is >2 inches (5 cm) or if it persists beyond age 2-3. As the legs begin to straighten the next stage is **genu valgum** in which the knees come together with the ankles separated. Children remain knock-kneed from about ages 2-5 although it may persist until age 7 in some children. It is clinically significant if the measured distance between the ankles (malleoli) is >3 inches (7.5 cm) or if it persists after about age 7, at which time the legs should straighten so the child can stand with the knees and ankles together.

LEGG-CALVÉ-PERTHES DISEASE

Legg-Calvé-Perthes disease is avascular necrosis of the femoral head resulting from compromised blood supply, which may result from genetic predisposition, traumatic injury, low birth weight, and exposure to environmental tobacco smoke. It is most common between 2-12 with peak incidence at 4-8, affecting boys 4 times more than girls. There are 5 **stages**:

1. Pre-necrotic injury interferes with blood supply.
2. Necrosis (3-6 months) is the avascular stage with mild pain or limp but normal radiograph.
3. Revascularization (1-4 years) with pain and limited movement and sometimes fractures of the femoral head. Necrotic bone is resorbed and new bone deposited.
4. Healing involves reossification of bone and decrease in pain.
5. Remodeling is the end of the healing process with no pain and improved function.

Treatment to prevent pain and deformity:

- Traction to maintain abduction followed by Petrie (abduction) casting
  OR
- Adductor tenotomy followed by Toronto (abduction) brace

SCOLIOSIS

Scoliosis is abnormal curvature of the spine. It can be congenital or caused by trauma, neuromuscular abnormalities, contractures of the hip or knee, or a leg length discrepancy, but most of the time there is no known cause. The curve will worsen during the growth spurts, but stabilize when the child stops growing. If the curve is bad enough, the child may have trouble breathing, leading to respiratory distress. Some cases go unnoticed for a while, until an observer notices the curve or that one shoulder is higher than the other. X-rays show the degree of curve. An MRI can diagnose any underlying diseases that can be causing the scoliosis. A brace may be required, which can cause emotional problems in the growing child. If surgery is needed, monitor for adequate neurological, cardiovascular, skin, and bowel and bladder functioning.

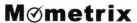

PROGRESSIVE INFANTILE MUSCULAR ATROPHY

Progressive infantile muscular atrophy (Werdnig-Hoffmann disease) is an autosomal recessive inherited disorder ("floppy infant syndrome") with progressive weakness and wasting of skeletal muscles caused by degeneration of anterior horn cells of the spinal cord and the motor nuclei of the brainstem. There are three different groups of the disorder, characterized by different onset and symptoms:

- **Group 1**: Most severe with onset ≤2 months. Children are alert with normal intellect but weak and inactive and have little movement of extremities except for fingers and toes. The motor skills do not progress, and the child usually dies by age 3.
- **Group 2**: Onset is 2-12 months and progresses from weakness of arms and legs to generalized. Pectus excavatum is prominent. Life expectancy ranges from 7 months to 7 years.
- **Group 3**: Onset in 2nd year with normal control of head but thigh and hip muscles are weak and there is lumbar lordosis, waddling gait, and protruding abdomen. Child is usually wheelchair bound between 10-20 years of age.

OSTEOMYELITIS

Musculoskeletal infections encompass a variety of different disorders with differing pathologies. Osteomyelitis, cellulitis, and septic arthritis are examples of musculoskeletal infections that can be both serious and debilitating in nature.

Osteomyelitis is an infection of the bone that can occur from an open fracture or an infection that has occurred somewhere else in the body. Osteomyelitis can also be caused by wounds or soft tissue infections that have progressed and extended to the bone. Signs and symptoms of osteomyelitis include pain, swelling, erythema and possible drainage at the site. The patient may also experience fever and chills. Diagnosis includes lab work including a complete blood count, erythrocyte sedimentation rate (ESR), C-reactive protein (CRP), and blood cultures, as well as radiologic testing that may include CT, MRI, x-ray, bone scan, or a bone biopsy. Treatment includes the administration of IV antibiotics. A needle aspiration may be performed to determine the organism and drain the area. Surgical irrigation and debridement may also be indicated.

FRACTURES

PEDIATRIC FRACTURES

Pediatric fracture types include the following:

- **Bend**: Children's flexible bones may bend up to 45° without breaking. While they will slowly straighten, they will not do so completely. Bends are most common in the ulna with fracture of the radius and in the fibula with fracture of the tibia.
- **Buckle**: When porous bone is compressed, a bulging occurs, usually near the metaphysis. Buckles are most common in younger children.
- **Complete**: The bone fragments are completely separated but may be attached on one side by a periosteal hinge.
- **Comminuted**: A comminuted fracture involves bone fragments chipping off from the broken bone and lying in the surrounding tissue. Because children's bones are more pliable than adults', comminuted fractures are rare but may occur in adolescents.
- **Greenstick**: This is an incomplete fracture on one side of a bone.
- **Spiral**: This spiraling, circular fracture goes around the bone shaft and often results from child abuse.

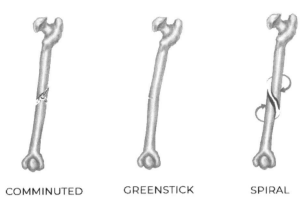

COMMINUTED   GREENSTICK   SPIRAL

DIAGNOSIS AND TREATMENT

Fractures and dislocations are commonly diagnosed by clinical examination, history, and radiographs. Careful inspection, observation of range of motion, palpation, and observation of abnormalities are important because pain may be referred. Neurovascular assessment should be done immediately to prevent vascular compromise. Radiographs should usually precede reduction of dislocations to ensure there are no fractures and follow reduction to ensure the dislocation is reduced. **Treatment** includes:

- Analgesia and sedation as indicated
- Application of cold compresses and elevation of fractured area to reduce edema
- Reduction of fracture: Steady and gradual longitudinal traction to realign bone
- Immobilization with brace, cast, sling, or splint indicated
- Reduction of dislocation: Varies according to area of dislocation
- Open fracture:
  - o Wound irrigation with NS
  - o Tetanus prophylaxis
  - o Antibiotic prophylaxis
  - o Referral to orthopedic specialist for open fractures, irreducible dislocations, and complications such as compartment syndrome or circulatory impairment

FRACTURED RIBS

Fractured ribs are usually an indication of severe injury in children because the elasticity of their ribs generally makes them resistant to fracture. Most fractures are the result of severe trauma, such as blunt force from a motor vehicle accident or physical abuse. Children presenting with rib fractures from "falls" or other vague reports of injury should be examined for signs of abuse and have a radionuclide bone scan that will show both new and old fractures. Since much force is required to fracture a child's ribs, underlying injuries should be expected according to the area of fractures.

- **Upper 4 ribs**: Injuries to trachea, bronchi, or great vessels
- **Middle ribs (5-9)**: Pneumothorax or hemothorax from penetration wounds
- **Lower ribs**: Trauma to liver, kidney, and/or spleen

Treatment is primarily supportive as rib fractures usually heal in about 6 weeks. Underlying injuries are treated according to the type and degree of injury. Supplemental oxygen is provided if indicated. Administer analgesia. Provide pulmonary physiotherapy.

FRACTURE OF THE CLAVICLE

Fracture of the clavicle is the most common pediatric fracture, with some associated with childbirth trauma and half occurring <age 7. There are three **classes**:

- **Middle third of clavicle** (80%): Usually from force on the lateral shoulder related to fall, motor vehicle accident, or sports injury. Treatment includes sling or figure-eight immobilization. Displaced fractures may be surgically repaired.
- **Lateral third** (15%): Usually from force on top of shoulder and may be nondisplaced (type I), displaced (type II), or involving the articular surface of the joint (type III). Treatment includes ice (initially) and sling. Displaced fractures usually require surgical repair.
- **Medial third** (5%): Usually from force against the anterior chest. Treatment includes ice (initially), reduction if displaced, sling, and close observation for intrathoracic injury.

Indications include pain, restricted movement of upper extremity, edema, deformity, and bruising. With compression of nerves or vasculature, circulatory compromise and numbness or weakness may be evident. In rare cases, pneumothorax may occur.

FRACTURE OF THE WRIST

A wrist fracture can occur in the distal radius (thumb side), ulna, or the wrist joint. The radius is the most commonly fractured, but both the radius and ulna may be fractured. Fracture usually occurs from falls with the weight falling on an outstretched hand, resulting in hyperextension, or direct blunt trauma. It is most common in sports such as football, soccer, hockey, skiing, and ice-skating. Pain is usually severe and deformity may be obvious. Mobility is often markedly decreased and the child has an inability to bear any weight on the wrist. Edema often begins immediately, and there may be tingling or numbness as nerves are compressed. Any bleeding should be controlled with compression and dressings applied to open wounds. The bones are aligned and wrist casted or splinted. If both bones are broken, internal fixation may be required.

ELBOW DISLOCATION/FRACTURE

Dislocation or fracture of an elbow may present with similar symptoms and radiograph may be needed for diagnosis. The injury usually results from fall or blunt trauma to the elbow. The child complains of severe pain, and muscle spasms may occur. Mobility is limited and there may be obvious deformity. Usually, edema begins immediately after injury. There may be pallor and coolness of the arm and hand distal to the injury. The child may exhibit signs of shock. Immediate care includes treating for shock, monitoring pulses, and splinting the elbow. No attempt should be made to change the position of the elbow as it may increase damage to nerves and vessels. It should be splinted as found and ice applied initially. Supracondylar fractures are common in children <8 while epicondylar fractures are common in children 9-14. Growth plate fractures may arrest growth. **Treatment** depends on degree and specific site of injury and may include manipulation; immobilization in sling, cast, or splint; or surgical repair.

FRACTURE OF THE TIBIA/FIBULA

Fracture of the tibia or fibula, or both bones, may occur as a result of a twisting injury at any point from the proximal to the distal ends. The fibula is more protected by tissue, and fracture of this bone alone may be more difficult to detect as the tibia provides a natural splint. There may be little obvious deformity, and the child may be able to walk. Tibia fractures are more likely to result in an open fracture because of proximity to the skin surface. If both bones are fractured, there is usually pronounced deformity and edema at the site of the fractures with severe pain and marked tenderness on palpation. Immediate treatment includes stopping blood flow with compression, monitoring pulses, applying dressing to an open wound, splinting the leg with rigid splints on each side of the leg to prevent the legs from rotating, and parenteral analgesia. **Treatment** may include immobilization with cast or splint or surgical fixation, depending on site and degree of injury.

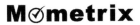

SPRAIN INJURIES

A sprain is damage to a joint, with a partial rupture of the supporting ligaments, usually caused by wrenching or twisting that may occur with a fall. The rupture can damage blood vessels, resulting in edema, tenderness at the joint, and pain on movement with pain increasing over 2–3 hours after injury. An avulsion fracture (bone fragment pulled away by a ligament) may occur with strain, so x-rays rule out fractures. Sprains may be **classified** according to severity.

- **1st degree**: This is a relatively mild degree of injury, usually associated with good range of motion and mild pain. Swelling may vary considerably, depending upon whether vessels are disrupted by the sprain.
- **2nd degree**: This comprises a wide range of signs and symptoms, as there is further injury and partial rupture of the ligaments. Usually range of motion is limited by pain. Edema and bruising are usually present but vary in degree. The joint may be somewhat unstable.
- **3rd degree**: This involves total rupture of the ligament with immediate marked pain (although sometimes less than with 2nd degree), bruising, edema, and decreased range of motion. The joint is usually markedly unstable.

MUSCLE STRAIN

A strain is an overstretching of a part of the musculature ("pulled muscle") that causes microscopic tears in the muscle or tendon, usually resulting from excess stress or overuse of the muscle. Strains may be caused by blunt trauma to a muscle or overstretching related to sports activities, such as field events, football, and soccer. Common sites for strains include the ankle, back, and hamstrings. Neglect of warm-up routines and fatigue may increase risk of strains. Onset of pain is usually sudden with local tenderness on use of the muscle.

Strains are **classified** according to severity of injury.

- **1st degree**: This injury is relatively mild, and symptoms, such as slight discomfort and tenderness to palpation, may be delayed until the following day, as the athlete may be unaware of the injury. Range of motion remains intact.
- **2nd degree**: This injury comprises a wide range of symptoms resulting from stretching or partial tearing of the muscle or tendon. Pain is usually felt on injury with tenderness on palpation and decreased passive and active range of motion, depending upon the site of injury. There may be signs of injury, such as edema and bruising. Pain increases with passive stretching or active contraction of injured muscles.
- **3rd degree**: The muscle or tendon is completely ruptured and pain occurs with injury. A defect may be palpable. Often there is extensive edema and bruising from injury to vasculature. While loss of function in affected muscle occurs, strength and loss of range of motion varies according to site of injury.

232

Hematologic Pathophysiology

THALASSEMIA

Thalassemia refers to a group of inherited blood disorders in which hemoglobin production is increased, resulting in destruction of RBCs. **Thalassemia minor** usually produces no symptoms and results in slight anemia. **Thalassemia major** produces symptoms starting at about 6 months of age, such as anemia, fever, loss of appetite and weight, and enlarged spleen. These symptoms are followed by hypoxia, damage to some major organs, jaundice, slow growth, thickened cranial bones and delayed sexual maturation. Over time, complications can include skeletal deformities of the face and head, fractures, splenomegaly, heart problems, enlarged liver and cirrhosis, gallstones, jaundice, growth delays and endocrine system abnormalities (diabetes). Hgb and Hct will be decreased. A complete blood count will show small red blood cells with varying sizes and shapes, spotted staining, nonspecific enlarged RBCs, and decreased reticulocytes.

HYPERBILIRUBINEMIA

Hyperbilirubinemia, excess of bilirubin in the blood, is characterized by jaundice. There are four basic types:

- **Physiologic**: Common in newborns and usually benign, resulting from immature hepatic function and increased RBC hemolysis. Onset is usually within 24-48 hours, peaking in 72 hours and declining within a week. Phototherapy is the indicated treatment.
- **Breast-feeding associated**: Relates to inadequate calories during early breast-feeding with onset in the first 2-3 days. More frequent feeding with caloric supplements is usually sufficient, but phototherapy may be used for bilirubin 18-20 mg/dL.
- **Breast milk jaundice**: May result from breast milk breaking down bilirubin and its being reabsorbed in the gut. Jaundice is characterized by less frequent stools and onset in the 4th or 5th day, peaking in 10-15 days, but it may persist for a number of weeks. Treatment involves discontinuing breastfeeding for 24 hours.
- **Hemolytic**: Caused by blood/antigen (Rh) incompatibility with onset in the first 24 hours. Preventive treatment is RhoGAM prenatally or post-natal exchange transfusion.

SCID

Severe combined immunodeficiency (SCID) ("bubble boy disorder") is a genetic disorder characterized by dysfunction of one or both of the T- and B-lymphocytes, essentially crippling the immune system so that the child has no immune response to pathogenic microorganisms. Many different molecular variations occur, but all have the lack of antibody formation. The disorder may be X-linked (50%) or autosomal recessive. Onset of **symptoms** is usually within the first 2 months and includes:

- Severe infection, especially pneumonia or sepsis from bacterial, herpetic, or fungal infections with associated fever, tachypnea, dyspnea, tachycardia
- Marked failure to thrive with retarded growth
- Chronic diarrhea and dehydration
- Fever, tachypnea

Without diagnosis and treatment, most children will die before 2 years of age.

Treatment:

- Prophylactic antibiotics: trimethoprim-sulfamethoxazole (Bactrim)
- Bone marrow/stem cell transplant
- Intravenous immunoglobulin replacement therapy (if B cells fail to graft)
- Gene therapy (experimental)

233

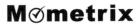

ANEMIA

Anemia occurs when there is an insufficient number of red blood cells to sufficiently oxygenate the body. As a result of the decreased level of oxygen being supplied to the organs, the body will attempt to compensate by increasing cardiac output and redistributing blood to the brain and heart. In return, the blood supply to the skin, abdominal organs, and kidneys is decreased. Anemia can occur from blood loss, increased destruction of red blood cells (hemolytic anemia), or as a result of a decreased production in red blood cells.

Signs and symptoms: Pallor, fatigue, hypotension, weakness, and mental status changes. As perfusion decreases and the body attempts to compensate for the lack of oxygenation, tachycardia, chest pain, and shortness of breath may occur. In hemolytic anemias, jaundice and splenomegaly may occur as the result of the breakdown of red blood cells and the excretion of bilirubin.

Diagnosis: A complete blood count, reticulocyte count, and iron studies may be used to diagnose anemia.

Treatment: The treatment of anemia is focused on treating the underlying cause. Parenteral iron may be given for patients with iron deficiency anemias caused from chronic blood loss, or inadequate iron intake or absorption. Blood transfusions are used to treat patients with active bleeding as well as those patients who are displaying significant clinical symptoms. Erythropoietin stimulating proteins may also be utilized to decrease the need for a transfusion.

SICKLE CELL DISEASE

Sickle cell disease is a recessive genetic disorder of chromosome 11, causing hemoglobin to be defective so that red blood cells (RBCs) are sickle-shaped and inflexible, resulting in their accumulating in small vessels and causing painful blockage. While normal RBCs survive 120 days, sickled cells may survive only 10-20 days, stressing the bone marrow that cannot produce fast enough and resulting in severe anemia. There are 5 variations of sickle cell disease, with sickle cell anemia the most severe. Different types of crises occur (aplastic, hemolytic, vaso-occlusive, and sequestrating), which can cause infarctions in organs, severe pain, damage to organs, and rapid enlargement of liver and spleen. Complications include anemia, acute chest syndrome, congestive heart failure, strokes, delayed growth, infections, pulmonary hypertension, liver and kidney disorders, retinopathy, seizures, and osteonecrosis. Sickle cell disease occurs almost exclusively in African Americans in the United States, with 8-10% carriers.

> **Review Video: What is Sickle Cell Disease?**
> Visit mometrix.com/academy and enter code: 603869

TREATMENT

Treatment for sickle cell disease includes:

- **Prophylactic penicillin** for children from 2 months to 5 years to prevent pneumonia
- **IV fluids** to prevent dehydration
- **Analgesics** (morphine) during painful crises
- **Folic acid** for anemia
- **Oxygen** for congestive heart failure or pulmonary disease
- **Blood transfusions** with chelation therapy to remove excess iron OR erythropheresis, in which red cells are removed and replaced with healthy cells, either autologous or from a donor
- **Hematopoietic stem cells transplantation** is the only curative treatment, but immunosuppressive drugs must be used and success rates are only about 85%, so the procedure is only used on those at high risk. It requires ablation of bone marrow, placing the patient at increased risk.
- **Partial chimerism** uses a mixture of the donor and the recipient's bone marrow stem cells and does not require ablation of bone marrow. It is showing good success.

VON WILLEBRAND DISEASE

Von Willebrand disease is a group of congenital bleeding disorders (inherited from either parent) affecting 1-2% of the population, associated with deficiency or lack of von Willebrand factor (vWF), a glycoprotein that is synthesized, stored, and secreted by vascular endothelial cells. This protein interacts with thrombocytes to create a clot and prevent hemorrhage; however, with von Willebrand disease, this clotting mechanism is impaired. There are three types:

- **Type I**: Low levels of vWF and also sometimes factor VIII (dominant inheritance)
- **Type II**: Abnormal vWF (subtypes a, b) may increase or decrease clotting (dominant inheritance)
- **Type III**: Absence of vWF and less than 10% factor VIII (recessive inheritance)

Symptoms vary in severity and include bruising, menorrhagia, recurrent epistaxis, and hemorrhage.

Treatment includes:

- **Desmopressin acetate** parenterally or nasally to stimulate production of clotting factor (mild cases)
- **Severe bleeding**: factor VIII concentrates with vWF, such as Humate-P

HEMOPHILIA

Hemophilia is an inherited disorder in which the person lacks adequate clotting factors. There are three types:

- **Type A**: lack of clotting factor VIII (90% of cases)
- **Type B**: lack of clotting factor IX
- **Type C**: lack of clotting factor XI (affects both sexes, rarely occurs in the United States)

Both Type A and B are usually X-linked disorders, affecting only males. The severity of the disease depends on the amount of clotting factor in the blood.

Symptoms:

- Bleeding with severe trauma or stress (mild cases)
- Unexplained bruises, bleeding, swelling, joint pain
- Spontaneous hemorrhage (severe cases), often in the joints but can be anywhere in the body
- Epistaxis, mucosal bleeding
- First symptoms often occur during infancy when the child becomes active, resulting in frequent bruises

Treatment:

- Desmopressin acetate parenterally or nasally to stimulate production of clotting factor (mild cases)
- Infusions of clotting factor from donated blood or recombinant clotting factors (genetically engineered), utilizing guidelines for dosing
- Infusions of plasma (Type C)

THROMBOCYTOPENIA

Thrombocytopenia is a deficiency of circulating platelets in the blood. It can be caused by a decrease in the production of platelets from the bone marrow or an increase in destruction of platelets. Thrombocytopenia may also be caused from the use of heparin. Heparin induced thrombocytopenia can occur after heparin therapy (average 4-14 days post therapy) and is characterized by a decrease in platelet count to less than 50% of baseline or the occurrence of an unexplained thrombolytic event. A decreased production of platelets within the bone marrow can occur as a result of malignancy, bone marrow failure, infection, alcohol abuse, or a nutritional deficiency. An increase in the destruction of platelets may occur in disseminated intravascular coagulation, vasculitis, thrombotic thrombocytopenic purpura, sepsis, or idiopathic thrombocytopenic purpura.

Signs and symptoms: Signs and symptoms may include petechiae, ecchymosis, bleeding from the mouth or gums, epistaxis, pallor, weakness, fatigue, splenomegaly, blood in the urine or stool, and jaundice.

Diagnosis: Physical exam and lab studies including complete blood count, partial thromboplastin time and prothrombin time may be used to diagnosis thrombocytopenia. A bone marrow biopsy may be indicated to determine the cause of the decreased production of platelets.

Treatment: Treatment of thrombocytopenia involves identifying and treating the underlying cause. Medications that decrease the platelet count should be held. Platelet transfusions may be administered to patients with extremely low counts (less than 50,000) or if spontaneous bleeding occurs. Platelet transfusions are contraindicated in patients with thrombotic thrombocytopenia purpura.

ITP

The autoimmune disorder **idiopathic thrombocytopenic purpura (ITP)** causes an immune response to platelets, resulting in decreased platelet counts. ITP affects primarily children and young women although it can occur at any age. The acute form primarily occurs in children, but the chronic form affects primarily adults. Platelet counts are usually 150,000–400,000 per mcL. With ITP, platelet levels are less than 100,000. Maintaining a platelet count of at least 30,000 is necessary to prevent intracranial hemorrhage, the primary concern. The cause of ITP is unclear and may be precipitated by viral infection, sulfa drugs, and conditions, such as lupus erythematosus. ITP is usually not life threatening and can be controlled. **Symptoms** include:

- Bruising and petechiae with hematoma in some cases
- Epistaxis
- Increased menstrual flow in post-puberty females

Treatment includes:

- Corticosteroids to depress immune response and increase platelet count
- Splenectomy may be indicated for chronic conditions
- Platelet transfusions
- Avoiding aspirin, ibuprofen, or other NSAIDs

HITTS

Heparin-induced thrombocytopenia and thrombosis syndrome (HITTS) occurs in patients receiving heparin for anticoagulation. There are two types:

- **Type I** is a transient condition occurring within a few days and causing depletion of platelets ($<100,000$ mm³), but heparin may be continued as the condition usually resolves without intervention.
- **Type II** is an autoimmune reaction to heparin that occurs in 3–5% of those receiving unfractionated heparin and also occurs with low-molecular-weight heparin. It is characterized by low platelets ($<50,000$ mm³) that are ≥50% below baseline. Onset is 5–14 days but can occur within hours of heparinization. Death rates are <30%. Heparin-antibody complexes form and release platelet factor 4 (PF4), which attracts heparin molecules and adheres to platelets and endothelial lining, stimulating thrombin and platelet clumping. This puts the patient at risk for thrombosis and vessel occlusion rather than hemorrhage, causing stroke, myocardial infarction, and limb ischemia with symptoms associated with the site of thrombosis. Treatment includes:
  - Discontinuation of heparin
  - Direct thrombin inhibitors (lepirudin, argatroban)
  - Monitor for signs/symptoms of thrombus/embolus

TRANSFUSION COMPONENTS

Blood components that are commonly used for transfusions include:

- **Packed red blood cells:** RBCs (250-300 mL per unit) should be warmed >30 °C (optimal 37 °C) before administration to prevent hypothermia and may be reconstituted in 50-100 mL of normal saline to facilitate administration. RBCs are necessary if blood loss is about 30% (1,500-2,000 mL lost; Hgb ≤7). Above 30% blood loss, whole blood may be more effective. RBCs are most frequently used for transfusions.

- **Platelet concentrates:** Transfusions of platelets are used if the platelet count is <50,000 cells/mm³. One unit increases the platelet count by 5,000-10,000 cells/mm³. Platelet concentrates pose a risk for sensitization reactions and infectious diseases. Platelet concentrate is stored at a higher temperature (20-24 °C) than RBCs. This contributes to bacterial growth, so it is more prone to bacterial contamination than other blood products and may cause sepsis. Temperature increase within 6 hours should be considered an indication of possible sepsis. ABO compatibility should be observed but is not required.

- **Fresh frozen plasma** (FFP) (obtained from a unit of whole blood frozen ≤6 hours after collection) includes all clotting factors and plasma proteins, so each unit administered increases clotting factors by 2-3%. FFP may be used for deficiencies of isolated factors, excess warfarin therapy, and liver-disease-related coagulopathy. It may be used for patients who have received extensive blood transfusions but continue to hemorrhage. It is also helpful for those with antithrombin III deficiency. FFP should be warmed to 37 °C prior to administration to avoid hypothermia. ABO compatibility should be observed if possible, but it is not required. Some patients may become sensitized to plasma proteins.

- **Cryoprecipitate** is the precipitate that forms when FFP is thawed. It contains fibrinogen, factor VIII, von Willebrand, and factor XIII. This component may be used to treat hemophilia A and hypofibrinogenemia.

TRANSFUSION ADMINISTRATION

Prior to the transfusion of any blood component, the nurse should obtain the patient's transfusion history along with a consent form. A type and crossmatch must be completed on the patient's blood and an IV in place for administration. An 18-gauge catheter is standard, but 22-gauge can also be used at a slower rate. Baseline vital signs need to be taken prior to starting the infusion, and then the patient should be under direct observation for at least the first 15 minutes. Vital signs should be monitored at 5 minutes, 15 minutes, and then at least every 30 minutes during the transfusion and one hour post-transfusion.

> **Review Video: Blood Transfusions**
> Visit mometrix.com/academy and enter code: 759682

TRANSFUSION-RELATED COMPLICATIONS

There are a number of transfusion-related complications, which is the reason that transfusions are given only when necessary. Complications include:

- **Infection:** Bacterial contamination of blood, especially platelets, can result in severe sepsis. A number of infective agents (viral, bacterial, and parasitic) can be transmitted, although increased testing of blood has decreased rates of infection markedly. Infective agents include HIV, hepatitis C and B, human T-cell lymphotropic virus, CMV, WNV, malaria, Chagas' disease, and variant Creutzfeldt-Jacob disease (from contact with mad cow disease).

- **Transfusion-related acute lung injury (TRALI):** This respiratory distress syndrome occurs ≤6 hours after transfusion. The cause is believed to be antileukocytic or anti-HLA antibodies in the transfusion. It is characterized by non-cardiogenic pulmonary edema (high protein level) with severe dyspnea and arterial hypoxemia. Transfusion must be stopped immediately and the blood bank notified. TRALI may result in fatality but usually resolves in 12-48 hours with supportive care.

- **Graft vs. host disease:** Lymphocytes cause an immune response in immunocompromised individuals. Lymphocytes may be inactivated by irradiation, as leukocyte filters are not reliable.
- **Post-transfusion purpura:** Platelet antibodies develop and destroy the patient's platelets, so the platelet count decreases about 1 week after transfusion.
- **Transfusion-related immunosuppression:** Cell-mediated immunity is suppressed, so the patient is at increased risk of infection, and in cancer patients, transfusions may correlate with tumor recurrence. This condition relates to transfusions that include leukocytes. RBCs cause a less pronounced immunosuppression, suggesting a causative agent is in the plasma. Leukoreduction is becoming more common to reduce transmission of leukocyte-related viruses.
- **Hypothermia**: This may occur if blood products are not heated. Oxygen utilization is halved for each 10 °C decrease in normal body temperature.

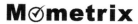

Immunologic/Oncologic Pathophysiology

HIV/AIDS

Children born to mothers with HIV/AIDS may show false positive or false negative results on antibody testing after birth because of passage of maternal immunoglobulin across the placenta; the mother's HIV antibodies may be present for up to 18 months. Therefore, virologic testing must be done. The HIV DNA polymerase chain reaction assay (PCR) or RNA assay is performed for infants at risk after birth, at 1-2 months, and at 3-6 month. Both tests are almost 100% effective by age 3 months. Many use PCR for initial diagnosis with confirmation by RNA assay. HIV antibody testing may be done at 18 months to confirm seroconversion to negative. Children with HIV positive status are started on treatment although some will progress to AIDS. Mortality rates have fallen over 80% with new treatments. **Symptoms** that indicate AIDS include:

- Failure to thrive and developmental abnormalities
- Hepatosplenomegaly
- Respiratory distress with chronic interstitial pneumonia, PCP
- Oral candidiasis
- Recurrent infections
- Lymphadenopathy, generalized

TREATMENT

Pediatric HIV treatment involves combination therapy with at least 3 anti-retroviral drugs: NRTIs, NNRTIs, PIs, and fusion inhibitors. Factors to be considered:

- Severity of disease and co-morbid conditions
- Short and long-term effects of treatment
- Initial treatment's effect on later treatment
- Compliance of child/parent with regimen
- Whether HIV acquired perinatally or through other means
- Stage of puberty (early puberty = pediatric regimen; late puberty = adult regimen) although puberty is often delayed
- Antiviral drug resistance testing to insure proper treatment

Treatment is based on CD4 counts, according to age, indicating the amount of immunosuppression:

Category	Level of detectable CD4 Suppression	CD4 Count Based on Age
Category 1	No detectable suppression	<1 yr: ≥1500 1-5 yrs: ≥1000 6-12 yrs: ≥500
Category 2	Moderate suppression	<1 yr: 750-1499 1-5 yrs: 500-999 6-12 yrs: 200-499
Category 3	Severe suppression	<1 yr: <750 1-5 yrs: <500 6-12 yrs: <200

COMMON TYPES OF CHILDHOOD CANCERS

Among children, the most common types of cancers include leukemia, brain cancer, and lymphoma:

- **Leukemia** is a cancer that causes abnormally high levels of white blood cells within the bone marrow, eventually prohibiting the body from producing other important blood cells, such as red blood cells and platelets. Leukemia may be classified as lymphocytic or myelogenous, depending on the type of blood cells affected.
- **Brain cancers** typically develop as brain tumors and may be considered slow-growing or aggressive. Brain tumors are also classified as localized or invasive; both descriptions define the course of treatment for the child.
- **Lymphoma** is a type of cancer that grows in the lymph system, which includes the lymph nodes, spleen, tonsils, and bone marrow. The condition is classified as either Hodgkin's lymphoma or non-Hodgkin's lymphoma, depending on the presence of certain types of cells.

> **Review Video: Lymphoma**
> Visit mometrix.com/academy and enter code: 513277

LEUKEMIA

Leukemia occurs when the bone marrow makes an overabundance of white blood cells that are abnormal. It is seen mostly in 3- to 5-year-olds and the most common type is **acute lymphocytic leukemia** (ALL). The red blood cells will be suppressed, causing the child to be tired, pale, and tachycardic. Suppression of platelets will cause bleeding. The immune system will be compromised from WBC suppression, causing infections. There may be bone pain, enlarged liver, spleen, and lymph nodes, headache, increased ICP, vomiting, and weight loss. Diagnosis is assisted by a CBC (abnormal WBC count, decreased RBCs and platelets), a bone marrow aspiration (leukemic cells), and a lumbar puncture (abnormal cells in the CSF).

AML AND ALL

Acute myeloid leukemia (AML) and acute lymphocytic leukemia (ALL) are the two most common types of leukemias that affect children.

- **AML** is also referred to as granulocytic, myelocytic, monocytic, myelogenous, monoblastic, and monomyeloblastic leukemia. It is caused by a defect in the stem cells that differentiate into all myeloid cells. It affects all ages, occurring in children and adults and often has a genetic component. Survival rates with adequate treatment are about 50%.
- **ALL** is also referred to as lymphatic, lymphocytic, lymphoblastic, or lymphoblastoid leukemia and is caused by a defect in the stem cells that differentiate into lymphocytes. This is the most common type of childhood leukemia, peaking between ages 2-5. The cause is not known. There are a number of different types of ALL, and treatment and survival relate to the type. Overall survival rates with adequate treatment are about 80%.

Some rare forms of leukemia are named for the cells involved, such as basophilic leukemia.

TREATMENT OPTIONS

Leukemia treatment depends upon the protocol established for each type of leukemia. Combined drugs are usually more effective than single. **Chemotherapy** usually includes three stages:

1. **Induction therapy**: The purpose is to induce remission to the point that the bone marrow is clear of disease and blood counts are normal. Chemotherapy is usually given for about 4-6 weeks, followed by transplantation or the next stage of chemotherapy. The chemotherapy is potent and suppresses blood elements, leaving the body at risk for serious infections and hemorrhage, so supportive care is critical.

2. **Consolidation therapy**: The goal is to kill any cells that may have escaped the induction stage. This stage lasts 4-8 months. Intrathecal chemotherapy may be administered concurrently as a prophylaxis to prevent CNS involvement.

3. **Maintenance therapy**: Treatment may continue for another 2-3 years, but with less intense chemotherapy to maintain the child in remission. Weekly blood counts monitor progress and side effects.

Sometimes after the three stages of chemotherapy are completed, the child will relapse and leukemic cells return. In that case, re-induction is carried out, usually using a different arsenal of drugs. Many drugs in use now, especially for relapses, are those in clinical trials. Clinical trials are ongoing for many chemotherapeutic agents to determine the best combination of drugs and duration of treatment. **Other treatments** may be instituted, depending on the severity of the disease:

- **Intrathecal chemotherapy** is administered into the spinal fluid for treatment of infiltration of the central nervous system.
- **Radiation** to the brain may be indicated in addition to intrathecal chemotherapy with severe disease but poses danger to brain development.
- **"Bone marrow" or cord blood transplant**, also known as hematopoietic stem cell transplantation (HCST), may be done if chemotherapy fails or after the first remission for AML, which has a lower cure rate.

BONE MARROW TRANSPLANTATION

Leukemia is a type of cancer found in the bone marrow, which ultimately impacts the ability to create healthy red and white blood cells and platelets. A **bone marrow transplant** (BMT) destroys the bone marrow, including that affected by leukemia, and replaces it with healthy bone marrow tissue, which allows children to create new blood cells. A bone marrow transplant requires a match from a donor; children may use their own bone marrow if the tissue is taken during a time of remission. Before the transplant, chemotherapy and radiation are administered to eliminate all cancerous cells. After receiving the bone marrow transplant, children must be isolated for a specified period to reduce the risk of infection; they then need time to recover from the procedure and are monitored to determine if remission occurs.

NURSING CARE OF CHILDREN UNDERGOING BMT AND OTHER NURSING CARE FOR CHILDREN WITH CANCER

BMT is undertaken to destroy leukemia cells and replace them with healthy cells, either from a donor or the child himself. Monitor for the following **complications** of BMT:

- Infection
- Anemia
- Bleeding
- GI problems
- Veno-occlusive disease (back up of blood in the liver leading to liver damage; signs are jaundice, weight gain, enlarged liver, pain in the area of the liver)
- Pneumonia
- Kidney problems
- Graft vs. host disease (rash, fever, high BP, jaundice, enlarged liver, infection)
- Graft rejection (infection, fever)

During any treatment, watch for and prevent tumor lysis (lethargy, nausea and vomiting, decreased urine output, flank pain, itching and twitching muscles), low WBC counts (respiratory distress, cyanosis, lethargy, visual problems), obstructed blood flow through the superior vena cava (cyanosis and edema of the chest and higher and bulging jugular veins), and infection. Watch for bleeding and handle the child gently to prevent bruising. Encourage good fluid intake and monitor I&O. Maintain adequate diet and mouth care. Provide pain relief as needed.

BRAIN TUMORS IN INFANTS AND CHILDREN

Any type of brain tumor can occur in children, but the most common are those that arise from immature (blast) cells or supportive (glial) tissue. The most common age group for children with brain tumors is ages 3-12.

- **Astrocytoma**: This arises from astrocytes, which are glial cells. It is the most common type of tumor. It can occur throughout the brain but is most common in the cerebellum of children. There are many types of astrocytomas, and most are slow growing. Some are operable; others are not. Radiation may be given after removal.
- **Brain stem glioma**: This may be fast or slow growing but is generally not operable because of location, although it may be treated with radiation or chemotherapy.
- **Craniopharyngioma**: This is a congenital, slow-growing, and benign cystic tumor, but it is difficult to resect and treated with surgery and radiation. They may be recurrent, especially if >5 cm, so early excision is important.
- **Ependymoma**: This is usually benign in a cerebral hemisphere. Surgical excision and radiation are done.
- **Ganglioglioma**: This can occur anywhere in the brain but 70% in children occur above the tentorium (the membrane separating the cerebellum from the occipital lobes). They are usually slow growing and benign.
- **Medulloblastoma**: There are many types of medulloblastoma. Most arise in the cerebellum, are malignant, and are fast growing. Surgical excision is done and often followed by radiation and chemotherapy although recent studies show using just chemotherapy controls recurrence with less neurological damage.
- **Oligodendroglioma**: This tumor most often occurs in the cerebrum, primarily the frontal or temporal lobes, involving the myelin sheath of the neurons.
- **Optical nerve glioma**: This slow growing tumor of the optic nerve is usually a form of astrocytoma. It is often associated with neurofibromatosis type I (NF1), occurring in 15-40%. Despite surgical, chemotherapy, or radiotherapy treatment, it is usually fatal.

SYMPTOMS AND MANAGEMENT

Brain tumors are lesions inside the cranium, seen mostly in children age 5-10 years. The hallmark **symptom** is a headache that comes and goes, occurring most often in the morning, or possibly with an increase in intracranial pressure (coughing, sneezing). Other symptoms can include projectile vomiting, changes in behavior, motor functions and speech. High BP, low pulse rate, visual disturbances and seizures may occur. The lesion may be seen on a CT scan and MRI. A lumbar puncture may be done to examine the cells, glucose, protein, and enzymes. The child should be monitored for increased ICP. Medications may include chemo and steroids. Surgery is needed to remove the tumor; the family should be counseled about the head shaving, post-op bandaging, edema, and headache. After surgery, the child will need frequent monitoring of vital signs, neuro checks, ICP, pain management, and for any signs of infection or seizures. The head should be elevated to promote drainage.

NEUROBLASTOMAS

Neuroblastoma is the most common childhood solid tumor occurring outside the brain, and the deadliest. It arises from neural crest cells, which are normally located along sympathetic nerve pathways. These tumors, therefore, can occur anywhere in the body that sympathetic nerves are found. The abdomen is the most common primary site (65%), especially involving the adrenal glands. Cervical and thoracic sites are also common, particularly in infants. Neuroblastoma accounts for about 10% of all childhood cancers and is primarily a disease of young children. About 33% of neuroblastomas are found in infancy, with nearly 90% of cases accounted for in children aged 5 and younger. The occurrence of neuroblastoma in children over 10 years old is quite rare. There are no discernible environmental risk factors for neuroblastoma. Prenatal and postnatal exposures have been investigated, but thus far, nothing conclusive has been identified. In about 20% of cases, however, an autosomal dominant genetic predilection has been described.

TYPICAL PRESENTATION

Symptoms of neuroblastoma are directly related to the site and extent of the tumor. Abdominal complaints are common and may include a feeling of fullness and subsequent discomfort. The associated tumor, then, is likely firm, fixed, and may cross mid-line. In primary liver tumors, respiratory obstruction can occur. In cases involving thoracic lesions, the tumor is often discovered incidentally during work-up for other causes. Cervical tumors may present with symptoms of Horner's syndrome (ptosis, myosis, and anhidrosis). Tumors can also occur within the subcutaneous tissue (almost always in infants); these nodules are usually nontender and have a blue coloring (blueberry muffin sign). Fever, fatigue, and irritability are also seen at presentation.

APPROPRIATE DIAGNOSTIC PROCEDURES

Physical exam should pay special attention to the size and location of any abdominal mass. Evaluation of lymph nodes, liver, and spleen are also important. A complete neurologic exam is necessary to ascertain the degree of any functional deficit. Lab studies should include a CBC, serum ferritin, and LDH levels. Urinary catecholamines typically reveal elevations in both vanillylmandelic acid and homovanillic acid. Bilateral BMA is recommended. Imaging studies should include CT or MRI with gadolinium (depending on the site), as well as bone scan and X-rays to investigate metastatic spread. Lastly, tumor biopsy will yield definitive information that will guide appropriate diagnosis and treatment.

TREATMENT PROTOCOL

Treatment of neuroblastoma will most often consist of a combination of surgery, chemotherapy, radiation therapy (RT), and/or bone marrow transplant (BMT). The degree to which any or all of these modalities are utilized is directly related to the disease stage and the child's age. Surgical treatment can include complete resection (which is curative in some cases) or debulking to diminish tumor burden. The agents most often used for chemotherapy include carboplatin, cisplatin, cyclophosphamide, ifosfamide, etoposide, doxorubicin, and vincristine. These are usually used in those with moderate to high risk. RT is administered directly to the tumor and will accompany chemotherapy and/or surgery. However, it can also be used to diminish tumor size in emergency settings or for palliation. Autologous BMT may be appropriate for patients with a poorer expected outcome. Here, autologous BMT is administered following high-dose, short-course chemotherapy.

RETINOBLASTOMA
EPIDEMIOLOGY AND ASSOCIATED PATHOLOGIC FEATURES

Retinoblastoma occurs almost exclusively in young children and accounts for about 3% of all cancer diagnoses in those under 15 years old, which translates to 200 new cases in the US annually. The median age at diagnosis is 2 years old, with 80% of diagnoses occurring by the age of 4; it is exceedingly rare in children over the age of 6. This malignancy may be either hereditary (40% of cases) or non-hereditary (60% of cases), the latter of which is predominantly unilateral. Retinoblastoma is a malignancy that arises from precursor cells that give rise to the sensory body of the eye. Histologically, the presence of Flexner-Wintersteiner rosettes is a common feature of retinoblastoma. However, other histological characteristics, such as Homer Wright rosettes, fleurettes, or a lack of rosettes altogether, can also occur. Retinoblastoma can exhibit endophytic or exophytic growth, whereby the tumor extends from the retina into either the vitreal cavity or out to the subretinal space respectively. These patterns can occur independently or simultaneously; rarely, widespread infiltration can also occur.

CLINICAL PRESENTATION AND DIAGNOSTIC TOOLS

The child with retinoblastoma is commonly brought to a healthcare provider for evaluation when a caregiver or family member notices ophthalmic changes. Leukocoria is the most common presenting sign of retinoblastoma and may be either unilateral or bilateral. Strabismus is also common. Other **signs and**

symptoms may include decreased visual acuity, heterochromia, rubeosis iridis, and hyphema. Additionally, symptoms of glaucoma (as a result of new blood vessel growth) may be present. Interestingly, pain is usually not a presenting feature, unless as a result or significant inflammation or glaucoma. In a child with any of the above features, a thorough history and physical exam are the first steps in definitive **diagnosis**. Funduscopic exam, while particularly challenging in the pediatric population, is essential. In the pediatric population, this is often performed under anesthesia. Under pupillary dilation, retinal mass, retinal detachment, hemorrhage, or other abnormalities can often be visualized. Diagnostic imaging methods, including ultrasound, CT, or MRI, are also necessary to determine any degree of extraretinal spread.

TREATMENT PROTOCOL

Treatment for retinoblastoma depends upon the tumor type and stage. There are several modalities currently used to treat retinoblastoma. These include enucleation, external beam radiation, cryotherapy, thermotherapy, laser photocoagulation, plaque radiation therapy, and chemotherapy. Enucleation is performed when visual function will not likely remain intact as a result of the extent of the disease. In cases of tumor extension into the sclera, exenteration may be performed. Patients with intraocular retinoblastoma will undergo chemotherapy. Those with bilateral familial retinoblastoma will also undergo chemotherapy; specific treatment includes vincristine, carboplatin, teniposide, and cyclophosphamide.

OSTEOSARCOMA
PRESENTING CHARACTERISTICS

Osteosarcoma is the single most common primary bone tumor in children. The presence of bone pain, especially at night, is practically universal in the presentation of osteosarcoma. This pain overlies the affected area, most commonly at the femur and tibia adjacent to the knee. A soft-tissue mass may or may not coincide with the pain. In general, osteosarcoma favors bone that is undergoing rapid growth. Therefore, the long bones of adolescents, particularly at the growth plates, are frequently the site of primary disease. Likewise, because this pain often affects the joints, and because adolescents are so active, the symptoms can be blamed on an injury. As a result, diagnosis is frequently delayed an average of 3 months from symptom onset. At the time of diagnosis, 15-20% of patients also have metastatic spread, usually in the lungs.

DIAGNOSTIC PROCEDURES

History of painful symptoms will be useful in determining the extent of disease. **Physical exam** should focus on aberrations in function within the affected limb(s). Additionally, physical assessment of the affected limb, including comparative measurements or signs of inflammation, will lend insight into the tumor. X-rays of the affected limb typically show areas of bone loss and scarring. However, such studies should also ascertain the presence of fractures. Information about the primary tumor itself should include MRI to determine tumor extent, arteriography to investigate tumor vascularity, and serum alkaline phosphatase to be utilized as a type of tumor marker. Biopsy is required for definitive diagnosis. Other imaging studies, such as chest x-ray, bone scan, or CT help to determine the presence and extent of metastases.

TREATMENT PROTOCOL

Osteosarcoma **treatment** will consist of chemotherapy followed by surgery followed by another round of chemotherapy. Chemotherapy is given on the basis that all patients with osteosarcoma are assumed to have some degree of metastatic disease. Treatment will usually include high-dose methotrexate, doxorubicin, or cisplatin; ifosfamide or etoposide may also be used. Surgical resection is aimed at complete removal of the tumor with a healthy cell margin of at least 0.5 cm around the cancer site. Surgical options may include limb salvage, arthrodesis, amputation, or rotationplasty. Radiation therapy is generally reserved for those with obvious metastatic disease or who are in end-stage care.

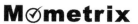

EWING SARCOMA FAMILY OF TUMORS
BIOLOGICAL DEFINITION AND ASSOCIATED EPIDEMIOLOGY

The Ewing sarcoma family of tumors (ESFT) includes neoplasms historically known as classical Ewing sarcoma of bone, extraskeletal Ewing sarcoma, and peripheral primitive neuroectodermal tumor, among others. However, advances in genetics found that nearly all these malignancies share the same genetic mutation [t(11,22)(q24,q12)] between chromosomes 11 and 22. Therefore, biopsies which reveal this aberration are definitively diagnosed as ESFT. It is exceedingly more common in children of European descent than in children of Asian or African descent with a mildly higher incidence in males. It is the second most common primary bone tumor, and occurs in 2.9 out of 1,000,000 children.

TYPICAL PRESENTATION

Like osteosarcoma, bone pain is the single most **common feature** in children with ESFT. Unlike osteosarcoma, however, the average time elapsed between symptom onset and diagnosis is 3-9 months. Bone pain typically overlies the affected structure, and although it tends to improve at night, it is usually never completely absent. Also, like osteosarcoma, the disease is frequently mistaken for trauma or overuse injury. Symptoms of pain lasting longer than one month, palpable mass, or other unusual corresponding features (e.g., fever) should prompt further investigation. X-rays will frequently reveal osteolysis of the affected bone. The pelvis is the most common site of primary ESFT, followed by femur, chest wall, and tibia. Metastatic spread favors the lungs, bone, and bone marrow and is present in 25% of patients at diagnosis.

RHABDOMYOSARCOMA
PATHOPHYSIOLOGY, INCIDENCE, AND ETIOLOGY

Rhabdomyosarcoma (RMS) falls under the category of small round blue-cell tumors. It is mesenchymal in origin, most often formed from immature skeletal muscle. Four main classifications exist: botryoid and spindle cell, embryonal, alveolar, and undifferentiated sarcoma. Both botryoid and spindle cell are considered embryonal as well. Primary sites involving the head and neck, bladder or vagina are most often seen in younger children; adolescents have a higher propensity for extremity tumors. Children aged 6 or younger account for about 66% of all new RMS cases. RMS occurs somewhat more frequently in males than females, and while the incidence is the same for African-American and Caucasian boys, in African-American girls it is about half that of Caucasian girls. The bulk of RMS cases occur at random. However, neurofibromatosis, Li-Fraumeni, and Beckwith-Wiedemann syndrome are all associated with a higher rate of RMS. Additionally, one large study showed a significant increased risk of RMS in children whose parents used marijuana, cocaine, or other illicit substances.

CLINICAL PRESENTATION

Like most solid tumors, signs and **symptoms present at diagnosis** are directly related to the location and size of the malignancy. About 40% of RMS tumors occur in the head and neck, 25% of which originate in the orbit. Orbital growths are nearly always embryonal and commonly produce proptosis; eye muscle paralysis may also occur. Other head and neck tumors may occur within the sinuses or nasopharynx. Here, symptoms include bloody or mucopurulent discharge; obstruction may also occur. About 25% of RMS tumors occur in the genitourinary tract, particularly at the bladder or prostate, and are most common in children under 4 years old. Symptoms may include hematuria, difficulty urinating (e.g., strangury), obstruction, constipation, or neoplastic extrusion. A pelvic mass may be found in prostate, cervical, and uterine cases. Testicular growths are most frequently unilateral and painless. In 20% of RMS cases, the primary site is an extremity. These are most often found in adolescents and are predominantly of alveolar histology. Symptoms are typically localized and may include pain, edema, erythema, or regional lymphatic inclusion.

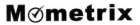

NON-RHABDOMYOSARCOMA SOFT TISSUE SARCOMAS OF CHILDHOOD

The non-rhabdomyosarcoma soft tissue sarcomas (NRSTSs) account for between 4-5% of all pediatric malignancies. Fibrosarcoma is categorized as either infantile or adult (IFS or AFS respectively); IFS is the most common NRSTS in infants. IFS occurs almost exclusively in children aged 2 or younger; AFS peaks between the ages of 10-15 years old. Clinically, children present with a rapidly enlarging mass, occurring in an extremity or on the trunk. Metastatic spread is uncommon in IFS. Synovial sarcoma is another relatively common NRSTS; pediatric cases account for 20-30% of occurrences. Presentation most frequently involves an enlarging mass occurring in the leg (thigh or knee) or upper extremity, although it can manifest in the trunk, head, or neck as well. Alveolar soft part sarcoma (ASPS) is a very rare NRSTS of undefined histology. It usually occurs in those aged 15-35 years old and presents as an extremity mass. Like synovial sarcoma, it occurs most commonly in the thigh. Metastatic disease may be present at diagnosis, with the lungs being the most common site of spread.

TREATMENT PROTOCOLS FOR ESFT, FIBROSARCOMA, GERM CELL TUMORS, AND RHABDOMYOSARCOMA

The treatment for the Ewing's sarcoma family of tumors will consist of both system and local treatment. Systemic therapy includes combination chemotherapy utilizing cyclophosphamide, ifosfamide, etoposide, dactinomycin, and doxorubicin. Local therapy will depend on the location of the tumor and its response to chemotherapy; both radiation and surgery may be used. Fibrosarcoma treatment will generally include surgical resection. In older patients, chemotherapy may be administered prior to surgical treatment. Similarly, children with germ cell tumors will often undergo pre-operative chemotherapy to diminish the tumor burden and surgical resection will round out the therapy. The preferred treatment for rhabdomyosarcoma is surgical resection; however, the size and location of the tumor may dictate other therapeutic modalities. Chemotherapy followed by radiation therapy 9 weeks later is administered to all children with this diagnosis except for those group I rhabdomyosarcoma. Chemotherapeutic agents most often used include vincristine, dactinomycin, doxorubicin, cyclophosphamide, ifosfamide, and etoposide. It is important to note that radiation therapy may be administered prior to other treatments in emergency cases.

WILMS' TUMOR

Wilms' tumor is a cancer of the kidney, usually on one side, occurring most often in children 2 to 3 years of age. Stage I refers to cancer in one kidney only; in stage V, the tumor is found in both kidneys. A mass in the abdomen is the hallmark sign, possibly with fever, pain, blood in the urine, and high BP. Diagnosis is by ultrasound or CT scan. The abdomen should not be palpated due to the risk of rupturing the tumor. Watch the child for high BP. Administer chemotherapy as prescribed. Post-op care involves monitoring and preventing bowel obstruction, infection, and pneumonia.

GRAFT VERSUS HOST DISEASE (GVHD)

Graft versus host disease (GVHD) is an immunological response to "foreign" tissue (such as a transplanted organ or non-irradiated blood transfusion). GVHD is one of the major causes of morbidity and mortality after transplantations, so immunosuppression is provided before, during, and after transplantations (usually about 6 months for allogenic stem cell transplantation and life-long for solid organs). GVHD may be acute (<100 days after transplantation) or chronic (>100 days after transplantation). **Symptoms** may involve many organs, such as the skin, the GI tract, and the liver. Patients may experience diffuse lacy maculopapular rash, nausea, vomiting, diarrhea, sloughing of mucosal tissue, and increasing bilirubin. GVHD is staged according to severity of symptoms related to the skin, GI system, and liver, with each system graded 1 to 4 depending upon severity. **Treatment** includes corticosteroids to suppress the immune response.

Endocrine Pathophysiology

DIABETES MELLITUS TYPES 1 AND 2

Diabetes mellitus is the most common metabolic disorder. Over 6% of adults have diabetes, but only 4% of adults are diagnosed. Insulin resistance tends to increase in older adults, so there is less ability to handle glucose. Type II is more common in older adults, with incidence increasing with age.

- **Type I:** Immune-mediated form with insufficient insulin production because of the destruction of pancreatic beta cells
  - o **Symptoms** include pronounced polyuria and polydipsia, short onset, obesity or recent weight loss, and ketoacidosis present on diagnosis.
  - o **Treatment** includes insulin as needed to control blood sugar, glucose monitoring 1–4 times daily, diet with carbohydrate control, and exercise.
- **Type II:** Insulin resistant form with defect in insulin secretion
  - o **Symptoms** include long onset, obesity with no weight loss or significant weight loss, mild or absent polyuria and polydipsia, ketoacidosis or glycosuria without ketonuria, androgen-mediated problems such as hirsutism and acne (adolescents), and hypertension.
  - o **Treatment** includes diet and exercise, glucose monitoring, and oral medications.

> **Review Video: <u>Diabetes Mellitus: Diet, Exercise, & Medications</u>**
> Visit mometrix.com/academy and enter code: 774388
>
> **Review Video: <u>Diabetes: Complications</u>**
> Visit mometrix.com/academy and enter code: 996788
>
> **Review Video: <u>Diabetes Mellitus</u>**
> Visit mometrix.com/academy and enter code: 501396

DIABETIC KETOACIDOSIS

Diabetic ketoacidosis is a complication of type 1 diabetes mellitus, usually related to noncompliance with treatment, stress, illness, or lack of awareness of having diabetes (this event often being the first time that diabetes is diagnosed). Inadequate production of insulin results in glucose being unavailable for metabolism, so lipolysis (breakdown of fat) produces free fatty acids (FFAs) as an alternate fuel source. Glycerol is converted to ketone bodies which are used for cellular metabolism less efficiently than glucose. Excess ketone bodies are excreted in the urine (ketonuria) or exhalations. Acidosis of any type causes potassium in cells to shift to the serum. The ketone bodies lower serum pH, leading to ketoacidosis.

Symptoms include:

- Kussmaul respirations: "Ketone breath," or fruity smelling breath; progresses to CNS depression with loss of airway
- Fluid imbalance, including loss of potassium and other electrolytes from cellular death resulting in dehydration and diuresis with excess thirst
- Dangerous cardiac arrhythmias, related to potassium loss; hypotension, chest pain, tachycardia
- GI: Nausea/vomiting, abdominal pain, loss of appetite
- Neurological: malaise, confusion/lethargy progressing to coma

Diagnosis is based on:

- Labs: Blood glucose >250 mg/dL, lower Na and elevated K (switches after treatment), elevated beta-hydroxybutyrate (byproduct of ketones)
- ABG: pH <7.3, HCO_3 <18 mEq/L
- Urine: + glucose, ketones

TREATMENT AND POTENTIAL COMPLICATIONS

Treatment of DKA:

- **Fluids**: Priority is fluid resuscitation with 1-2 liters of isotonic fluids given in the first hour, up to 8 liters in the first 24 hours. Potassium will be added to the fluids when levels begin to fall.
- **Insulin**: Continuous drip IV, with/without loading dose. Will usually begin at 0.1 unit/kg/ hour (5-7 units an hour generally), with a goal of decreasing blood glucose 50–75 mg/dL an hour. Blood glucose is checked every hour, and when levels are < 200 mg/dL, add dextrose to IV fluids to prevent rebound hypoglycemia.
- **Potassium**: Watch carefully, as fluids and insulin will cause rapid fall in serum levels. When K <5 mEq/L, it should be added to the IV fluids (Per liter: 20 mEq for K 4-5, 40 mEq for K 3–4). If potassium falls below 3, stop insulin drip and give 10–20 an hour until >3.5.
- **Sodium and Magnesium**: Na has an inverse relationship with potassium, and will increase as potassium falls. If sodium levels rise above 150 mEq, switch fluids to 0.45 NS. Low magnesium levels prevent potassium uptake, so replace as necessary.
- **Electrolytes**: Continue to monitor electrolytes and anion gap during ICU stay. When ABG and electrolytes normalized, transition to SQ insulin.

Potential complications include:

- Sudden electrolyte shifts (potassium) leading to catastrophic arrythmias, cerebral edema, and other complications
- Vomiting and decreased LOC leading to aspiration/ARDS
- Mechanical ventilation stops respiratory alkalosis and increases acidosis

HHNK

Hyperglycemic hyperosmolar nonketotic syndrome (HHNK) occurs in people without history of diabetes or with mild type 2 diabetes, resulting in persistent hyperglycemia leading to osmotic diuresis. Fluid shifts from intracellular to extracellular spaces to maintain osmotic equilibrium, but the increased glucosuria and dehydration results in hypernatremia and increased osmolarity. This condition is most common in those 50–70 years old and often is precipitated by an acute illness, such as a stroke, medications (thiazides), or dialysis treatments. HHNK differs from ketoacidosis because, while the insulin level is not adequate, it is high enough to prevent the breakdown of fat. Onset of symptoms often occurs over a few days. Glucose levels are often higher than those in DKA due to the gradual increase over time (often greater than 600), and the body living in a state of hyperglycemia, therefore the individual is not symptomatic until the blood glucose level is at an extreme high.

Symptoms: Polyuria, dehydration, hypotension, tachycardia, changes in mental status, seizures, hemiparesis.

Diagnosis: Increased glucose, Na, osmolality (urine and serum), BUN/Creatinine.

Treatment is similar to that for ketoacidosis:

- Insulin drip with frequent (hourly) blood sugar monitoring.
- Intravenous fluids and electrolytes.
- Correct blood glucose and other labs.

ACUTE HYPOGLYCEMIA

Acute hypoglycemia (hyperinsulinism) may result from pancreatic islet tumors or hyperplasia, increasing insulin production, or from the use of insulin to control diabetes mellitus. Hyperinsulinism can cause damage to the central nervous and cardiopulmonary systems, interfering with functioning of the brain and causing neurological impairment. Other causes may include: genetic defects (chromosome 11: short arm), severe infections, and toxic ingestion of alcohol or drugs (salicylates).

Symptoms include:

- Blood glucose <50-60 mg/dL
- Central nervous system: seizures, altered consciousness, lethargy, and poor feeding with vomiting, myoclonus, respiratory distress, diaphoresis, hypothermia, and cyanosis
- Adrenergic system: diaphoresis, tremor, tachycardia, palpitation, hunger, and anxiety

Diagnosis: Blood work, patient history, presentation.

Treatment depends on underlying cause:

- Glucose/Glucagon administration to elevate blood glucose levels
- Diazoxide (Hyperstat) to inhibit release of insulin
- Somatostatin (Sandostatin) to suppress insulin production
- Careful monitoring

DIABETES INSIPIDUS

Diabetes insipidus (DI) is caused by a deficiency of the antidiuretic hormone (ADH), or vasopressin. DI may develop secondary to head trauma, primary brain tumor, meningitis, encephalitis, or surgical ablation or irradiation of the pituitary gland, or metastatic tumors. This is different from congenital nephrogenic diabetes insipidus, in which production of ADH is normal but the renal tubules do not respond.

Symptoms:

- Polydipsia—enormous quantities of fluid may be ingested (3-30 L/day)
- Polyuria—large volumes of very dilute urine is excreted (3-30 L/day); nocturia almost always occurs
- Dehydration and hypovolemia can develop quickly if urinary losses are not continuously replaced

Diagnosis: A water deprivation test is the most reliable diagnostic test, but should only be done while the patient is under constant supervision. The test measures urine production, blood electrolyte levels, and weight over about 12 hours, during which the person is not allowed to drink. At the end of the 12 hours, vasopressin is given and a diagnosis of DI is confirmed if the person's excessive urination stops, BP rises to normal, and HR is normal.

Treatment includes:

- **Hormonal drugs**—Desmopressin, a synthetic analog of vasopressin, has prolonged antidiuretic activity, lasting 12 to 24 hours in most patients, and may be given intranasally, SQ, IV, or orally. Overdosage can lead to water intoxication, so monitor neurological status.
- **Nonhormonal drugs**—Three groups of nonhormonal drugs can reduce polyuria:
  - Diuretics, primarily thiazides (hydrochlorothiazide)
  - Vasopressin-releasing drugs (chlorpropamide or carbamazepine)
  - Prostaglandin inhibitors (indomethacin)

SIADH

Syndrome of inappropriate secretion of antidiuretic hormone (SIADH) is related to hypersecretion of the posterior pituitary gland. This causes the kidneys to reabsorb fluids, resulting in fluid retention, and triggers a decrease in sodium levels (dilutional hyponatremia), resulting in production of only concentrated urine. This syndrome may result from central nervous system disorders, such as brain trauma, surgery, or tumors. It may also be triggered by other disorders, such as tumors of various organs, pneumothorax, acute pneumonia, and other lung disorders. Some medications (vincristine, phenothiazines, tricyclic antidepressants, and thiazide diuretics) may also trigger SIADH.

Symptoms: Edema, dyspnea, crackles on auscultation, anorexia with nausea and vomiting, irritability, stomach cramps, alterations of personality, stupor, and seizures (related to progressive sodium depletion).

Diagnosis: Increased urine specific gravity, decreased Na and serum osmolality.

Treatment includes: (treat underlying cause)

- Correct fluid volume excess and electrolytes.
- Monitor urine output continuously: <0.5-1 mL/kg/hour is cause for concern.
- Seizure precautions.
- With SIADH expect low serum sodium and serum osmolality with high urine osmolality.

CHRONIC ADRENAL INSUFFICIENCY (ADDISON'S DISEASE)

Adrenal/Adrenocortical insufficiency (Addison's disease) is caused by damage to the adrenal cortex related to a variety of causes, such as autoimmune disease or genetic disorders, but it may relate to destructive lesions or neoplasms. Without treatment the condition is life threatening.

Symptoms may be vague and the condition undiagnosed until 80–90% of the adrenal cortex has been destroyed:

- Chronic weakness and fatigue
- Abdominal distress with nausea and vomiting
- Salt or licorice craving as a result of aldosterone deficiency
- Pigmentary changes in skin and mucous membranes, hyperpigmentation
- Hypotension
- Hypoglycemia
- Recurrent seizures (more common in children)

Treatment includes hormone replacement therapy with glucocorticoids (cortisol) and mineralocorticoids (aldosterone), which may be taken orally or by monthly parenteral injections. Androgen replacement is sometimes recommended for women.

Note: During times of stress or illness, the demand for glucocorticoids may increase, and dosages up to 3 times the normal dosage may be needed to prevent an acute crisis.

ACUTE ADRENAL INSUFFICIENCY (ADRENAL CRISIS)

Acute adrenal insufficiency (adrenal crisis) is a sudden, life-threatening condition resulting from an exacerbation of primary chronic adrenal insufficiency (Addison's disease), often precipitated by sepsis, surgical stress, adrenal hemorrhage related to septicemia, anticoagulation complications, and cortisone withdrawal related to a decreased or inadequate dose to compensate for stress. Acute adrenal insufficiency may occur in those who do not have Addison's disease, such as those who have received cortisone for various reasons, usually a minimum of 20 mg daily for at least 5 days.

Symptoms:

- Fever
- Nausea and vomiting
- Abdominal pain
- Weakness and general fatigue
- Disorientation, confusion
- Hypotensive shock
- Dehydration
- Electrolyte imbalance with hyperkalemia, hypercalcemia, hypoglycemia, and hyponatremia

Treatment:

- IV fluids in large volume
- Glucocorticoid
- 50% dextrose if indicated (hypoglycemia)
- Mineralocorticoid may be needed after intravenous solutions
- The precipitating cause must be identified and treated as well

HYPERTHYROIDISM

Hyperthyroidism (thyrotoxicosis) usually results from excess production of thyroid hormones (Graves' disease) from immunoglobulins providing abnormal stimulation of the thyroid gland. Other causes include thyroiditis and excess thyroid medications.

Symptoms vary and may be non-specific, especially in the elderly:

- Hyperexcitability
- Tachycardia (100-160) and atrial fibrillation
- Increased systolic (but not diastolic) BP
- Poor heat tolerance, skin flushed and diaphoretic
- Dry skin and pruritis (especially in the elderly)
- Hand tremor, progressive muscular weakness
- Exophthalmos (bulging eyes)
- Increased appetite and intake but weight loss

Treatment includes:

- Radioactive iodine to destroy the thyroid gland. Propranolol may be used to prevent thyroid storm. Thyroid hormones are given for resultant hypothyroidism.
- Antithyroid medications, such as Propacil or Tapazole to block conversion of T4 to T3.
- Surgical removal of thyroid is used if patients cannot tolerate other treatments or in special circumstances, such as large goiter. Usually one-sixth of the thyroid is left in place and antithyroid medications are given before surgery.

Review Video: 7 Symptoms of Hyperthyroidism
Visit mometrix.com/academy and enter code: 923159

Review Video: Graves' Disease
Visit mometrix.com/academy and enter code: 516655

Review Video: Thyroid and Antithyroid
Visit mometrix.com/academy and enter code: 666133

THYROTOXIC STORM

Thyrotoxic storm is a severe type of hyperthyroidism with sudden onset, precipitated by stress such as injury or surgery, in those un-treated or inadequately treated for hyperthyroidism. If not promptly diagnosed and treated, it is fatal. Incidence has decreased with the use of antithyroid medications but can still occur with medical emergencies or pregnancy. Diagnostic findings are similar to hyperthyroidism and include increased T3 uptake and decreased TSH.

Symptoms:

- Increase in symptoms of hyperthyroidism
- Increased temperature >38.5 °C
- Tachycardia >130 with atrial fibrillation and heart failure
- Gastrointestinal disorders such as nausea, vomiting, diarrhea, and abdominal discomfort
- Altered mental status with delirium progressing to coma

Treatment:

- Controlling production of thyroid hormone through antithyroid medications such as propylthiouracil and methimazole
- Inhibiting release of thyroid hormone with iodine therapy (or lithium)
- Controlling peripheral activity of thyroid hormone with propranolol
- Fluid and electrolyte replacement
- Glucocorticoids, such as dexamethasone
- Cooling blankets
- Treatment of arrhythmias as needed with antiarrhythmics and anticoagulation

HYPOTHYROIDISM

Hypothyroidism occurs when the thyroid produces inadequate levels of thyroid hormones. Conditions may range from mild to severe myxedema. There are a number of **causes**:

- Chronic lymphocytic thyroiditis (Hashimoto's thyroiditis)
- Excessive treatment for hyperthyroidism
- Atrophy of thyroid
- Medications such as lithium and iodine compounds
- Radiation to the area of the thyroid
- Diseases that affect the thyroid such as scleroderma
- Iodine imbalances

Symptoms may include chronic fatigue, menstrual disturbances, hoarseness, subnormal temperature, low pulse rate, weight gain, thinning hair, thickening skin. Some dementia may occur with advanced conditions. Clinical findings may include increased cholesterol with associated atherosclerosis and coronary artery disease. Myxedema may be characterized by changes in respiration with hypoventilation and CO_2 retention resulting in coma.

Treatment involves hormone replacement with synthetic levothyroxine (Synthroid) based on TSH levels, but this increases the oxygen demand of the body, so careful monitoring of cardiac status must be done during early treatment to avoid myocardial infarction while reaching euthyroid (normal) level.

HYPERPARATHYROIDISM

Hyperparathyroidism occurs when there is **overproduction of parathyroid hormone (PTH)**. Normal range is 10-55 pg/mL. This occurs more often in women and those over 50 years old. Hypercalcemia (total Ca^{++} >10.4 mg/dL) is the most common finding in hyperparathyroidism. Patients may complain signs of hypercalcemia

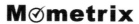

which can be easily remembered with *bones, stones, groans, and moans.* This includes **bone pain** due to demineralization, **kidney stones**, **abdominal groans** (nausea, vomiting, constipation, loss of appetite), and **psychiatric moans** (nervous system issues: muscle weakness, fatigue, lethargy, depression, confusion). Polyuria can occur with renal failure. Cardiac arrhythmias, hypertension, and even coma can occur. Ca^{++} levels >12 mg/dL may be due to cancer, and therefore cancer must be ruled out, especially if Ca^{++} levels rise rapidly. Hyperparathyroidism is treated with parathyroidectomy of affected glands.

HYPOPARATHYROIDISM

Hypoparathyroidism is the **deficiency of PTH**. This is more common in women and is usually due to accidental damage during thyroid/neck surgery, radioactive iodine treatment for hyperthyroidism, radiation, or due to autoimmune causes. As Ca^{++} levels drop, patients may complain of paresthesia of the fingers, toes, and perioral area. Patients will show other signs of neuromuscular irritability with muscle aches, hyperreflexia, carpopedal spasm (tetany), laryngospasm, and facial grimacing. A positive Chvostek sign (unilateral spasm of the facial muscles when the facial nerve is tapped) and a positive Trousseau sign (carpal spasm when upper arm is compressed with a blood pressure cuff) may be present. Irritability, confusion, fatigue, seizures, brittle hair and nails, and personality changes may occur. Diagnose with an ionized Ca^{++} level (<4.7 mg/dL), reduced PTH, and elevated phosphate. Treat with Ca^{++} and vitamin D supplements. Patients with renal failure must also reduce the amount of phosphate in their diet. Patients with tetany are treated with IV calcium gluconate.

CUSHING SYNDROME AND CUSHING'S DISEASE

Cushing syndrome results when **cortisol levels** are increased. Most commonly, this is due to steroid treatment with **prednisone**. Endogenous causes include a pituitary adenoma producing excess amounts of adrenocorticotropic hormone (ACTH) which leads to elevated cortisol (termed **Cushing's disease**) or a primary tumor of the adrenal gland causing increased cortisol secretion. Forms of cancer (e.g., lung, carcinoid) can present with ectopic sources of ACTH secretion. Patients will develop proximal muscle weakness, muscular atrophy, truncal obesity with thin arms and legs, round facies, buffalo hump, and purple striae usually across the abdomen. Patients may bruise easily, have non-healing sores, and women may be affected with hirsutism and oligomenorrhea/amenorrhea. Osteoporosis can occur as can glucose intolerance. For diagnosis a patient should be screened with one of the following: 24-hour urine free cortisol x3, low dose (1 mg) dexamethasone suppression test, midnight serum or salivary cortisol. Once Cushing syndrome is established, determine the cause using an ACTH and simultaneous cortisol measurement (elevated = adrenal adenoma or carcinoma) or a high-dose (8 mg overnight, or 2-day) dexamethasone suppression test (differentiates between pituitary cause and ectopic ACTH cause). Patients should be weaned off prednisone if possible. Removal of a pituitary adenoma can decrease ACTH production. Removal of an adrenal adenoma or other ectopic source of hormone secretion can decrease cortisol levels. Complications include hypertension, CV disease, DM, osteoporosis, risk of adrenal crisis, and psychosis.

HYPERALDOSTERONISM

Hyperaldosteronism leads to hypokalemia and hypernatremia (and often resulting hypertension). In fact, patients with untreated hypertension and potassium <2.8meq/dL often have primary hyperaldosteronism:

- **Aldosterone-producing adenoma** (Conn's syndrome) accounts for most primary hyperaldosteronism and affects women more often than men.
- **Idiopathic hyperaldosteronism** accounts for about 30% of primary hyperaldosteronism and has no identifiable changes on imaging.
- **Glucocorticoid suppressible hyperaldosteronism** is familial and rare.
- **Aldosterone-producing adrenocortical carcinoma** is another rare cause and presents with hyperandrogenism.

Diagnosis of hyperaldosteronism requires diastolic hypertension without edema, low renin levels that do not respond to volume depletion, and high aldosterone levels that fail to drop with saline boluses. An adrenal CT scan is performed to distinguish between Conn's syndrome and idiopathic hyperaldosteronism. **Treatment**

253

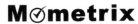

includes spironolactone or eplerenone to block the mineralocorticoid receptor, normalizing potassium and improving blood pressure. Adrenalectomy is indicated for unilateral hyperplasia or Conn's syndrome.

PHEOCHROMOCYTOMA

Pheochromocytoma is a rare tumor of chromaffin tissue. Ninety percent of these occur in the adrenal medulla, 10% are bilateral, and 10% are malignant. These tumors produce epinephrine and norepinephrine, leading to episodic symptoms of headaches, chest pain, palpitations, diaphoresis, tremor, nausea, vomiting, weight loss, and constipation. Initial diagnosis requires a 24-hour urine test to check for metanephrine, VMA, and catecholamines. These are always elevated with pheochromocytoma. If associated with a multiple endocrine neoplasia (MEN) syndrome, then one must check serum free metanephrine. Then one should begin imaging with CT or MRI scanning of the adrenals. If the adrenals appear normal, a radiolabeled iodine (called MIBG-metaiodobenzylguanidine scintigraphy) scan can localize extra-adrenal pheochromocytoma tissue or metastases. This scan uses a compound that concentrates in the adrenals to highlight the pheochromocytoma tissue. **Treatment** is surgical. But first, phenoxybenzamines are used to block the catecholamines, and then beta-blockers are used to control heart rate. Surgery has a 90% cure rate. Urinary catecholamines should be followed for at least 10 years.

PAGET'S DISEASE

Paget's disease is a disease of high bone turnover and disorganized osteoid formation. It is most prevalent in patients in the northeast US or of European descent and in older patients. The disease is usually asymptomatic, being detected on radiographs. However, it may present with bone pain, fractures, and bony deformities. Commonly involved bones include the skull, femur, tibia, pelvis, and humerus. Specifically, with skull involvement, the patient may note frequent headaches and increasing hat size, sometimes associated with deafness. Examination findings include frontal bossing, bowed legs, and superficial erythema and warmth, due to the increased vascularity of the bones. This disease is **diagnosed** with increased alkaline phosphatase, and elevated urinary hydroxyproline. Calcium and phosphorous are often normal. Imaging reveals hyperdense and enlarged bones in some regions and erosions in others. Bone scanning reveals increased uptake in certain areas. **Treatment** includes bisphosphonate and management of complications, including CHF, spinal cord compression, or nerve entrapment.

HYPOPITUITARISM RELATED TO DEFICIENT GROWTH HORMONE

Hypopituitarism may affect production of one or multiple hormones because of organic defects or idiopathic ideology, but deficiency in somatotropin, or growth hormone, (GH) is the primary disorder, which may be associated with other disorders. A decrease in GH causes a condition known as hypopituitary dwarfism, with **symptoms** characterized by:

- Normal growth in the first year but below 5th percentile in year 2
- Height retarded to a greater extent than weight
- Well-nourished with proportional skeleton
- Inactive as infants and children
- Primary teeth normal but permanent teeth delayed and overcrowded because of lack of adequate development of the jaw
- Sexual development delayed

Treatment:

- Identify any organic causes, such as tumors, and treat them accordingly.
- Biosynthetic GH administration can more than double growth rate, but the degree of benefit depends upon the age the treatments are started and the individual response.
- Provide sex hormone therapy during adolescence.

254

CONGENITAL AND JUVENILE HYPOTHYROIDISM

Hypothyroidism is caused by a deficiency in production of the thyroid hormones (TH) T4 and T3. It may be congenital or acquired from a lack of adequate dietary iodine, rare in the United States because salt is iodized. A number of disorders can cause hypothyroidism: congenital hypoplasia, partial or complete thyroidectomy, irradiation for Hodgkin's disease or other cancers, and infections. **Congenital hypothyroidism** (formerly called cretinism) may manifest at birth or be delayed for years, but severe early onset can result in profound neurological deficit and intellectual disability if undiagnosed and treated:

- **Neonates**: Widened posterior fontanel, hypothermia ≤95 °F, edema, respiratory distress, feeding difficulties, lethargy, delayed passage of meconium, prolonged physiologic jaundice, and vomiting
- **≤3 months of age**: Umbilical hernia, dry skin, constipation, enlarged tongue, lethargy, and minimal crying
- **Childhood**: Short stature with infantile proportions of trunk relative to legs, obesity, short forehead, broad nose, enlarged protruding tongue, dry skin and hair, and intellectual deficit

The brain is developed by age 2-3, and the onset of symptoms with **juvenile hypothyroidism** usually occurs after this time, so the condition is not associated with intellectual disability or neurological impairment. This form of hypothyroidism is most commonly caused by Hashimoto's thyroiditis, an autoimmune disease in which the immune system attacks the thyroid. **Symptoms** vary according to age of onset and include:

- Deceleration of growth
- Sensitivity to cold
- Constipation
- Muscle cramps
- Lethargy
- Mental decline
- Dry skin, thinning hair, and puffy face
- Goiter (swelling of the thyroid gland) may occur in some

Treatment for all types of hypothyroidism includes:

- Oral TH replacement therapy. Prompt initiation of therapy is critical for congenital hypothyroidism in order to prevent developmental abnormalities. If symptoms of hypothyroidism are severe, therapy to reach appropriate levels of TH is initially given gradually over 3-4 weeks to avoid hyperthyroidism.

PRECOCIOUS PUBERTY

Precocious puberty is the onset of puberty before age 7 in girls and 9 in boys. It can result from disorders of the gonads, the adrenal gland, or the hypothalamic-pituitary-gonad axis, producing gonadotropin hormones (GH) that cause early maturing of secondary sexual characteristics. It is much more common in girls than boys. Symptoms of **complete precocious puberty** include:

- Breast development and menstruation in girls
- Enlargement of testes and penis in boys with deepening of voice
- Development of pubic and axillary hair in both and facial hair in boys
- Acne
- Rapid increase in height for age
- Production of perspiration and odor

Partial precocious puberty presents similarly but results from overproduction of sex hormones, often because of a tumor of the ovary or testes, hyperplasia of the adrenal gland, or exogenous sources of hormones.

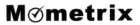

Treatment:

- Identifying and treating underlying causes
- If caused by GH, parenteral synthetic analog of luteinizing hormone-releasing hormone until puberty to slow development

INBORN ERRORS OF METABOLISM

Inborn errors of metabolism comprise a wide range of genetic metabolic disorders, usually related to defects in gene coding for enzymes, resulting in toxic accumulations that interfere with metabolism. Disorders are **classified** according to the type of metabolic disorder and include:

- Carbohydrate (glycogen storage disease, fructose intolerance)
- Proteins (clotting defects, sickle cell, thalassemia, osteogenesis imperfecta, Marfan)
- Amino acids (phenylketonuria, hyperammonemia)
- Organic acid (alcaptonuria)
- Cholesterol/lipoprotein (hyperlipoproteinemia, hypoproteinemia)
- Mitochondrial (Kearns-Sayre syndrome)
- Porphyrin (porphyria)
- Defective DNA repair (xeroderma pigmentosum)

Symptoms relate to the specific defect. Some symptoms are present in the neonate but others appear in childhood or adulthood. Some diseases are life-threatening, and others slowly progress. **Symptoms** common to many metabolic disorders may include:

- Encephalopathy with poor feeding, lethargy, tachypnea
- Metabolic acidosis and/or hyperammonemia
- Hypoglycemia
- Hepatic dysfunctions with jaundice
- Dysmorphism (structural anomalies)
- Abnormal body odor or urine odor

Infectious Diseases

PEDIATRIC INFECTIOUS DISEASE RISKS
TODDLERS AND PRESCHOOLERS

These children will still put toys in their mouths, which can transmit infections. Toilet training is still in the early stages, and their hand washing may need more practice, leading to transmitting fecal-oral germs. Toddlers and preschoolers are at risk for infections from animal scratches and bites, such as ringworm of the body. Daycare centers can be breeding grounds for germs, and these children are very susceptible to any infections in their environment. Day care workers should wear gloves and clean diaper changing areas with a disinfectant each time a diaper is changed. Children should be assisted in hand washing (after toileting, before and after eating, and after coughing or sneezing) and should be educated in these areas.

SCHOOL AGE CHILDREN

School environments are similar to daycare centers. Children may not always use good hand washing after toileting and before meals. They tend to share personal objects, which can lead to the spread of lice, scabies, tinea corporis, tinea capitis, and pinworms. Children with respiratory illnesses who don't cover their mouth and nose when coughing or sneezing and don't wash their hands afterwards can spread common illnesses. Pneumonia in this age group is usually caused by Mycoplasma pneumoniae and is very contagious. Fifth's disease is also common, very contagious, and causes a lacy rash that can come and go for up to a month. The child is contagious before the rash appears.

ADOLESCENTS

Adolescents are normally fairly healthy individuals and so aren't often seen at the doctor's office. This puts them at risk of skipping any needed immunizations or boosters. Without the boosters, they will be susceptible to measles, mumps, rubella, hepatitis B, and chickenpox. The MMR vaccine should not be given to females who may be pregnant. Sexually active teens are at risk for sexually transmitted infections and HIV. Adolescents tend to believe they won't get infections from their partners and that they won't get pregnant. Teens using crack cocaine are at higher risk for becoming infected with STIs and HIV. Teens should be given a private room, away from parents, when visiting the doctor so that an accurate portrayal of the teen's knowledge of STIs and sexual behaviors can be gleaned.

VIRAL INFECTIONS
HERPES SIMPLEX VIRUS INFECTIONS

There are 2 types of the herpes simplex virus (HSV), human herpesvirus 1 and 2. **HSV-1** usually causes a **gingivostomatitis** (often referred to as "cold sores" or "fever blisters") and is transmitted through **close contact. HSV-2** usually causes painful **genital lesions** through **sexual contact**. Either may be found in other areas of the body.

- **Incubation** period is around 2-12 days.
- The primary infection is usually more severe (causes systemic **symptoms**) than the reactivated infection, but it may be asymptomatic. After the primary infection, the virus remains dormant in the nerve ganglia, and can be reactivated especially during times of stress, illness, immunosuppression, or sun exposure. While patients are most contagious during times of active lesions, the disease may be spread while asymptomatic. The frequency of the outbreaks usually decreases over time.
- HSV **lesions** are grouped vesicles with an erythematous base. They are usually painful, and a prodrome of tingling, pain, or burning sensations may be felt hours to a couple days before the eruption. Lesions last for approximately 2-3 weeks in primary infection (up to 4 weeks with genital HSV), and 1-2 weeks in recurrent infections.
- HSV is **diagnosed** clinically and confirmed with a + culture, PCR test, or HSV antibody tests (HSV-1 or HSV-2: IgM= active or recent infection; IgG= previous infection).

- Symptomatic **treatment**, proper wound care, and antivirals (acyclovir, valacyclovir, or famciclovir) may be given.
- **Complications** include perinatal infection, keratitis, herpetic whitlow, herpes gladiatorum, secondary infections, and encephalitis.

EPSTEIN-BARR INFECTION

Epstein-Barr virus (EBV) is a **herpesvirus** (human herpesvirus 4) and is responsible for causing **infectious mononucleosis**. After the initial infection, it remains latent in B cells and epithelial cells. It has been linked to certain epithelial and lymphatic neoplasms (e.g., nasopharyngeal carcinoma, Burkitt lymphoma, Hodgkin lymphoma).

- EBV is **transmitted** through **body fluids** like saliva, so it is sometimes referred to as the kissing disease. It is most common in teenagers and college-age young adults
- **Incubation** period is typically 30-50 days.
- **Symptoms** of EBV infection range from being asymptomatic to swollen painful lymph nodes, pharyngitis (can mimic strep pharyngitis), extreme fatigue, fever, and possibly hepatosplenomegaly. The WBC count is elevated (~10,000-20,000 cells/mL) with 10-30% atypical lymphocytes in the differential.
- Confirm **diagnosis** with a Mono Spot test or EBV antibody serology tests.
- **Treatment** is supportive, and antibiotics are not helpful in treating this viral infection. Therefore, avoid unnecessary antibiotics in those with EBV, especially since administration of ampicillin or amoxicillin is often associated with a pruritic, maculopapular rash. Analgesics, warm salt water gargles, increased fluid intake, and rest will help to relieve some of the symptoms. Symptoms may last for several weeks and fatigue may last even longer. Patients should avoid contact sports for up to 2 months.
- **Complications** include hepatitis, cytopenias (e.g., thrombocytopenia), Guillain Barré syndrome, and splenic rupture.

MEASLES, MUMPS, AND RUBELLA

Measles (rubeola) virus is highly contagious, is spread through **respiratory secretions** (incubation is 7-14 days), and peaks in late winter to spring. It causes a prodrome of high fever (4-7 days), cough, congestion, conjunctivitis; then Koplik spots (pathognomonic), and finally a maculopapular rash (spreads cephalocaudally). Report suspected cases immediately to the health dept. **Diagnose** with a + IgM antibody test (collected after 3 days of rash), viral culture, or PCR. **Treatment** is supportive.

Mumps (parotitis) is a viral infection that is spread via **saliva** (incubation is 12-24 days), and often occurs during winter and spring. It causes painful swelling of the salivary glands (parotid). Report to health dept. Supportive **treatment**. Complications include orchitis (infertility), pancreatitis, and meningitis.

Rubella (German measles) is a virus that spreads via **respiratory droplets** (incubation is 2-3 weeks), and peaks in the spring. There is a mild prodrome (fever, aches, sore throat, conjunctivitis, swollen nodes [esp. suboccipital, postauricular, & posterior cervical]), then a maculopapular rash (face first, then down). Report to health dept. Confirm with rubella antibodies IgM or IgG. Symptomatic care.

INFLUENZA

Influenza is a highly contagious viral infection that affects the entire **respiratory system** from the nose to the lungs. There are 3 types of **influenza virus**: **A** (causes epidemics), **B** (only in humans), and **C**. Types A and B are seen most often and are the strains that the annual flu vaccine is most effective against; and type C is not as common and much less severe.

- Prevention is key and annual, age-appropriate influenza **vaccines** should be given to those ≥6 months; 2 vaccines are required in first-time vaccine patients if 6 mo. through 8-year-olds (separated by 28 days).
- **Incubation** period is 1-4 days and it is spread via respiratory droplets.
- Though **symptoms** can be very similar, the flu and the common cold differ in that the flu has a very sudden onset. Symptoms of influenza include a high fever (may last up to 5 days), headache, myalgias, dry cough, rhinorrhea, and fatigue. There may also be vomiting and diarrhea, although children are more prone to this.
- Clinical judgment, community patterns, and rapid influenza tests (high specificity, but lower sensitivity) aid in **diagnosis**, but RT-PCR or viral culture definitively confirm the diagnosis; pulse oximetry and CXR as needed for pulmonary issues.
- Antibiotic **treatment** is not effective unless there is a secondary bacterial infection (e.g., pneumonia). Look for signs of secondary infections (e.g., dyspnea, cyanosis, fever that goes away and returns, confusion/lethargy). Supportive treatment with rest, fluids, and analgesics. Antivirals should be considered in those who are at high risk (<5 years old, elderly, pregnant, chronic conditions). These are most effective if initiated within 24-48 hours of symptom onset. The neuraminidase inhibitors (oseltamivir, zanamivir) treat type A, type B, and avian H5N1. There is extensive resistance to the adamantanes (amantadine, rimantadine) so they are rarely used.
- **Complications** include pneumonia, ARDS, and death.

CORONAVIRUS

A coronavirus is a common virus that causes cold-like symptoms, including a cough, runny nose, sore throat, and congestion. Most cases of coronavirus are not dangerous and are often given little attention or go entirely unnoticed. However, specific coronavirus strains have led to two worldwide pandemics. The first, **severe acute respiratory syndrome (SARS)**, appeared in China in 2002 and quickly spread worldwide. Presenting symptoms of SARS were fever, cough, dyspnea, and general malaise. It was extremely virulent, spreading easily from person to person through close contact by way of contaminated droplets produced by coughing or sneezing. SARS was also very deadly, with a case fatality rate of nearly 10%. High rates of infection occurred in health care workers and others in contact with infected patients, so prompt diagnosis and proper isolation were essential. By 2004, there were no longer any documented active cases of SARS.

The most recent coronavirus outbreak was the **COVID-19** strain, which first appeared in December of 2019, in the Chinese city of Wuhan, and quickly became a global pandemic. Presentation of COVID-19 was similar to that of SARS, with the notable additional symptom of acute loss of taste/smell as a unique identifier. Much is still unknown about this strain, including exact transmission methods (though droplet transmission is suspected), effective treatment protocols, and long-term effects.

Precautions to take when treating patients with pandemic coronavirus include the following:

- Contact and droplet precautions, including eye protection and appropriate personal protection equipment.
- Airborne precautions (recommended by the CDC), especially with aerosol-producing procedures (ventilators, nebulizers, intubation).
- Immediate notification of public health authorities and institution of contact tracing.
- Activity restrictions of exposed health care workers planned in coordination with public health officials.

CYTOMEGALOVIRUS

Cytomegalovirus (CMV) is a herpes virus, occurring in most people by the time they are adults.

- **Transmission** can occur through secretions during personal contact and from mother to baby before, during or after birth.
- Most cases have no **symptoms**, although a few infants will have fetal damage, such as jaundice, hepatitis, brain damage, or growth retardation.
- **Treatment** for those with severe infections is with ganciclovir, an antiviral drug.

RESPIRATORY SYNCYTIAL VIRUS

Respiratory syncytial virus (RSV) is a virus that infects the respiratory tract, causing symptoms of nasal congestion, cough, sore throat, and headache. Severe cases can lead to high fever, breathing difficulties, severe cough, and cyanosis.

- Respiratory syncytial virus may **manifest** as a cold in adults and older children; however, there are some children who are more at risk of developing complications.
- **Transmission** is through contact with droplets from an infected person's nose or throat, generally through coughing and sneezing.
- Infants born prematurely, children with chronic lung disease, children with cystic fibrosis, and children who are in an immunocompromised state because of surgery or illness are at **high risk** of breathing difficulties, poor oxygenation, and even death from RSV.

FIFTH DISEASE

Fifth disease, or **erythema infectiosum**, is a viral illness caused by parvovirus B19. It is most prevalent in the spring, with outbreaks in preschools, daycares, and elementary schools.

- The **incubation** period is 4-20 days, and it may be communicable for several days before the rash appears.
- **Transmission** occurs through oral and nasal secretions and possibly blood.
- **Symptoms** are possible fever, headache, nasal congestion, general unwell feeling, and rash starting on the cheeks (slapped cheek appearance). The rash typically spreads to the rest of the body as a lacy red rash that may come and go for up to a month.
- Use over-the-counter fever medications as needed and provide **supportive care**.
- The virus can cause fetal death if contracted during pregnancy. There is no vaccine for fifth disease, and because it is a viral infection, it is not treated with antibiotics.

CHICKENPOX

Chickenpox (Varicella) is a viral infection, most prevalent in the late winter and early spring in children under 10 years of age.

- It has an **incubation** period of 10-21 days and is communicable from 1-2 days before the rash appears to after all lesions have dried up.
- **Transmission** is through direct contact and contact with respiratory droplets.
- **Symptoms** are low fever and feeling unwell, followed by the itchy rash (raised red bumps that develop vesicles which then ooze and crust over).
- The patient should be isolated until all lesions are dry. Aveeno baths and Benadryl help with the itching. Ibuprofen or acetaminophen can be used for the fever, and acyclovir is indicated in some cases. Encourage the patient not to scratch the lesions to prevent secondary infections. Provide supportive care as indicated.

ROSEOLA

Roseola is a viral illness, most prevalent in children 6-24 months of age.

- The **incubation** period is about 9 days.
- **Transmission** may be through oral and nasal.
- The illness begins with a high fever for 3-5 days; the patient appears well otherwise. The fever drops and then the rash appears. The rash is a light pink maculopapular rash which lasts 1-2 days.
- Parents should **treat the fever** as needed with anti-inflammatory medications.

POLIOMYELITIS

Poliomyelitis (commonly referred to as **polio**) is caused by an enterovirus and occurs most often in babies and young children.

- The **incubation** period is 3-14 days, and transmission occurs through direct contact with respiratory secretions and the oral-fecal route.
- The **symptoms** are slight fever, sore throat, general malaise, nausea and vomiting, headache, stomach ache, and constipation, but there can be severe pain, muscular weakness, and then paralysis.
- There are no drug therapies for polio. Observe for respiratory distress, provide general support measures, and provide for physical therapy.

ROTAVIRUS

Rotavirus is a viral illness that causes diarrhea, fever, and vomiting in children.

- It can be extremely **contagious** within groups where large numbers of children are present, such as in daycare centers, preschools, pediatric offices, clinics, and children's units in hospitals.
- Rotavirus can be prevented through **immunization** with a vaccine, as recommended by the American Academy of Pediatrics. Immunization can prevent up to 98% of severe cases of the illness.
- Children should wash their hands before eating and after using the bathroom to avoid spreading the disease. Caregivers should wash their hands before preparing food, after changing diapers, and after using the bathroom; they should avoid letting small children place toys or other items in their mouths and should disinfect surfaces after use.

BACTERIAL INFECTIONS

DIPHTHERIA

Diphtheria, caused by ***Corynebacterium diphtheriae***, is most prevalent in fall and winter.

- The **incubation** period is 2-7 days, possibly longer, and transmission is through direct contact with nasal, eye, and oral secretions.
- The **symptoms** are slight fever, nasal discharge, sore throat, feeling unwell, poor appetite, and swelling of the airway.
- If the disease is severe, death can result. The patient requires isolation, bed rest, fluids, antibiotics, medication for fever, and an antitoxin. The patient may also require oxygen therapy and tracheostomy if the airway is obstructed.

TETANUS

Tetanus, caused by ***Clostridium tetani***, occurs all over the world. The spores formed by the bacillus are present in soil, dust, and the GI tracts of animals and humans.

- The **incubation** period is 3-21 days.
- **Symptoms** start with headache, irritability, jaw muscle spasms, and inability to open the mouth. This is followed by severe back muscle spasms, seizures, incontinence, and fever.

- **Treatment** requires human tetanus immune globulin, penicillin G, Valium, and placement on a ventilator. The environment should be kept quiet because the spasms are initiated by stimuli.

SCARLET FEVER

Scarlet fever, caused by **group A beta-hemolytic streptococci**, is most prevalent in school-age children during the fall, winter, and spring.

- The **incubation** period is 1-7 days, and transmission occurs through direct or indirect contact with oral and nasal secretions.
- The illness begins with a high fever, very sore throat, headache, malaise, chills and possibly vomiting and stomach pain. A rash appears in about 12 hours as sandpapery red pinpoints in creases of the skin, flushed face and then a strawberry tongue.
- Antibiotics will be prescribed, but patients should be isolated until taking the antibiotic for 24 hours. Analgesics are needed to bring down the fever and the patient should be encouraged to drink plenty of fluids.

WHOOPING COUGH

Whooping cough, caused by ***Bordetella pertussis* bacillus**, is most prevalent in infants and children who were not immunized.

- The **incubation** period is 6-20 days, and transmission occurs through direct contact with oral and nasal secretions.
- The **symptoms** are cold symptoms for 1-2 weeks, when the cough will worsen and progress to a whoop sound, usually occurring at night. Vomiting will usually follow an episode of intense coughing. As the patient recovers, the coughing will subside. In babies, a mucus plug or apnea can result in death by respiratory arrest. Hospitalization is usually required for infants less than 6 months of age and those with a severe case of pertussis.
- The patient needs isolation and bed rest, with a calm, quiet environment to limit coughing spells. Fluid intake needs to be monitored and humidified air will help.
- Watch for signs of respiratory distress and give antibiotic and pertussis immune globulin as prescribed.

IMPETIGO

Impetigo is a skin infection that is most commonly seen in preschool children or those in young childhood.

- Impetigo causes blister-like sores on skin areas that may already be compromised, such as under the nose, on the hands or neck, or in the diaper area. It is caused by a bacterial infection, most commonly *Staphylococcus aureus* or group A *Streptococcus*. The sores may itch or the patient may already have irritation at the site, such as a diaper rash.
- To **prevent the spread of infection**, children and caregivers should wash their hands frequently and avoid scratching the sores and then touching items. Isolation by staying home from school or daycare may be necessary until the sores have crusted over. Treating skin irritations, such as poison ivy or eczema, can also prevent infection from spreading to impetigo.

FUNGAL INFECTIONS

CRYPTOCOCCOSIS

Cryptococcosis is an infection resulting from inhaling the **fungus** *Cryptococcus neoformans,* which is found worldwide in soil (can be associated with bird droppings), or *Cryptococcus gattii,* which is associated with certain trees in the Northwest.

- Cryptococcosis is most often due to *C. neoformans.* It is often found among those with compromised immune systems and is an **AIDS-defining opportunistic infection**.
- Healthy patients may be asymptomatic and the only finding may be pulmonary lesions on CXR that resolve spontaneously. The fungus can disseminate and cause meningitis, encephalitis, cutaneous lesions, and affect long bones and other tissues. **Symptoms** are based on the area of involvement. Patients may experience cough, pleuritic chest pain, weight loss, and fever if there is pulmonary involvement; headache, double vision, light sensitivity, N/V, and confusion if CNS involvement; cutaneous lesions (papules, pustules, nodules, ulcers) if the skin is involved.
- **Diagnosis** includes microscopic analysis, culture (gold standard), or an antigen test (highly sensitive; good for detecting early infection) for *Cryptococcus* using CSF, tissue, sputum, blood, or urine. Check CSF by India ink (limited sensitivity) or culture so meningitis can be ruled out. Confirm that no mass lesion is present by CT or MRI before LP is performed.
- Mild cases may only require monitoring to ensure that the infection does not spread. In more advanced cases, the infection is treated with different antifungal medications (e.g., fluconazole for pulmonary infections, amphotericin B ± flucytosine for meningitis). The patient should also be monitored for CNS infection and medication side effects. AIDS patients may need lifelong antifungals.
- **Complications** include cryptococcal meningitis, neural deficits, optic nerve damage, and hydrocephalus.

HISTOPLASMOSIS

Histoplasmosis is an infection caused by inhalation of **spores** from the fungus *Histoplasma capsulatum* that is found in soil and is associated with bird and bat droppings (e.g., chicken coops, caves).

- Healthy patients are usually asymptomatic and those with symptoms are typically immunocompromised or those who've had a heavy exposure to spores. The primary **pulmonary infection** occurs 3-17 days after exposure and can present with flu-like symptoms. It is typically self-limited but may become chronic. Histoplasmosis can also spread through the **blood** and can cause progressive disseminated disease in the immunocompromised (high mortality rate); this is an **AIDS-defining illness**.
- **Diagnose** through antigen tests (urine, serum), histopathology, or cultures; order a CXR. Mild and even moderate acute pulmonary histoplasmosis may resolve on its own.
- If needed, **treat** mild to moderate infections with itraconazole and severe illness with amphotericin B.

PNEUMOCYSTIS

Pneumocystis jiroveci is a **fungus** (previously known as *Pneumocystis* carinii) that causes **pneumonia** (PJP, previously PCP) in the immunocompromised. Most people have been exposed to this by the age of 3 or 4.

- **Symptoms** of PJP include a dry nonproductive cough, fever, dyspnea, and weight loss.
- CXR may show diffuse bilateral infiltrates or it may be normal; and pulse oximetry may be low, especially on exertion. **Diagnosis** is confirmed with sputum histopathology using sputum induction or bronchoalveolar lavage.

- **Treat** immediately with TMP-SMX (trimethoprim/sulfamethoxazole) for 21 days if HIV + and for 14 days in other cases. Steroids may be added for HIV patients with severe PJP. HIV/AIDS patients with CD4 counts <200/μL should receive PJP prophylaxis with TMP-SMX. Dapsone and pentamidine are alternatives.
- **Complications** include ARDS and death.

CANDIDAL INFECTIONS

Candida is a type of yeast that may cause a variety of infections:

- **Oral thrush** is commonly seen in diabetic patients and those who are immunosuppressed (HIV or underlying neoplasm). Patients often complain of burning on the tongue or in the mouth, associated with "curd-like" white patches that can be scraped away leaving reddish tissue underneath. Diagnosis is with KOH prep. Treatment is with oral or topical antifungals, including nystatin (swish and swallow or troches).
- **Candida esophagitis** also occurs in the immunosuppressed population, and patients may complain of dysphasia, odynophagia, and chest pain. This is diagnosed on EGD and may be treated with oral or IV antifungals (ketoconazole).
- **Candidal intertrigo**, or diaper rash, presents with beefy-red lesions at skin fold areas as well as satellite lesions. Treatment is with topical antifungals.
- **Candidemia** is diagnosed with fungal blood cultures and may lead to osteomyelitis, endocarditis, and other complications. Treatment is with IV antifungals.

RINGWORM

Ringworm is caused by an infection from the ***Tinea* fungus**, which produces patches on the skin that have normal centers, giving the appearance of a ring.

- The fungus can cause hair loss and patches of scaly skin that may develop blisters that ooze or crust.
- It is **transmitted** by touching the affected skin or through objects that have touched the affected skin.
- Ringworm may be **diagnosed** by viewing the skin section under a Wood's lamp. Skin cultures may also be taken for examination to identify the fungus. A potassium hydroxide (KOH) exam involves scraping the affected skin and placing the skin sample in KOH to test for the presence of the fungus.

VECTOR-BORNE AND PARASITIC INFECTIONS

MALARIA

Malaria is a **blood-borne disease** caused by a **parasite** from the genus *Plasmodium and* found in tropical areas. There are 4 known to cause disease in humans (*P. malariae*, *P. vivax*, *P. ovale*, and *P. falciparum*). These protozoa are transmitted by the **female *Anopheles* mosquito**. They travel to the **liver** where they multiply, are released, and then infect the RBCs, where they continue to multiply. Incubation time can be as little as 9 days or as much as multiple years depending on the species of the infecting parasite.

- **Signs and symptoms** include headache, high fever with shaking chills and sweating (rigors; occurs when merozoites, an immature form of the parasite, are released from RBCs), jaundice, anemia, and hepatosplenomegaly. Take a thorough history including recent travel.
- **Diagnose** with 3 thin and thick blood smears (gold standard) stained with Giemsa (preferred) and obtained 12-24 hours apart. Labs typically show elevated LDH, thrombocytopenia, and atypical lymphocytes. Rapid antigen tests are also available as well as PCR.
- **Treat** with chloroquine. If travelling, chemoprophylaxis depends on the area of travel due to species and resistance patterns, and may include chloroquine, primaquine, mefloquine, Malarone, or doxycycline. Report infections to your local or state health department.
- **Complications** include severe anemia and hemolysis, organ failure (liver, spleen, kidneys), cerebral malaria, ARDS, and death.

LYME DISEASE

Lyme disease occurs from a bite from a **deer tick** (blacklegged tick) infected with the **spirochete bacterium** *Borrelia burgdorferi*. It is the most common tick-borne disease in the US and is more prevalent in heavily wooded areas. Adult ticks are more active during colder times whereas the nymphs (<2 mm in size) are more active in the warm, spring or summer months. Once the tick bites, it stays attached; however, it takes about 36-48 hours for nymphs and about 48-72 hours for adult ticks before the spirochete is transmitted to the person. **Incubation** period is 3-30 days. There are 3 stages to this disease: early localized, early disseminated, and chronic disseminated.

- At **Stage 1**, 75% have the characteristic expanding red rash (erythema migrans; can be large, ~30cm) which can progress to have central clearing (bull's eye), headache, fever, chills, myalgias, and fatigue.
- **Stage 2** occurs weeks to months after initial infection and involves systemic symptoms (flu-like), neck stiffness, headaches, migrating pain in muscles and joints, rashes, paresthesias, Bell's palsy, confusion, fatigue, myocarditis, and heart palpitations.
- **Stage 3** occurs months to years after initial infection and involves neurologic (e.g., encephalitis) and rheumatologic issues, especially arthritis of large joints (e.g., knee).

> **Review Video: Lyme Disease**
> Visit mometrix.com/academy and enter code: 505529

DIAGNOSIS AND TREATMENT OF LYME DISEASE

Diagnose Lyme disease using 2-tiered testing: antibodies (IgM, IgG), then Western blot. Antibiotic treatment for localized Lyme disease involves 2-3 weeks of doxycycline, amoxicillin, or cefuroxime axetil is started immediately after diagnosis. IV antibiotics may be needed for severe disease (e.g., IV ceftriaxone). Prevention is key by wearing clothes covering the skin, using tick repellents, showering soon after being outdoors in tick-prone areas, and thoroughly checking for ticks (especially in hard to see areas by using a mirror). The Lyme vaccine is no longer available and previous vaccine recipients are still at risk of contracting the disease as protection decreases over time. Complications are prevalent with untreated Lyme disease and include chronic arthritis, fatigue, chronic musculoskeletal issues, acrodermatitis chronica atrophicans, and memory and concentration issues. Report cases to the local health dept.

ROCKY MOUNTAIN SPOTTED FEVER

Rocky Mountain spotted fever is a tick-borne illness caused by **Rickettsia rickettsii**. It tends to occur in spring and summer throughout the United States.

- **Incubation** period is about one week.
- **Symptoms** include headache, fever, nausea, vomiting, loss of appetite, muscle pain, and rash on the ankles and wrists.
- **Treatment** requires an antibiotic, usually Vibramycin.

ZIKA VIRUS IN PREGNANT WOMEN

Zika virus is a **flavivirus** that is transmitted by the *Aedes* mosquito and through sexual contact. This virus can be passed on to an unborn baby causing severe congenital defects while causing mild or no disease in the mother. It is advised that all pregnant women avoid traveling to areas with the Zika virus (e.g., Central and South America, Mexico, Caribbean, Africa).

- **Incubation** period is 3-14 days and symptoms may last 4-7 days. The virus has been found to remain longer in semen than in other body fluids.
- If **symptoms** are present, they may include fever, headache, myalgias, arthralgias, a maculopapular rash, and conjunctivitis. Congenital defects include severe microcephaly, severe brain abnormalities, macular scarring, hearing loss, motor disabilities (e.g., hypertonia), and contractures. Women should be screened for Zika exposure at each prenatal visit.

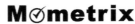

- **Diagnostic** testing is recommended for all asymptomatic pregnant women who have continued exposure to Zika and for all symptomatic pregnant women who have possibly been exposed to the Zika virus. Testing includes RNA NAT testing on serum and urine, and serum IgM Zika antibody testing. Prenatal ultrasound helps determine if the effects of Zika are present. Report cases to the state health department; and the CDC can be consulted.
- There is **no treatment** or cure for the Zika virus.

HELMINTH INFESTATIONS

Helminth infestations (worms) include **roundworms** [nematodes: *Ascaris*, hookworms (cause anemia), **filariae** (cause elephantiasis)] and **flatworms** [tapeworms (cause weight loss); **flukes** (intestinal or liver)]. **Pinworms** are a type of roundworm that cause enterobiasis and is the most common helminth infestation. Pinworms are more prevalent in warmer areas of the country and infestations occur more frequently in children. The worms lay eggs within the digestive tract and then travel to the anal area where they are usually found. Pinworms are highly contagious. As a patient itches the anal area where the eggs are located, the eggs cling to the fingers and can easily be transmitted to other people either directly or through food or surfaces. The eggs can survive for 2-3 weeks on inanimate objects.

- Patients may be asymptomatic or have intense anal itching that is usually worse at night and can cause insomnia. Abdominal pain, nausea, and vomiting can also occur.
- **Diagnose** with the "tape test" which involves pressing cellophane tape over the perianal area to pick up eggs or worms and examine under the microscope. Most other helminth infestations can be diagnosed with a stool sample for ova and parasites; filariasis requires a blood smear or antigen test.
- Anthelmintic medications are given in a single dose and repeated in 2 weeks to kill the pinworms and their larvae (mebendazole, albendazole, or pyrantel pamoate). The entire family and close contacts should be treated simultaneously since pinworms are so contagious.

GIARDIA LAMBLIA

Giardia lamblia is a **protozoan** that infects water supplies and spreads to children through the fecal-oral route. It is the most common cause of non-bacterial diarrhea in the United States, causing about 20,000 cases of infection each year in all ages.

- Children often become infected after swallowing recreational waters (pools, lakes) while swimming or putting contaminated items into the mouth. *Giardia* live and multiply within the small intestine where cysts develop.
- **Symptoms** occur 7-14 days after ingestion of 1 or more cysts and include diarrhea with greasy floating stools (rarely bloody), stomach cramps, nausea, and flatulence, lasting 2-6 weeks. A chronic infection may develop that can last for months or years.
- **Treatment** includes Furazolidone 5-8 mg/kg/day in 4 doses for 7-10 days or Metronidazole 40 mg/kg/day in 3 doses for 7-10 days. Chronic infections are often very resistant to treatment.

TOXOPLASMOSIS

Toxoplasmosis is an infection caused by the **parasite *Toxoplasma gondii***, which is commonly found in soil. It is widespread and transmitted through cat feces; however, it also may be contracted by eating undercooked meat (especially pork, lamb, or venison) or poorly washed vegetables. Toxoplasmosis can cause serious disease and can affect various organs; and immunocompromised and pregnant women and their unborn babies are especially likely to have side effects of the disease (the "T" in congenital TORCH infections).

- Healthy patients are usually asymptomatic; however, once infected the parasite can remain latent until the patient becomes immunocompromised and the parasite is reactivated causing **symptoms**. The disease can cause a flu-like illness with fever, myalgias, and lymphadenopathy. More serious effects include retinochoroiditis, brain lesions, and encephalitis. Congenital toxoplasmosis may cause retinochoroiditis, microcephaly, hydrocephalus, intellectual disability, and possibly miscarriage or stillbirth.
- **Diagnose** with serology for *Toxoplasma* antibodies IgM and IgG. Also, PCR may be used to test amniotic fluid, CSF, or tissue.
- **Treat** with pyrimethamine (preferred) plus folinic acid or sulfadiazine plus folinic acid. Pregnant women should avoid high-risk practices like changing the cat litter and should avoid sand boxes.

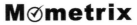

Multisystem Pathophysiology

RANGE OF SEVERE INFECTION

There are a number of terms used to refer to severe infections which are often used interchangeably. It is important to know these terms to properly perform the continuum of care.

- **Bacteremia** is the presence of bacteria in the blood without systemic infection.
- **Septicemia** is a systemic infection caused by pathogens (usually bacteria or fungi) present in the blood.
- **Systemic inflammatory response syndrome** (SIRS) is a generalized inflammatory response affecting many organ systems. It may be caused by infectious or non-infectious agents, such as trauma, burns, adrenal insufficiency, pulmonary embolism, and drug overdose. If an infectious agent is identified or suspected, SIRS is an aspect of sepsis. Infective agents include a wide range of bacteria and fungi, including *Streptococcus pneumoniae* and *Staphylococcus aureus*. SIRS includes 2 of the following:
  - Elevated (>38 °C) or subnormal rectal temperature (<36 °C)
  - Tachypnea or $PaCO_2$ <32 mmHg
  - Tachycardia
  - Leukocytosis (>12,000) or leukopenia (<4000)
- **Sepsis** is the presence of infection either locally or systemically in which there is a generalized life-threatening inflammatory response (SIRS). It includes all the indications for SIRS as well as one of the following:
  - Changes in mental status
  - Hypoxemia without preexisting pulmonary disease
  - Elevation in plasma lactate
  - Decreased urinary output <5 mL/kg/hr for ≥1 hour
- **Severe sepsis** includes both indications of SIRS and sepsis as well as indications of increasing organ dysfunction with inadequate perfusion and/or hypotension.
- **Septic shock** is a progression from severe sepsis in which refractory hypotension occurs despite treatment. There may be indications of lactic acidosis.
- **Multi-organ dysfunction syndrome** (MODS) is the most common cause of sepsis-related death. Cardiac function becomes depressed, acute respiratory distress syndrome (ARDS) may develop, and renal failure may follow acute tubular necrosis or cortical necrosis. Thrombocytopenia appears in about 30% of those affected and may result in disseminated intravascular coagulation (DIC). Liver damage and bowel necrosis may occur.

> **Review Video: <u>Multiple Organ Dysfunction Syndrome</u>**
> Visit mometrix.com/academy and enter code: 394302

SHOCK

There are a number of different types of shock, but there are general characteristics that they have in common. In all types of shock, there is a marked decrease in tissue perfusion related to hypotension, so that there is insufficient oxygen delivered to the tissues and inadequate removal of cellular waste products, causing injury to tissue:

- Hypotension (systolic below 90 mmHg); this may be somewhat higher (110 mmHg) in those who are initially hypertensive
- Decreased urinary output (<0.5 mL/kg/hr), especially marked in hypovolemic shock
- Metabolic acidosis
- Peripheral/cutaneous vasoconstriction/vasodilation resulting in cool, clammy skin
- Alterations in level of consciousness

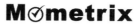

Types of shock are as follows:

- **Distributive:** Preload decreased, CO increased, SVR decreased
- **Cardiogenic:** Preload increased, CO decreased, SVR increased
- **Hypovolemic:** Preload decreased, CO decreased, SVR increased

SEPTIC SHOCK

Septic shock is caused by toxins produced by bacteria and cytokines that the body produces in response to severe infection, resulting in a complex syndrome of disorders. **Symptoms** are wide-ranging:

- **Initial**: Hyper- or hypothermia, increased temperature (>38 °C) with chills, tachycardia with increased pulse pressure, tachypnea, alterations in mental status (dullness), hypotension, hyperventilation with respiratory alkalosis ($PaCO_2$ ≤30 mmHg), increased lactic acid, unstable BP, and dehydration with increased urinary output
- **Cardiovascular**: Myocardial depression and dysrhythmias
- **Respiratory**: Acute respiratory distress syndrome (ARDS)
- **Renal**: Acute kidney injury (AKI) with decreased urinary output and increased BUN
- **Hepatic**: Jaundice and liver dysfunction with an increase in transaminase, alkaline phosphatase, and bilirubin
- **Hematologic**: Mild or severe blood loss (from mucosal ulcerations), neutropenia or neutrophilia, decreased platelets, and DIC
- **Endocrine**: Hyperglycemia, hypoglycemia (rare)
- **Skin**: Cellulitis, erysipelas, and fasciitis, acrocyanotic and necrotic peripheral lesions

DIAGNOSIS AND TREATMENT

Septic shock is most common in newborns, those >50, and those who are immunocompromised. There is no specific test to confirm a diagnosis of septic shock, so **diagnosis** is based on clinical findings and tests that evaluate hematologic, infectious, and metabolic states: Lactic acid, CBC, DIC panel, electrolytes, liver function tests, BUN, creatinine, blood glucose, ABGs, urinalysis, ECG, radiographs, blood and urine cultures.

Treatment must be aggressive and includes:

- Oxygen and endotracheal intubation as necessary
- IV access with 2-large bore catheters and central venous line
- Rapid fluid administration at 0.5L NS or isotonic crystalloid every 5-10 minutes as needed (to 4-6 L)
- Monitoring urinary output to optimal >30 mL/hr (>0.5-1 mL/kg/hr)
- Inotropic or vasoconstrictive agents (dopamine, dobutamine, norepinephrine) if no response to fluids or fluid overload
- Empiric IV antibiotic therapy (usually with 2 broad spectrum antibiotics for both gram-positive and gram-negative bacteria) until cultures return and antibiotics may be changed
- Hemodynamic and laboratory monitoring
- Removing source of infection (abscess, catheter)

DISTRIBUTIVE SHOCK

Distributive shock occurs with adequate blood volume but inadequate intravascular volume because of arterial/venous dilation that results in decreased vascular tone and hypoperfusion of internal organs. Cardiac output may be normal or blood may pool, decreasing cardiac output. **Distributive shock** may result from anaphylactic shock, septic shock, neurogenic shock, and drug ingestions.

Symptoms include:

- Hypotension (systolic <90 mmHg or <40 mmHg below normal), tachypnea, tachycardia (>90) (may be lower if patient receiving β-blockers)
- Hypoxemia
- Skin initially warm, later hypoperfused
- Hyper- or hypothermia (>38 °C or <36 °C)
- Alterations in mentation
- Decreased urinary output
- Symptoms related to underlying cause

Treatment includes:

- Treating underlying cause while stabilizing hemodynamics
- Oxygen with endotracheal intubation if necessary
- Rapid fluid administration at 0.25-0.5 L NS or isotonic crystalloid every 5-10 minutes as needed to 2-3 L
- Vasoconstrictive and inotropic agents (dopamine, dobutamine, norepinephrine) if necessary, for patients with profound hypotension

NEUROGENIC SHOCK

Neurogenic shock is a type of distributive shock that occurs when injury to the CNS from trauma resulting in acute spinal cord injury (from both blunt and penetrating injuries), neurological diseases, drugs, or anesthesia, impairs the autonomic nervous system that controls the cardiovascular system. The degree of symptoms relates to the level of injury with injuries above T1 capable of causing disruption of the entire sympathetic nervous system and lower injuries causing various degrees of disruption. Even incomplete spinal cord injury can cause neurogenic shock.

Symptoms include:

- Hypotension and warm dry skin related to lack of vascular tone that results in hypothermia from loss of cutaneous heat
- Bradycardia (common but not universal)

Treatment includes:

- ABCDE (airway, breathing, circulation, disability evaluation, exposure)
- Rapid fluid administration with crystalloid to keep mean arterial pressure at 85-90 mmHg
- Placement of pulmonary artery catheter to monitor fluid overload
- Inotropic agents (dopamine, dobutamine) if fluids don't correct hypotension
- Atropine for persistent bradycardia

HYPOVOLEMIC SHOCK/VOLUME DEFICIT

Hypovolemic shock occurs when there is inadequate intravascular fluid. The loss may be *absolute* because of an internal shifting of fluid or an external loss of fluid, as occurs with massive hemorrhage, thermal injuries, severe vomiting or diarrhea, and internal injuries (such as ruptured spleen or dissecting arteries) that interfere with intravascular integrity. Hypovolemia may also be *relative* and related to vasodilation, increased capillary membrane permeability from sepsis or injuries, and decreased colloidal osmotic pressure that may occur with loss of sodium and some disorders, such as hypopituitarism and cirrhosis.

Hypovolemic shock is **classified** according to the degree of fluid loss:

- **Class I:** <750 mL or ≤15% of total circulating volume (TCV)
- **Class II:** 750-1500 mL or 15-30% of TCV
- **Class III:** 1500-2000 mL or 30-40% of TCV
- **Class IV:** >2000 mL or >40% of TCV

SYMPTOMS AND TREATMENT

Hypovolemic shock occurs when the total circulating volume of fluid decreases, leading to a fall in venous return that in turn causes a decrease in ventricular filling and preload, indicated by ↓ in right atrial pressure (RAP) and pulmonary artery occlusion pressure (PAOP). This results in a decrease in stroke volume and cardiac output. This in turn causes generalized arterial vasoconstriction, increasing afterload (↑ systemic vascular resistance), causing decreased tissue perfusion.

Symptoms: Anxiety, pallor, cool and clammy skin, delayed capillary refill, cyanosis, hypotension, increasing respirations, weak, thready pulse.

Treatment is aimed at identifying and treating the cause:

- Administration of blood, blood products, autotransfusion, colloids (such as plasma protein fraction), and/or crystalloids (such as normal saline)
- Oxygen—intubation and ventilation may be necessary
- Medications may include vasopressors, such as dopamine. **Note: Fluids must be given before starting vasopressors**!

ANAPHYLACTIC SHOCK

Anaphylactic reaction or anaphylactic shock may present with a few symptoms or a wide range of potentially lethal effects.

Symptoms may recur after the initial treatment (biphasic anaphylaxis), so careful monitoring is essential:

- Sudden onset of weakness, dizziness, confusion
- Severe generalized edema and angioedema; lips and tongue may swell
- Urticaria
- Increased permeability of vascular system and loss of vascular tone leading to severe hypotension and shock
- Laryngospasm/bronchospasm with obstruction of airway causing dyspnea and wheezing
- Nausea, vomiting, and diarrhea
- Seizures, coma, and death

Treatments:

- Establish patent airway and intubate if necessary, for ventilation
- Provide oxygen at 100% high flow
- Monitor VS
- Administer epinephrine (Epi-pen or solution)
- Albuterol per nebulizer for bronchospasm
- Intravenous fluids to provide bolus of fluids for hypotension
- Diphenhydramine if shock persists
- Methylprednisolone if no response to other drugs

BURN INJURIES
TYPES AND CLASSIFICATIONS

Burn injuries may be chemical, electrical, or thermal, and are assessed by the area, percentage of the body burned, and depth:

- **First-degree burns** are superficial and affect the epidermis, causing erythema and pain.
- **Second-degree burns** extend through the dermis (partial thickness), resulting in blistering and sloughing of epidermis.
- **Third-degree burns** affect underlying tissue, including vasculature, muscles, and nerves (full thickness).

Burns are classified according to the **American Burn Association's criteria**:

- **Minor**: Less than 10% body surface area (BSA). 2% BSA with third degree without serious risk to face, hands, feet, or perineum.
- **Moderate**: 10-20% combined second- and third-degree burns (children younger than 10 years or adults older than 40 years). 10% or less full thickness without serious risk to face, hands, feet, or perineum.
- **Major**: 20% BSA; at least 10% third-degree burns. All burns to face, hands, feet, or perineum that will result in functional/cosmetic defect. Burns with inhalation or other major trauma.

SYSTEMIC COMPLICATIONS

Burn injuries begin with the skin but can affect all organs and body systems, especially with a major burn:

- **Cardiovascular**: Cardiac output may fall by 50% as capillary permeability increases with vasodilation and fluid leaks from the tissues.
- **Urinary**: Decreased blood flow causes kidneys to increase ADH, which increases oliguria. BUN and creatinine levels increase. Cell destruction may block tubules, and hematuria may result from hemolysis.
- **Pulmonary**: Injury may result from smoke inhalation or (rarely) aspiration of hot liquid. Pulmonary injury is a leading cause of death from burns and is classified according to the degree of damage:
    - *First*: Singed eyebrows and nasal hairs with possible soot in airways and slight edema
    - *Second*: (At 24 hours) Stridor, dyspnea, and tachypnea with edema and erythema of upper airway, including area of vocal cords and epiglottis
    - *Third*: (At 72 hours) Worsening symptoms if not intubated and if intubated, bronchorrhea and tachypnea with edematous, secreting tissue
- **Neurological**: Encephalopathy may develop from lack of oxygen, decreased blood volume and sepsis. Hallucinations, alterations in consciousness, seizures, and coma may result.
- **Gastrointestinal**: Ileus and ulcerations of mucosa often result from poor circulation. Ileus usually clears within 48-72 hours, but if it returns it is often indicative of sepsis.
- **Endocrine/metabolic:** The sympathetic nervous system stimulates the adrenals to release epinephrine and norepinephrine to increase cardiac output and cortisol for wound healing. The metabolic rate increases markedly. Electrolyte loss occurs with fluid loss from exposed tissue, especially phosphorus, calcium, and sodium, with an increase in potassium levels. Electrolyte imbalance can be life-threatening if burns cover >20% of BSA. Glycogen depletion occurs within 12-24 hours and protein breakdown and muscle wasting occurs without sufficient intake of protein.

MANAGEMENT

Management of burn injuries must include both wound care and systemic care to avoid complications that can be life threatening. **Treatment** includes:

- Establishment of airway and treatment for inhalation injury as indicated:
  - Supplemental oxygen, incentive spirometry, nasotracheal suctioning
  - Humidification
  - Bronchoscopy as needed to evaluate bronchospasm and edema
  - β-Agonists for bronchospasm, followed by aminophylline if ineffective
  - Intubation and ventilation if there are indications of respiratory failure (This should be done prior to failure. Tracheostomy may be done if ventilation >14 days.)
- Intravenous fluids and electrolytes, based on weight and extent of burn. Parkland formula: Fluid replacement (mL) in first 24 hours = (mass in kg) × (body % burned) × 400
- Enteral feedings, usually with small lumen feeding tube into the duodenum
- NG tube for gastric decompression to prevent aspiration
- Indwelling catheter to monitor urinary output. Urinary output should be 0.5-2 mL/kg/hr
- Analgesia for reduction of pain and anxiety
- Topical and systemic antibiotics
- Wound care with removal of eschar and dressings as indicated

CHEMICAL BURNS

Chemical burns may result from contact with acid or alkali substances. The pH scale ranges from 0 to 14 with 7 being neutral, 0 being extremely acidic, and 14 being extremely alkaline. Alkali burns tend to be more severe because acid burns denature proteins, resulting in formation of eschar that prevents deeper penetration of the acid. Alkaline burns, however, both denature proteins and hydrolyze fats, allowing for deeper penetration and tissue damage because of liquefaction necrosis. Hydrofluoric acid is similar to alkaline substances in that it also causes liquefaction necrosis. Symptoms vary depending on the substance, strength, and site of injury but often includes severe pain, tissue blistering and sloughing, and bleeding. Initial treatment includes removal of contaminated clothing and copious wound irrigation with water. If substances contain Na, K, Mg, or metallic lithium, then the burn area should be covered with mineral oil rather than irrigated. If hydrofluoric acid, copious water irrigations and soft-tissue injection or IV infusion of calcium gluconate may help reduce pain and tissue destruction. Patients may need fluid resuscitation and skin grafting. Complications include disfigurement, infection, and electrolyte imbalance.

ELECTRICAL BURNS

Electrical injuries result from electricity passing through the body from contact with live wires, lighting strikes, and short-circuiting equipment. Injuries may be high voltage (≥1000 volts) or low voltage (<1000 volts). Electrical injuries can result in extensive subdermal burns. The injury severity correlates with resistance of tissue and current amperage (AC usually causes more damage than DC). Tissue with the highest degree of resistance tends to suffer the most damage with low voltage injury, but high voltage injury can destroy all tissue. Tissue resistance (highest to lowest) include bone >fat >tendons >skin >muscles >vessels > nerves.

- **Low voltage** injuries may cause cardiac dysrhythmias (VF), external burns, tissue damage, fractures and dislocations from muscle contractions, respiratory arrest, or oral burns (children particularly). Treatment includes monitoring and cardiac care as needed, topical antimicrobials, and excision and grafting if necessary.
- **High voltage** injuries may result in additional symptoms of myonecrosis, thrombosis, compartment syndrome, nerve entrapment syndrome. Treatment may include fluid resuscitation, wound debridement, fasciotomy, and amputation, topical antibiotics, systemic antibiotics, and analgesia.

THERMAL BURNS

Thermal burns are caused by heat (hot iron, stove, sun exposure) or fire. Burn injuries begin with the skin but can affect all organs and body systems, especially with a major burn. Management of burn injuries must include both wound care and systemic care to avoid complications that can be life threatening. Patients may experience open blistering wounds and severe pain. **Treatment** varies according to severity and may include:

- Establishment of airway and treatment for inhalation injury if necessary
- Cleansing of burned areas, flushing
- Debridement of open blisters (no needle aspiration)
- Tetanus immunization if needed
- Intravenous fluids and electrolytes, based on weight and extent of burn
- Enteral feedings, usually with small lumen feeding tube into the duodenum
- NG tube for gastric decompression to prevent aspiration
- Indwelling catheter to monitor urinary output. Urinary output should be 0.5-2 mL/kg/hr
- Analgesia for reduction of pain and anxiety
- Topical (usually silver sulfadiazine) and systemic antibiotics
- Wound care with removal of eschar and dressings as indicated
- Skin grafting

Complications include scarring, disfigurement, contractures, and infection.

RADIATION INJURIES

Radiation injuries may be caused by direct radiation in which waves pass through the body (locally or to the entire body), which can result in acute radiation illness and genetic damage. **Contamination** usually occurs from radioactive dust or liquid contacting the skin. It can be absorbed into the tissues (eventually causing chronic illnesses, such as cancer) or contaminate others who contact it. Contaminated material may also be ingested. The lethal dose of 50% of those exposed within 60 days (LD50/60) is 4.5 Gy with immediate intensive treatment.

Diagnosis for direct radiation is symptomatic as there is no specific test; however, contamination can be measured by Geiger counter.

Syndromes of **acute radiation sickness** vary according to exposure:

- **Hematopoietic:** (at least 2 Gy exposure) affects blood cell production. 2-12 hours after exposure: anorexia, nausea, vomiting, lethargy. Symptom-free week during which blood cell production decreases causing decreased WBC and platelet count, resulting in infection and hemorrhage with weakness and dyspnea. Recovery begins in 4-5 weeks if patient survives.
- **GI:** (at least 4 Gy exposure)
  - 2-12 hours after exposure: nausea, vomiting, diarrhea, dehydration. 4-5 days, fewer symptoms but lining of GI tract sheds, leaving ulcerated tissue.
  - Severe diarrhea (bloody) and dehydration and systemic infections
- **Cerebrovascular:** (20-30 Gy exposure) always fatal
  - Alterations in mental status, nausea, vomiting, and diarrhea (bloody), progressing to shock, seizures, coma, and death

Treatment includes:

- Decontamination if contamination irradiation or if source of irradiation not clear
- Complete history of event, including source of radiation

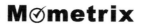

- Protocol for decontamination and securing of area should be followed, including use of individual dosimeters and protective coverings
- **Localized**: burn care and analgesia
- **Internal**: gastric decontamination, collection of urine and feces for 4 days to monitor rate of radioisotopes excretion, and collection of body fluids for bioassay
- **Whole body irradiation**: supportive treatment and prophylactic measures to combat opportunistic infections, hematopoietic growth factor for bone marrow depression

HEAT-RELATED ILLNESS

Children and the elderly are particularly vulnerable to heat-related illness, especially when heat is combined with humidity. Heat-related illnesses occur when heat accumulation in the body outpaces dissipation, resulting in increased temperature and dehydration, which can then lead to thermoregulatory failure and multiple organ dysfunction syndromes. Each year in the United States, about 29 children die from heat stroke after being left in automobiles. At temperatures of 72-96 °F, the temperature in a car rises 3.2 °F every 5 minutes, with 80% of rise within 30 minutes. Temperatures can reach 117 °F even on cool days. There are three **types of heat-related illness**:

- **Heat stress**: Increased temperature causes dehydration. Patient may develop swelling of hands and feet, itching of skin, sunburn, heat syncope (pale moist skin, hypotension), heat cramps, and heat tetany (respiratory alkalosis). Treatment includes removing from heat, cooling, hydrating, and replacing sodium.
- **Heat exhaustion**: Involves water or sodium depletion, with sodium depletion common in patients who are not acclimated to heat. Heat exhaustion can result in flu-like aching, nausea and vomiting, headaches, dizziness, and hypotension with cold, clammy skin and diaphoresis. Temperature may be normal or elevated to less than 106 °F. Treatment to cool the body and replace sodium and fluids must be prompt in order to prevent heat stroke. Careful monitoring is important and reactions may be delayed.
- **Heat stroke**: Involves failure of the thermoregulatory system with temperatures that may be more than 106 °F and can result in seizures, neurological damage, multiple organ failures, and death. Exertional heat stroke often occurs in young athletes who engage in strenuous activities in high heat. Young children are susceptible to nonexertional heat stroke from exposure to high heat. Treatment includes evaporative cooling, rehydration, and supportive treatment according to organ involvement.

HYPOTHERMIA

Hypothermia occurs with exposure to low temperatures that cause the core body temperature to fall below 95 °F (35 °C). Hypothermia may be associated with immersion in cold water, exposure to cold temperature, metabolic disorders (hypothyroidism, hypoglycemia, hypoadrenalism), or CNS abnormalities (head trauma, Wernicke disease). Many patients with hypothermia are intoxicated with alcohol or drugs.

Symptoms of hypothermia include pallor, cold skin, drowsiness, alterations in mental status, confusion, and severe shivering. The patient can progress to shock, coma, dysrhythmias (T-wave inversion and prolongation of PR, QRS, and QT) including atrial fibrillation and AV block, and cardiac arrest.

Diagnosis requires low-reading thermometers to verify temperature.

Treatment includes:

- Passive rewarming if cardiac status stable
- Active rewarming (external) with immersion in warm water or heating blankets at 40 °C, radiant heat
- Active rewarming (internal) with warm humidified oxygen or air inhalation, heated IV fluids, and internal (bladder, peritoneal pleural, GI) lavage

- Warming with extracorporeal circuit, such as arteriovenous or venovenous shunt that warms the blood
- Supportive treatment as indicated

LOCALIZED COLD INJURIES

Frostnip is a superficial freeze injury that is reversible. Frostbite is damage to tissue caused by exposure to freezing temperatures, most often affecting the nose, ears, and distal extremities. As frostbite develops, the affected part feels numb and aches or throbs, becoming hard and insensate as the tissue freezes, resulting in circulatory impairment, necrosis of tissue, and gangrene. There are **three zones of injury:**

- **Coagulation** (usually distal): severe, irreversible cellular damage
- **Hyperemia** (usually proximal): minimal cellular damage
- **Stasis** (between other 2 zones): severe but sometimes reversible damage

Symptoms vary according to the degree of freezing:

- **Partial freezing** with erythema and mild edema, stinging, burning, throbbing pain
- **Full-thickness freezing** with increased edema in 3-4 hours, edema and clear blisters in 6-24 hours, desquamation with eschar formation, numbness, and then aching and throbbing pain
- Prognosis is very good for **first-degree** and good for **second-degree** frostbite
- Full-thickness and into **subdermal tissue** freezing with cyanosis, hemorrhagic blisters, skin necrosis, and "wooden" feeling, severe burning, throbbing, and shooting pains
- Freezing extends into **subcutaneous tissue**, including muscles, tendons, and bones with mottled appearance, non-blanching cyanosis, and eventual deep black eschar

Prognosis is poor for **third-degree** and **fourth-degree** freeze injuries. Determining the degree of injury can be difficult because some degree of thawing may have occurred prior to admission to the hospital.

Treatment includes:

- Rapid rewarming with warm water bath (40-42 °C [104-107.6 °F]) 10-30 minutes or until the frostbitten area is erythematous and pliable
- Treatment for generalized hypothermia

Treatment **after warming**:

- Debridement of clear blisters but not hemorrhagic blisters
- Aloe vera cream every 6 hours to blistered areas
- Dressings, separating digits
- Tetanus prophylaxis
- Ibuprofen 12 mg/kg daily in divided doses
- Antibiotic prophylaxis if indicated (penicillin G 500,000 units IV every 6 hours for 24 to 72 hours)

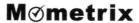

Respiratory Acute and Chronic Care

NON-INVASIVE VENTILATION
NASAL CANNULA

A nasal cannula can be used to deliver supplemental oxygen to a patient, but it is only useful for flow rates ≤6 L/min as higher rates are drying of the nasal passages. As it is not an airtight system, some ambient air is breathed in as well so oxygen concentration ranges from about 24-44%. The nasal cannula does not allow for control of respiratory rate, so the patient must be able to breathe independently.

NON-REBREATHER MASK

A non-rebreather mask can be used to deliver higher concentrations (60-90%) of oxygen to those patients who are able to breathe independently. The mask fits over the nose and mouth and is secured by an elastic strap. A 1.5 L reservoir bag is attached and connects to an oxygen source. The bag is inflated to about 1 liter at a rate of 8-15 L/min before the mask is applied as the patient breathes from this reservoir. A one-way exhalation valve prevents most exhaled air from being rebreathed.

NON-INVASIVE POSITIVE PRESSURE VENTILATORS

Non-invasive positive pressure ventilators provide air through a tight-fitting nasal or face mask, usually pressure cycled, avoiding the need for intubation and reducing the danger of hospital-acquired infection and mortality rates. It can be used for acute respiratory failure and pulmonary edema. There are 2 types of non-invasive positive pressure ventilators:

- **CPAP (Continuous positive airway pressure)** provides a steady stream of pressurized air throughout both inspiration and expiration. CPAP improves breathing by decreasing preload for patients with congestive heart failure. It reduces the effort required for breathing by increasing residual volume and improving gas exchange.
- **Bi-PAP (Bi-level positive airway pressure)** provides a steady stream of pressurized air as CPAP but it senses inspiratory effort and increases pressure during inspiration. Bi-PAP pressures for inspiration and expiration can be set independently. Machines can be programmed with a backup rate to ensure a set number of respirations per minute.

NEVER place a patient in wrist restraints while wearing these devices. If the patient vomits, they need to be able to remove the mask to prevent aspiration.

FACE MASK

Ensuring that a face mask (Ambu bag) is the correct fit and type is important for adequate ventilation, oxygenation, and prevention of aspiration. Difficulties in management of face mask ventilation relate to risk factors: >55 years, obesity, beard, edentulous, and history of snoring. In some cases, if dentures are adhered well, they may be left in place during induction. The face mask is applied by lifting the mandible (jaw thrust) to the mask and avoiding pressure on soft tissue. Oral or nasal airways may be used, ensuring that the distal end is at the angle of the mandible. There are a number of steps to prevent mask airway leaks:

- Increasing or decreasing the amount of air to the mask to allow better seal
- Securing the mask with both hands while another person ventilates

- Accommodating a large nose by using the mask upside down
- Utilizing a laryngeal mask airway if excessive beard prevents seal

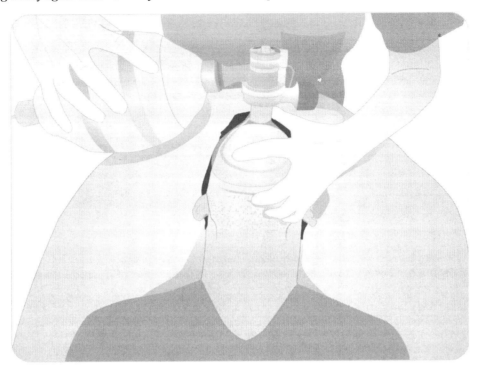

HIGH AND LOW FLOW OXYGEN DELIVERY

High flow oxygen delivery devices provide oxygen at flow rates higher than the patient's inspiratory flow rate at specific medium to high FiO_2, up to 100%. However, a flow of 100% oxygen actually provides only 60-80% FiO_2 to the patient because the patient also breathes in some room air, diluting the oxygen. The actual amount of oxygen received depends on the type of interface or mask. Additionally, the flow rate is actually less than the inspiratory flow rate upon actual delivery. High flow oxygen delivery is usually not used in the sleep center. Humidification is usually required because the high flow is drying.

Low flow oxygen delivery devices provide 100% oxygen at flow rates lower than the patient's inspiratory flow rate, but the oxygen mixes with room air, so the FiO_2 varies. Humidification is usually only required if flow rate is >3L/min. Much oxygen is wasted with exhalation, so a number of different devices to conserve oxygen are available. Interfaces include transtracheal catheters and cannulae with reservoirs.

AIRWAY DEVICES
OROPHARYNGEAL, NASOPHARYNGEAL, AND TRACHEOSTOMY TUBES

Airways are used to establish a patent airway and facilitate respirations:

- **Oropharyngeal**: This plastic airway curves over the tongue and creates space between the mouth and the posterior pharynx. It is used for anesthetized or unconscious patients to keep tongue and epiglottis from blocking the airway.
- **Nasopharyngeal** (trumpet): This smaller flexible airway is more commonly used in conscious patients and is inserted through one nostril, extending to the nasopharynx. It is commonly utilized in patients who need frequent suctioning.
- **Tracheostomy tubes**: Tracheostomy may be utilized for mechanical ventilation. Tubes are inserted into the opening in the trachea to provide a conduit and maintain the opening. The tube is secured with ties around the neck. Because the air entering the lungs through the tracheostomy bypasses the warming and moistening effects of the upper airway, air is humidified through a room humidifier or through the delivery of humidified air through a special mask or mechanical ventilation. If the tracheostomy is going to be long-term, eventually a stoma will form at the site, and the tube can be removed.

LARYNGEAL MASK AIRWAY

The laryngeal-mask airway (LMA) is an intermediate airway allowing ventilation but not complete respiratory control. The LMA consists of an inflatable cuff (the mask) with a connecting tube. It may be used temporarily before tracheal intubation or when tracheal intubation can't be done. It can also be a conduit for later blind insertion of an endotracheal tube. The head and neck must be in neutral position for insertion of the LMA. If the patient has a gag reflex, conscious sedation or topical anesthesia (deep oropharyngeal) is required. The LMA is inserted by sliding along the hard palate, using the finger as a guide, into the pharynx, and the ring is inflated to create a seal about the opening to the larynx, allowing ventilation with mild positive-pressure. The ProSeal LMA has a modified cuff that extends onto the back of the mask to improve seal. LMA is contraindicated in morbid obesity, obstructions or abnormalities of oropharynx, and non-fasting patients, as some aspiration is possible even with the cuff seal inflated.

ESOPHAGEAL-TRACHEAL COMBITUBE

The esophageal tracheal Combitube (ETC) is an intermediate airway that contains two lumens and can be inserted into either the trachea or the esophagus (≤91%). The twin-lumen tube has a proximal cuff providing a seal of the oropharynx and a distal cuff providing a seal about the distal tube. Prior to insertion, the Combitube cuffs should be checked for leaks (15 mL of air into distal and 85 mL of air into proximal). The patient should be non-responsive and with absent gag reflex with head in neutral position. The tube is passed along the tongue and into the pharynx, utilizing markings on the tube (black guidelines) to determine depth by aligning the ETC with the upper incisors or alveolar ridge. Once in place the distal cuff is inflated (10-15 mL) and then placement in the trachea or esophagus should be determined, so the proper lumen for ventilation can be used. The proximal cuff is inflated (usually to 50-75 mL) and ventilation begun. A capnogram should be used to confirm ventilation.

THORACENTESIS

A thoracentesis (aspiration of fluid or air from pleural space) is done to make a diagnosis, relieve pressure on the lung caused by pleural effusion, or instill medications. A chest x-ray is done prior to the procedure. A sedative may be given. The patient is in a sitting position, leaning onto a padded bedside stand, straddling a chair with head supported on the back of the chair, or lying on the opposite side with the head of the bed elevated 30-45° to ensure that fluid remains at the base. The patient should avoid coughing or moving during the procedure. The chest x-ray or ultrasound determines needle placement. After a local anesthetic is administered, a needle (with an attached 20-mL syringe and 3-way stopcock with tubing and a receptacle) is advanced intercostally into the pleural space. Fluid is drained, collected, examined, and measured. The needle is removed and a pressure dressing applied. A chest x-ray is done to ensure there is no pneumothorax. The patient is monitored for cough, dyspnea, and hypoxemia.

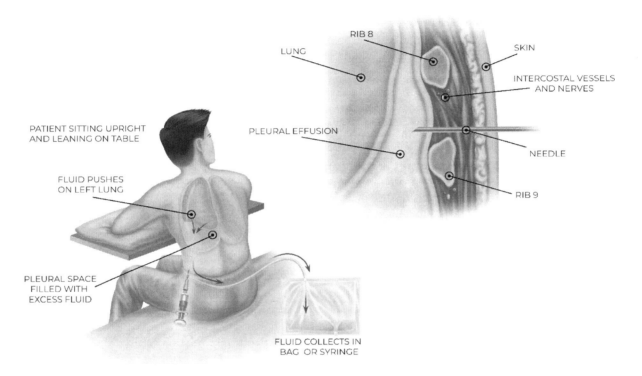

BRONCHOSCOPY

Bronchoscopy utilizes a thin, flexible fiberoptic bronchoscope to inspect the larynx, trachea, and bronchi for diagnostic purposes. It is also used to collect specimens, obtain biopsies, remove foreign bodies or secretions, treat atelectasis, and to excise lesions. The patient is in supine position during the procedure. The Mallampati classification may be used to determine difficulty of airway. The patient receives local anesthesia to the nares (lidocaine gel) and oropharynx (lidocaine gel, spray, or nebulizer), and usually receives a benzodiazepine (commonly midazolam or lorazepam), an opioid (fentanyl or meperidine), or propofol. Medications are usually given in small incremental doses throughout the procedure and may be combined. Over-sedation may cause physiologic depression, but undersedation may result in recall and agitation with sympathetic activation. The tube is advanced through the nares and down the trachea to the bronchi. Airway patency, respiratory rate, and oxygen saturation must be constantly monitored. Complications can include bleeding, arrhythmias, obstruction, laryngospasm, and respiratory failure.

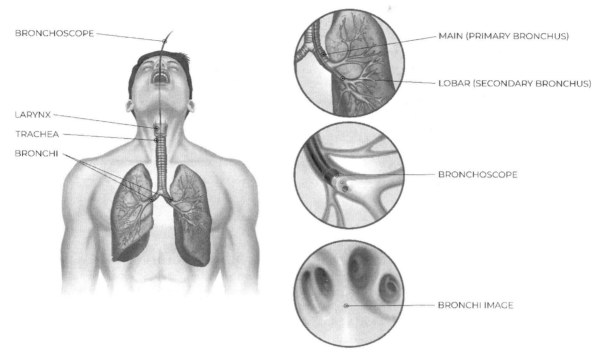

AHA Pediatric Advanced Life Support Guidelines for Respiratory Emergencies
Respiratory Distress/Arrest

According to the PALS guidelines, if a child experiences respiratory distress and arrest, the **ABC protocol** is recommended:

- **Airway**: Open and support the airway. Begin CPR with 2 respirations. Insert OPA/NPA if necessary.
- **Breathing**: monitor oxygen saturation, provide oxygen as needed and endotracheal intubation, ventilation as needed.
- **Circulation**: Monitor heartrate, rhythm, and BP and place IV. Begin standard CPR with chest compressions if cardiac arrest occurs.

The type of respiratory problem must be identified and treatment instituted:

- **Upper airway obstruction** (croup, RSV, epiglottitis, anaphylaxis, foreign body): Treatment depends on the cause. For example, epinephrine and corticosteroids for croup and epinephrine, albuterol, antihistamines, and corticosteroids for anaphylaxis.
- **Lower airway obstruction**: For bronchiolitis, nasal suctioning and bronchodilator and for asthma, albuterol and ipratropium, corticosteroids, epinephrine, $MgSO_4$, and terbutaline.
- **Disordered work of breathing**: Manage ICP, provide ventilatory support, and provide antidote in the case of poison/overdose.
- **Lung-tissue disease**: For pulmonary edema provide ventilatory support, a diuretic, and vasoactive support. For pneumonia provide albuterol, antibiotics, and CPAP.

HEIMLICH MANEUVER FOR CHILDREN <1 YEAR

Indications of choking in infants of less than one year include lack of breathing, gasping, cyanosis, and inability to cry. Procedures for the **Heimlich chest thrusts** include:

- Position the infant in prone (face down) position along the forearm with the infant's head lower than the trunk, being sure to support the head so the airway is not blocked.
- Using the heel of the hand, deliver 5 forceful upward blows between the shoulder blades.
- Sandwich the child between the two arms and turn the infant into supine position and drape over thigh with head lower than trunk and head supported.
- Using two fingers (as for CPR compressions), give up to 5 thrusts (about 1.5 inches deep) to lower third of sternum.
- Only do finger sweep and remove foreign object if the object is visible. Repeat 5 back blows followed by 5 chest thrusts until the foreign body is ejected or emergency personnel take over.
- If the infant loses consciousness, begin CPR. If a pulse is noted but spontaneous respirations are absent, continue ventilation only.

HEIMLICH MANEUVER FOR CHILDREN ≥1 YEAR

The universal sign of choking is when a person clutches the throat and appears to be choking or gasping for breath. If the person can speak ("Can you speak?") or cough, a **Heimlich maneuver** is not usually necessary. The Heimlich maneuver can be done with the victim sitting, standing, or supine. The Heimlich procedure for children (≥1 year) and adults:

- Wrap arms around the victim's waist from the back if sitting or standing. Make a fist and place the thumb side against the victim's abdomen slightly above the umbilicus. Grasp this hand with the other and thrust sharply upward to force air out of the lungs.
- Repeat as needed and call 911 if no response.
- If the victim loses consciousness, ease into supine position on the floor, place hands similarly to CPR but over the abdomen while sitting astride the victim's legs. Repeat upward compressions 5 times. If no ventilation occurs, attempt to sweep the mouth and ventilate lungs, mouth to mouth. Repeat compressions and ventilations until recovery or until emergency personnel arrive.

PHARMACOLOGICAL AGENTS USED FOR ASTHMA

Numerous pharmacological agents are used for control of asthma, some that are long-acting to prevent attacks and others that are short-acting to provide relief for acute episodes. Listed with each are the standard med and dosage used for urgent care:

- **β-Adrenergic agonists** include both long-acting and short-acting preparations used for relaxation of smooth muscles and bronchodilation, reducing edema, and aiding clearance of mucus. Medications include salmeterol (Serevent), sustained-release albuterol (Volmax ER) and short-acting albuterol (Proventil), and levalbuterol (Xopenex). Albuterol 2.5-5.0 mg every 20 minutes, 3 doses by nebulizer.
- **Anticholinergics** aid in preventing bronchial constriction and potentiate the bronchodilating action of β-Adrenergic agonists. The most commonly used medication is ipratropium bromide (Atrovent) 500 mcg every 20 minutes, 3 doses by nebulizer.
- **Corticosteroids** provide anti-inflammatory action by inhibiting immune responses and decreasing edema, mucus, and hyper-responsiveness. Because of numerous side effects, glucocorticosteroids are usually administered orally or parenterally for ≤5 days (prednisone, prednisolone, methylprednisolone) and then switched to inhaled steroids. If a person receives glucocorticoids for more than 5 days, then dosages are tapered. Methylprednisolone 60-125 mg IV is the standard dose for respiratory failure. The Global Initiative for Asthma (GINA) recommends daily inhaled corticosteroids for all individuals with severe asthma to reduce the risk of exacerbations.
- **Methylxanthines** are used to improve pulmonary function and decrease the need for mechanical ventilation. Medications include aminophylline and theophylline.

- **Magnesium sulfate** is used to relax smooth muscles and decrease inflammation. If administered intravenously, it must be given slowly to prevent hypotension and bradycardia. When inhaled, it potentiates the action of albuterol. Standard dosage: 2 g (8 mmol), 1 dose by IV over 20 minutes.
- **Heliox** (helium-oxygen) is administered to decrease airway resistance with airway obstruction, thereby decreasing respiratory effort. Heliox improves oxygenation of those on mechanical ventilation.
- **Leukotriene inhibitors** are used to inhibit inflammation and bronchospasm for long-term management. Medications include montelukast (Singulair).

ADDITIONAL PULMONARY PHARMACOLOGY

There is a wide range of agents used for pulmonary pharmacology, depending upon the type and degree of pulmonary disease. Agents include:

- **Opioid analgesics:** Used to provide both pain relief and sedation for those on mechanical ventilation to reduce sympathetic response. Medications may include fentanyl (Sublimaze) or morphine sulfate (MS Contin).
- **Neuromuscular blockers:** Used for induced paralysis of those who have not responded adequately to sedation, especially for intubation and mechanical ventilation. Medications may include pancuronium (Pavulon) and vecuronium (Norcuron). However, there is controversy about the use of such blockers, as induced paralysis has been linked to increased mortality rates, sensory hearing loss (pancuronium), atelectasis, and ventilation-perfusion mismatch.
- **Human B-type natriuretic peptides:** Used to reduce pulmonary capillary wedge pressure. Medications include nesiritide (Natrecor).
- **Surfactants**: Reduces surface tension to prevent the collapse of alveoli. Beractant (Survanta) is derived from bovine lung tissue and calfactant (Infasurf) from calf lung tissue. They are administered as inhalants.
- **Alkalinizers**: Used to treat metabolic acidosis and reduce pulmonary vascular resistance by achieving an alkaline pH. Medications include sodium bicarbonate and tromethamine (THAM).
- **Pulmonary vasodilator (inhaled nitric oxide):** Used to relax the vascular muscles and produce pulmonary vasodilation. Some studies show it reduces the need for extracorporeal membrane oxygenation (ECMO).
- **Methylxanthines:** Used to stimulate muscle contractions of the chest and stimulate respirations. Medications include aminophylline (Aminophylline), caffeine citrate (Cafcit), and doxapram (Dopram).
- **Diuretics**: Used to reduce pulmonary edema. Medications include loop diuretics such as furosemide (Lasix) and metolazone (Mykrox).
- **Nitrates**: Used for vasodilation to reduce preload and afterload, which in turn reduces myocardial need for oxygen. Medications include nitroglycerin (Nitro-Bid) and nitroprusside sodium (Nitropress).
- **Antibiotics**: Used for treatment of respiratory infections, including pneumonia. Medications are used according to the pathogenic agent and may include macrolides such as azithromycin (Zithromax) and erythromycin (E-Mycin).
- **Antimycobacterials**: Used for treatment of TB and other mycobacterial diseases. Medications include isoniazid (Laniazid, Nydrazid), ethambutol (Myambutol), rifampin (Rifadin), streptomycin sulfate, and pyrazinamide.
- **Antivirals**: Used to inhibit replication of a virus early in a viral infection. Effectiveness decreases as time passes because the replication process has already begun. Medications include ribavirin (Virazole) and zanamivir (Relenza).

NEBULIZERS

Nebulizers are used to provide respiratory treatments for conditions that can cause respiratory distress or wheezing, such as asthma. A nebulizer comes with several different parts, which often need to be assembled, depending on the model. The compressor works to power the machine to deliver the medication. Oxygen tubing is connected to the compressor, which travels from the machine to the patient. The other end of the oxygen tubing may be connected to either a mask that fits over the patient's mouth and nose or a mouthpiece that an older child may hold. Respiratory medication is available through vials or small, plastic bullets, which are emptied into a cup near the mouthpiece. Air flows from the compressor through the tubing to change the liquid into a mist that the patient can breathe during treatment.

INHALERS FOR CHILDREN

Inhalers used by children are typically one of two types: metered-dose inhalers or dry-powder inhalers.

- **Metered-dose inhalers** have a set amount of medication that is delivered with each use. The patient places the mouthpiece in his mouth and compresses the inhaler while breathing in the medication at the same time. For young children, a spacer may be added (**shown below**), which holds the medication for the patient to inhale at his or her own pace. This may also be connected to a mask, which makes breathing the medication easier for young children.

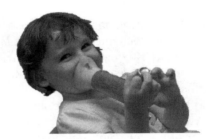

- With **dry-powder inhalers**, medication is inhaled in powdered form. The prescribed amount of medication is available in the inhaler, which is then inhaled at the patient's pace, without having to coordinate compressing the device and taking a breath.

Cardiovascular Acute and Chronic Care

CARDIOVERSION AND EMERGENCY DEFIBRILLATION DOSES FOR CHILDREN

The initial dose for cardioversion in a pediatric patient is 0.5–1.0 J/kg, doubled for subsequent doses if ineffective. The timing must be precise in order to prevent ventricular tachycardia or ventricular fibrillation. Sometimes, drug therapy is used in conjunction with cardioversion; for example, antiarrhythmics may be given before the procedure to slow the heart rate. Complications include dysrhythmias, burns, and injury to the myocardium. If ventricular fibrillation occurs, asynchronous shock is used.

The initial dose for emergency defibrillation in children is 2 J/kg, causing depolarization of myocardial cells, which can then repolarize to regain a normal sinus rhythm. Defibrillation delivers an electrical discharge usually through paddles applied to both sides of the chest. If the first shock and 2 minutes of CPR are ineffective, the dose is increased to 4 J/kg and 2 minutes of CPR and repeated if it is still ineffective.

AHA PEDIATRIC ADVANCED LIFE SUPPORT GUIDELINES FOR CARDIAC EMERGENCIES
CARDIAC ARREST

AHA Pediatric Advanced Life Support guidelines for **cardiac arrest** include:

- **Begin CPR** (30:2 for single rescuer and 15:2 for multiple) at rate of 100-120 compressions/minute and ventilate with oxygen if available. Maintain airway. Obtain IV/IO access when possible. If arrest is witnessed, obtain an AED/defibrillator immediately. If unwitnessed, begin first with compressions (CAB protocol) for 2 minutes and then obtain the AED/defibrillator and use it as soon as possible.
- **Shockable rhythm**: Defibrillate at 2 J/kg and resume CPR for 2 minutes, check rhythm, if necessary, defibrillate at 4 J/kg and continue CPR for 2 minutes. Obtain IV/IO access. Administer epinephrine 0.01 mg/kg IV/OI of a concentration of 1 g per 10,000 mL (1:10,000) every 3-5 minutes during resuscitative efforts. Continue to alternate CPR and defibrillation. The nurse may administer amiodarone 5 mg/kg up to two dosage or lidocaine 1 mg/kg.
- **Non-shockable rhythm**: Continue CPR at rate of 30 compressions:2 breaths (single rescuer) or 15:2 (multiple rescuers) and administer epinephrine 0.01 mg/kg IV/IO of 1:10,000 every 3-5 minutes.

If possible, identify the cause of the cardiac arrest and attempt treatment to reverse.

SYMPTOMATIC TACHYCARDIA

Treatment for pediatric tachycardia depends on the type of tachycardia. The child's airway should be maintained, and respirations should be assisted with oxygen and ventilation as needed and application of cardiac monitoring, vital signs, and oxygen saturation as well as IV/IO access. A 12-lead ECG should be obtained as soon as possible although treatment should not be delayed in order to obtain the ECG:

- **Probable sinus tachycardia** (P waves normal, variable R-R, PR constant, heart rate <220 for infants and <180 for children): Identify and treat cause.
- **Probable supraventricular tachycardia** (P waves missing/abnormal, heartrate ≥220 for infants and ≥180 for children): If IV/IO is available, adenosine per rapid bolus 0.1 mg/kg (maximum 6 mg); second dose 0.2 mg/kg (maximum 12 mg). If IV/IO is unavailable or medications are ineffective, use synchronized cardioversion.
- **Possible ventricular tachycardia with cardiopulmonary compromise** (hypotension, signs of shock, altered mental status): Synchronized cardioversion is indicated. If cardiopulmonary compromise is not evident and rhythm is regular and QRS is monomorphic, then one may administer adenosine IO/IV as for probable supraventricular tachycardia.

If synchronized cardioversion carried out, it should begin with 0.5-1.0 J/kg, increasing to 2 J/kg if ineffective.

SYMPTOMATIC BRADYCARDIA

When a child presents with symptomatic bradycardia, the first step is to maintain a patent airway and assist with respirations as needed, including administration of oxygen and ventilation and application of cardiac monitoring, vital signs, and oxygen saturation as well as IV/IO access. A 12-lead ECG should be obtained as soon as possible, although treatment should not be delayed in order to obtain the ECG. Indications of cardiopulmonary compromise include hypotension, signs of shock (pallor, cool clammy skin), and altered mental status. If heart rate persists below 60 beats per minute with continued poor perfusion despite interventions, then medications should be administered:

- Epinephrine (IV/IO) 0.01 mg/kg of 1:10,000 concentration. May repeat every 3-5 minutes. Alternately, if IV/IO access is unavailable and an ET is in place, then epinephrine may be administered per the ET tube at 0.1 mg/kg of 1:1000 concentration.
- Atropine (IV/IO) 0.02 mg/kg (minimum dose 0.2 mg and maximum single dose 0.5 mg). May repeat one time. Indicated for increased vagal tone or primary atrioventricular block.

For pulseless arrest, treatment for cardiac arrest is instituted.

ANTI-HYPERTENSIVE MEDICATIONS

The classes of anti-hypertensive medications are as follows: Diuretics, sympatholytics, vasodilators, calcium channel blockers, and angiotensin-converting enzyme inhibitors (ACE inhibitors).

- Diuretics include hydrochlorothiazide, chlorthalidone, chlorothiazide, indapamide, metolazone, amiloride, spironolactone, triamterene, furosemide, bumetanide, ethacrynic acid, and torsemide.
- Sympatholytics are clonidine, methyldopa, guanabenz, guanadrel, guanethidine, reserpine, labetalol, prazosin, and terazosin.
- Vasodilators include diazoxide, hydralazine, minoxidil, and nitroprusside sodium.
- Calcium channel blockers include amlodipine, nimodipine, isradipine, nicardipine, nifedipine, bepridil, diltiazem, and verapamil.
- ACE inhibitors include benazepril, captopril, enalapril, fosinopril, lisinopril, moexipril, quinapril, ramipril, and losartan.

DIURETICS

Diuretics increase **renal perfusion and filtration**, thereby reducing preload and decreasing peripheral and pulmonary edema, hypertension, CHF, diabetes insipidus, and osteoporosis. There are different types of diuretics: loop, thiazide, and potassium sparing.

LOOP DIURETICS

Loop diuretics inhibit the reabsorption of sodium and chloride (primarily) in the ascending loop of Henle. They also cause increased secretion of other electrolytes, such as calcium, magnesium, and potassium, and this can result in imbalances that cause dysrhythmias. Other side effects include frequent urination, postural hypotension, and increased blood sugar and uric acid levels. They are short-acting so are less effective than other diuretics for control of hypertension.

- **Bumetanide** (Bumex) is given intravenously after surgery to reduce preload or orally to treat heart failure.
- **Ethacrynic acid** (Edecrin) is given intravenously after surgery to reduce preload.
- **Furosemide** (Lasix) is used for the control of congestive heart failure as well as renal insufficiency. It is used after surgery to decrease preload and to reduce the inflammatory response caused by cardiopulmonary bypass (post-perfusion syndrome).

Review Video: Diuretics
Visit mometrix.com/academy and enter code: 373276

THIAZIDE DIURETICS

Thiazide diuretics inhibit the **reabsorption of sodium and chloride** primarily in the early distal tubules, forcing more sodium and water to be excreted. Thiazide diuretics increase secretion of potassium and bicarbonate, so they are often given with supplementary potassium or in combination with potassium-sparing diuretics. Thiazide diuretics are the first line of drugs for treatment of **hypertension**. They have a long duration of action (12-72 hours, depending on the drug) so they are able to maintain control of hypertension better than short-acting drugs. They may be given daily or 3–5 days per week. There are numerous thiazide diuretics, including:

- Chlorothiazide (Diuril)
- Bendroflumethiazide (Naturetin)
- Chlorthalidone (Hygroton)
- Trichlormethiazide (Naqua)

Side effects include, dizziness, lightheadedness, postural hypotension, headache, blurred vision, and itching, especially during initial treatment. Thiazide diuretics cause sensitivity to sun exposure, so people should be counseled to use sunscreen.

POTASSIUM-SPARING DIURETICS

Potassium-sparing diuretics inhibit the **reabsorption of sodium** in the late distal tubule and collecting duct. They are weaker than thiazide or loop diuretics, but do not cause a reduction in potassium level; however, if used alone, they may cause an increase in potassium, which can cause weakness, irregular pulse, and cardiac arrest. Because potassium-sparing diuretics are less effective alone, they are often given in a combined form with a thiazide diuretic (usually chlorothiazide), which mitigates the potassium imbalance. Typical side effects include dehydration, blurred vision, nausea, insomnia, and nasal congestion, especially in the first few days of treatment.

- **Spironolactone** (Aldactone) is a synthetic steroid diuretic that increases the secretion of both water and sodium and is used to treat congestive heart failure. It may be given orally or intravenously.
- **Eplerenone** is an antimineralocorticoid similar to spironolactone but with fewer side effects.

ANTIDYSRHYTHMIC DRUGS

Antidysrhythmic drugs include a number of drugs that act on the conduction system, the ventricles and/or the atria to control dysrhythmias. There are four classes of drugs that are used as well as some that are unclassified:

- **Class I:** 3 subtypes of sodium channel blockers (quinidine, lidocaine, procainamide)
- **Class II:** β-receptor blockers (esmolol, propranolol)
- **Class III:** Slows repolarization (amiodarone, ibutilide)
- **Class IV:** Calcium channel blockers (diltiazem, verapamil)
- **Unclassified:** Miscellaneous drugs with proven efficacy in controlling arrhythmias (adenosine, electrolyte supplements)

SMOOTH MUSCLE RELAXANTS

Smooth muscle relaxants decrease peripheral vascular resistance, but may cause hypotension and headaches.

- Sodium nitroprusside (Nipride) dilates both arteries and veins; rapid-acting and used for reduction of hypertension and afterload reduction for heart failure.
- Nitroglycerin (Tridil) primarily dilates veins and is used sublingual or IV to reduce preload for acute heart failure, unstable angina, and acute MI. Nitroglycerin may also be used prophylactically after PCIs to prevent vasospasm.
- Hydralazine (Apresoline) dilates arteries and is given intermittently to reduce hypertension.

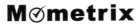

CALCIUM CHANNEL BLOCKERS

Calcium channel blockers are primarily arterial vasodilators that may affect the peripheral and/or coronary arteries.

- Side effects: Lethargy, flushing, edema, ascites, and indigestion:
- Nifedipine (Procardia) and nicardipine (Cardene) are primarily arterial vasodilators, used to treat acute hypertension. Diltiazem (Cardizem) and Verapamil (Calan, Isoptin) dilate primarily coronary arteries and slow the heart rate, thus are used for angina, atrial fibrillation, and SVT. *Note:* Nifedipine (Procardia) should be avoided in older adults due to increased risk of hypotension and myocardial ischemia.

> **Review Video: Ca Channel Blockers**
> Visit mometrix.com/academy and enter code: 942825

ADDITIONAL VASODILATORS

B-type natriuretic peptide (BNP) (Nesiritide [Natrecor]) is type of vasodilator (non-inotropic), which is a recombinant form of a peptide of the human brain. It decreases filling pressure, vascular resistance, and increases U/O.

- May cause hypotension, headache, bradycardia, and nausea. It is used short term for worsening decompensated CHF; contraindicated in SBP<90, cardiogenic shock, contrictive pericarditis, or valve stenosis.

Alpha-adrenergic blockers block alpha receptors in arteries and veins, causing vasodilation.

- May cause orthostatic hypotension and edema from fluid retention.
- Labetalol (Normodyne) is a combination peripheral alpha-blocker and cardiac β-blocker that is used to treat acute hypertension, acute stroke, and acute aortic dissection.
- Phentolamine (Regitine) is a peripheral arterial dilator that reduces afterload. It is used for HTN crisis in patients with pheochromocytoma, as well as a subcutaneous injection for extravasation of vessicants.

Selective specific dopamine DA-1-receptor agonists:

- Fenoldopam (Corlopam) is a peripheral dilator affecting renal and mesenteric arteries and can be used for patients with renal dysfunction or those at risk of renal insufficiency.

INOTROPIC AGENTS

Inotropic agents are drugs used to increase cardiac output and improve contractibility. IV inotropic agents may increase the risk of death, but may be used when other drugs fail. Oral forms of these drugs are less effective than intravenous. Inotropic agents include:

- **β-Adrenergic agonists**:
  - **Dobutamine** improves cardiac output, treats cardiac decompensation, and increases blood pressure. It helps the body to utilize norepinephrine. Side effects include increased or labile blood pressure, increased heart rate, PVCs, N/V, and bronchospasm.
  - **Dopamine** improves cardiac output, blood pressure, and blood flow to the renal and mesenteric arteries. Side effects include tachycardia or bradycardia, palpitations, BP changes, dyspnea, nausea and vomiting, headache, and gangrene of extremities.

- **Phosphodiesterase III inhibitors**:
  - o **Milrinone** (Primacor) increases strength of contractions and cause vasodilation. Side effects include ventricular arrhythmias, hypotension, and headaches.
- **Digoxin (Lanoxin)** increases contractibility and cardiac output and prevents arrhythmias.

MEDICATIONS FOR HEART FAILURE

A patient with heart failure may be prescribed with one or multiple of the drugs below:

- **ACE inhibitors:** Captopril (Capoten), enalapril (Vasotec), and lisinopril (Prinivil). Decrease afterload/preload and reverse ventricular remodeling; they also prevent neuropathy in DM. Contraindicated with renal insufficiency, renal artery stenosis, and pregnancy.
  - o Side effects include cough (#1), hyperkalemia, hypotension, angioedema, dizziness, and weakness.
- **Angiotensin receptor blockers (ARBs):** Losartan (Cozaar) and valsartan (Diovan). Decrease afterload/preload and reverse ventricular remodeling, causing vasodilation and reducing blood pressure. They are used for those who cannot tolerate ACE inhibitors.
  - o Side effects include cough (less common than with ACE inhibitors), hyperkalemia, hypotension, headache, dizziness, metallic taste, and rash.
- **β-Blockers:** Metoprolol (Lopressor), carvedilol (Coreg) and esmolol (Brevibloc). Slow the heart rate, reduce hypertension, prevent dysrhythmias, and reverse ventricular remodeling. Contraindicated in bradyarrythmias, decompensated HF, uncontrolled hypoglycemia/diabetes mellitus, and airway disease.
  - o Side effects: bradycardia, hypotension, bronchospasm, may mask signs of hypoglycemia.
- **Aldosterone agonist:** Spironolactone (Aldactone). Decreases preload and myocardial hypertrophy and reduces edema and sodium retention but may increase serum potassium.
- **Furosemide (Lasix)** is used for the control of congestive heart failure as well as renal insufficiency. It is used after surgery to decrease preload and to reduce the inflammatory response caused by cardiopulmonary bypass (post-perfusion syndrome).

> **Review Video: What are the Side Effects of ACE Inhibitors and ARBs?**
> Visit mometrix.com/academy and enter code: 525864

DIGOXIN (LANOXIN)

Digitalis drugs, most commonly administered in the form of digoxin (Lanoxin), are derived from the foxglove plant and are used to increase myocardial contractility, left ventricular output, and slow conduction through the AV node, decreasing rapid heart rates and promoting diuresis. Digoxin does not affect mortality, but increases tolerance to activity and reduces hospitalizations for heart failure. Therapeutic levels (0.5-2.0 ng/mL) should be maintained to avoid digitalis toxicity, which can occur even if digoxin levels are within therapeutic range, so observation of symptoms is critical. Because patients with heart failure are often on diuretics which decrease potassium levels, they are at increased risk for toxicity.

Symptoms of toxicity are as follows:

- Early signs: Increasing fatigue, lethargy, depression, and nausea and vomiting; progress to severe diarrhea, blurred vision/yellow or green halos around lights, fatigue/weakness
- Arrythmias: SA or AV block, VT/VF, PVCs, and bradycardia

Treatment consists of the following:

- Monitor serum levels and symptoms.
- Digoxin immune FAB (Digibind) may be used to bind to digoxin and inactivate it if necessary.

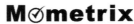

GLYCOPROTEIN IIB/IIIA INHIBITORS

Glycoprotein IIB/IIIA Inhibitors are drugs that are used to inhibit platelet binding and prevent clots prior to and following invasive cardiac procedures, such as angioplasty and stent placement. These medications are used in combination with anticoagulant drugs, such as heparin and aspirin for the following:

- Acute coronary syndromes (ACS), such as unstable angina or myocardial infarctions
- Percutaneous coronary intervention (PCI), such as angioplasty and stent placement

These medications are contraindicated in those with a low platelet count or active bleeding:

- **Eptifibatide (Integrilin)**: Used with both heparin and aspirin for ACS and PCI and affects platelet binding for 6-8 hours after administration. Should not be used in patients with renal problems.
- **Tirofiban (Aggrastat)**: Used with heparin for PCI patients with reduced dosage for those with renal problems and affects platelet binding for only 4-8 hours after administration.

PHARMACOLOGIC MEASURES TO MAXIMIZE PERFUSION

The primary focus of pharmacologic measures to **maximize perfusion** is to reduce the risk of **thromboses**:

- **Antiplatelet agents**, such as aspirin, Ticlid, and Plavix, which interfere with the function of the plasma membrane, interfering with clotting. These agents are ineffective to treat clots but prevent clot formation.
- **Vasodilators** may divert blood from ischemic areas, but some may be indicated, such as Pletal, which dilates arteries and decreases clotting, and is used for control of intermittent claudication.
- **Antilipemic**, such as Zocor and Questran, slow progression of atherosclerosis.
- **Hemorheologic agents**, such as Trental, reduce fibrinogen, reducing blood viscosity and rigidity of erythrocytes; however, clinical studies show limited benefit. It may be used for intermittent claudication.
- **Analgesics** may be necessary to improve quality of life. Opioids may be needed in some cases.
- **Thrombolytics** may be injected into a blocked artery under angiography to dissolve clots.
- **Anticoagulants**, such as Coumadin and Lovenox, prevent blood clots from forming.

ADMINISTRATION OF FIBRINOLYTIC (THROMBOLYTIC) INFUSIONS FOR MI

Fibrinolytic infusion is indicated for acute myocardial infarction under these conditions:

- Symptoms of MI, <6-12 hours since onset of symptoms
- ≥1 mm elevation of ST in ≥2 contiguous leads
- No contraindications and no cardiogenic shock

Fibrinolytic agents should be administered as soon as possible, within 30 minutes is best. All agents convert plasminogen to plasmin, which breaks down fibrin, dissolving clots:

- Streptokinase and anistreplase (1st generation)
- Alteplase or tissue plasminogen activator (tPA) (2nd generation)
- Reteplase and tenecteplase (3rd generation)

Contraindications

- Present or recent bleeding or history of severe bleeding
- History of intracranial hemorrhage
- History of stroke (<3 months unless within 3 hours)
- Aortic dissection or pericarditis
- Intracranial/intraspinal surgery or trauma within 3 months or neoplasm, aneurysm, or AVM

Relative contraindications

- Active peptic ulcer
- >10 minutes of CPR
- Advanced renal or hepatic disease
- Pregnancy
- Anticoagulation therapy
- Acute uncontrolled hypertension or chronic poorly controlled hypertension
- Recent (2–4 weeks) internal bleeding
- Non-compressible vascular punctures

Gastrointestinal Acute and Chronic Care

NG Tubes, Sump Tubes, and Levin Tubes

Nasogastric **(NG) tubes** are plastic or vinyl tubes inserted through the nose, down the esophagus, and into the stomach. **Sump tubes** are radiopaque with a vent lumen to prevent a vacuum from forming with high suction. **Levin tubes** have no vent lumen and are used only with low suction. NG tubes drain gastric secretions, allow sampling of secretions, or provide access to the stomach and upper GI tract. They are used for lavage after medication overdose, for decompression, and for instillation of medications or fluids. NG tubes are contraindicated with obstruction proximal to the stomach or gastric pathology, such as hemorrhage.

Tube-insertion length is estimated: earlobe to xiphoid + earlobe to nose tip + 15 cm.

The tube is inserted through the naris with the patient upright, if possible, and swallowing sips of water. Vasoconstrictors and topical anesthetic reduce gag reflex. Placement is checked with insufflation of air or aspiration of stomach contents and verified by x-ray. The NG is secured and drainage bag provided. Tubes attached to continuous low or intermittent high suction must be monitored frequently.

Levin Tube

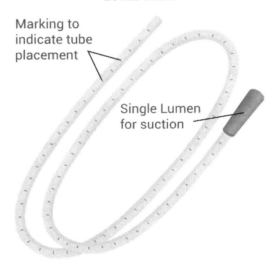

Marking to indicate tube placement

Single Lumen for suction

PEG Tube

Percutaneous endoscopic gastrostomy (PEG), used for tube feedings, involves intubation of the esophagus with the endoscope and insertion of a sheathed needle with a guidewire through the abdomen and stomach wall so that a catheter can be fed down the esophagus, snared, and pulled out through the opening where the needle was inserted and secured. The PEG tube should not be secured to the abdomen until the PEG is fully healed, which usually takes 2-4 weeks, because tension caused by taping the tube against the abdomen may cause the tract to change shape and direction. The tract should be straight to facilitate insertion and removal of catheters. Once the tract has healed, the original PEG tube can generally be replaced with a balloon gastrostomy tube. External stabilizing devices can be applied to the skin to hold the tube in place but should be placed 1-2 cm above the skin surface to prevent excessive tension that may result in buried bumper syndrome (BBS) in which the internal fixation device becomes lodged in the mucosal lining of the gastric wall, resulting in ulceration.

DRAINS

The following are different types of drains a patient may have, including pertinent nursing considerations:

- **Simple drains** are latex or vinyl tubes of varying sizes/lengths. They are usually placed through a stab wound near the area of involvement.
- **Penrose drains** are flat, soft rubber/latex tubes placed in surgical wounds to drain fluid by gravity and capillary action.

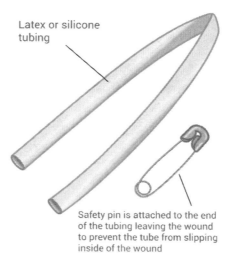

Latex or silicone tubing

Safety pin is attached to the end of the tubing leaving the wound to prevent the tube from slipping inside of the wound

- **Sump drains** are double-lumen or tri-lumen tubes (with a third lumen for infusions). The multiple lumens produce venting when air enters the inflow lumen and forces drainage out of the large lumen.
- **A percutaneous drainage catheter** is inserted into the wound to provide continuous drainage for infection/fluid collection. Irrigation of the catheter may be required to maintain patency. Skin barriers and pouching systems may also be necessary.

SAFE PERCUTANEOUS DRAINAGE KIT

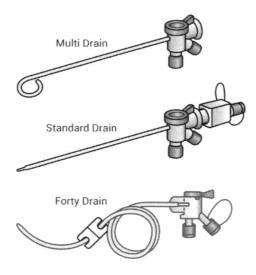

Multi Drain

Standard Drain

Forty Drain

- **Closed drainage systems** use low-pressure suction to provide continuous gravity drainage of wounds. Drains are attached to collapsible suction reservoirs that provide negative pressure. The nurse must remember to always re-establish negative pressure after emptying these drains. There are two types in frequent use:
  - **Jackson-Pratt** is a bulb-type drain that is about the size of a lemon. A thin plastic drain from the wound extends to a squeeze bulb that can hold about 100 mL of drainage.

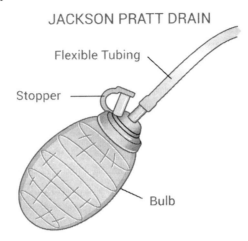

JACKSON PRATT DRAIN

Flexible Tubing

Stopper

Bulb

  - **Hemovac** is a round drain with coiled springs inside that are compressed after emptying to create suction. The device can hold up to 500 mL of drainage.

ENTERAL FEEDINGS

Caloric and nutritional needs for **enteral feedings** are assessed according to the age of the child, size, and stress factors. Breast milk is the optimal nutrition for infants. Feedings may be adjusted because of needs associated with diseases; for example, children with HF may require fluid restriction. Formula usually contains 24–30 calories per ounce. **Caloric requirements** are based on the recommended daily allowance (RDA) and resting energy expenditure (REE), the calories needed for a child at rest.

Age	RDA (kcal/kg/day)	REE (kcal/kg/day)	Protein (g/kg/day)
6-12 months	80	55	2.0-2.5
1-3 years	80-100	50-57	1.2-3.0
4-6 years	70-90	45-48	1.1-3.0
7-10 years	60-70	40	1.0-3.0
11-13 years	45-55	28-32	1.0-2.5
14-18 years	36-45	25-27	0.8-1.2

Total energy expenditure (TEE) is calculated by multiplying the REE by stress factors:

Maintenance: 0.2
Activity: 0.1-0.25
Fever: 0.13 per degree >38 °C
Burns: 0.5-1.0

Simple trauma: 0.2
Sepsis/major trauma: 0.4-1.5
Ventilation/sedation: 1.2-1.3
Growth: 0.5

NASOGASTRIC AND OROGASTRIC ENTERAL FEEDING TUBES

Nasogastric/orogastric enteral feeding tubes can be inserted quickly and nonsurgically but are usually reserved for short-term (<3 months) enteral feedings. A weighted or non-weighted catheter (5-8 Fr) is used. The length of insertion can be calculated using age-related height-based measurement or measuring the distance from the nose tip to the earlobe and from the earlobe to the midpoint between the xiphoid process and the umbilicus.

1. Mark the insertion length on the tube.
2. Explain the procedure in age-appropriate terms.
3. Check nares for patency, assess gag reflex, and note any contraindications (such as basal skull fracture with NG tubes).
4. Secure the child in supine position (swaddling, holding) with head elevated to 30–45°.
5. Lubricate tube or dip in water for pre-lubricated tubes.
6. Insert the tube into the mouth or nostril, aiming posteriorly and inferiorly.
7. When the NG/OG tube is in the pharynx, instruct the child to swallow or stimulate swallowing with use of pacifier.
8. Insert to the marking on the tube and temporarily secure.
9. Verify placement with radiograph.

GASTROINTESTINAL FEEDING TUBES PLACEMENT

Feeding tubes can be placed surgically, endoscopically, or radiologically:

- **Surgical placement**: There are both open and laparoscopic surgical techniques for placing tubes to the stomach or jejunum. The three most common methods are the Janeway, the Stamm, and the Witzel techniques.
- **Endoscopic placement**: Percutaneous endoscopic gastrostomy (PEG) involves intubation of the esophagus with the endoscope and insertion of a sheathed needle with a guidewire through the abdomen and stomach wall so that a catheter can be fed down the esophagus, snared, and pulled out through the opening where the needle was inserted and secured. Similar endoscopic procedures can be done in the jejunum.
- **Radiologic placement**: Through fluoroscopy, ultrasound and/or CT, a gastrostomy tube is inserted through the epigastrium and secured with a balloon and external bumper or disk. Insertion into the jejunum is done in a similar manner through the duodenum into the jejunum. A gastrojejunostomy tube, which both drains the stomach and feeds the jejunum, is another procedure.

PREVENTING DISPLACEMENT OF ENTERAL FEEDING TUBES

The displacement of an enteral feeding tube is usually the result of inadequate stabilization. Foley catheters must be marked where they exit the stoma to check for migration. Gastrostomy tubes with an internal balloon or mushroom tip, measured markings, and an external disk are easier to stabilize, but the internal device should be checked daily by gently pulling until resistance is felt. External stabilizing devices can be applied to the skin to hold the tube in place. The tube may also be taped to the abdomen or secured with a binder. Sometimes surgeons suture the tube in place, especially those with no balloon, such as jejunostomy tubes, which can become easily dislodged. A solid skin barrier with the tube fed through an anchored baby nipple is an inexpensive stabilizer. The position and length of the tube should be carefully documented. Balloon volume should be checked weekly to insure there are no leaks. Skin beneath disks/bumpers should be checked frequently.

PREVENTING AND TREATING OCCLUSION OF ENTERAL FEEDING TUBES

Prevention of occlusion of enteral feeding tubes involves proper administration of medications and feedings, and maintaining a regular schedule of flushing. Tubes should be flushed with 5–30 ml of water (depending on the age and size of the child) at least every 4 hours as well as before and after feedings and administration of medications. Medications should be in liquid form or crushed completely and enteric-coated or delayed release preparations should be avoided. Feeding solutions should be liquid consistency. The child should be positioned with head elevated for feedings.

Flushing of an occluded tube involves first checking for kinks or obvious problems, attaching a 20–30 mL syringe and aspirating fluid. Then, 5–10 mL of water or carbonated beverage (ginger ale, cola) can be slowly instilled (over about a minute) and aspirated a number of times to try to loosen the occlusion. After clamping for 10–15 minutes, the flushing procedure can be repeated with warm water/carbonated beverage. If the water or carbonated beverage fails, a multi-enzyme cocktail or Pancrease and sodium bicarbonate solution may succeed. If all flushing fails, the physician should be notified.

ADDITIONAL COMPLICATIONS

Additional complications of enteral feedings include:

Complication	Causes	Solutions
Vomiting/aspiration	Tube incorrectly placed Delayed gastric emptying Contaminated formula Increased residual volume	Check tube position Elevate head of bed 30-45° or have the child sit in a chair Refrigerate formula, check dates, and discard after 24 hours Delay feeding one hour and check residual volume before resuming
Diarrhea	Rapid feeding Medications (e.g., antibiotics) Contaminated formula Distal movement of tube Lactose intolerance Low-fiber/hypertonic formula	Slow rate of feeding or use continuous drip Change tubing every 24 hours and avoid hanging feedings for more than 4 hours Evaluate medications Check position of tube before feedings Change formula (add fiber, decrease sodium)
Constipation	Inadequate fluids Fecal impaction Medications Formula	Increase fluids, according to age/size Manual examination for fecal impaction Evaluate medications Consult dietitian regarding formula
Dehydration	Diarrhea/vomiting High protein formula Poor fluid intake Hyperosmotic diuresis	Treat same as for diarrhea/vomiting Consult dietitian for change in formula Increase fluids Monitor blood glucose levels

TOTAL PARENTERAL NUTRITION

Total parenteral nutrition (TPN) is an intravenous hypertonic solution containing glucose, fat emulsion, protein, minerals, and vitamins. Long PICCs may be inserted in the basilic or cephalic veins and advanced into central circulation for short-term TPN. Central venous catheters are usually inserted into the subclavian or jugular vein and advanced to the tip of the superior vena cava for long-term TPN. Central solutions are more hypertonic than peripheral. **Precautions**:

- Use aseptic technique for feedings and dressing changes
- Use micropore filter (solutions without fat emulsion)
- Use 1.2-micron filter (solutions with fat emulsion)
- Change filters and IV tubing every 24 hours
- Monitor VS every 4 hours
- Check daily weight
- Perform laboratory tests daily initially, 3 times weekly until stable, and then weekly (Glucose, electrolytes, CBC, urea nitrogen, and hepatic enzymes)

- Check triglyceride level every 4 hours after intralipid (fats and EFAs) infusion is begun to ensure level is ≤200 mg/dL
- Check label and ingredients before administration
- Discard cloudy solutions (contamination)
- Change solution at 24 hours
- Check for infection

INITIATION

Commercially-prepared TPN solutions contain dextrose and protein (amino acids), but electrolytes, vitamins, and trace elements are individualized. A total nutrient admixture that contains fat emulsion, dextrose, and amino acids is widely used although fat emulsion may be administered separately. Peripheral TPN for children allows a dextrose solution of ≤12.5% while central TPN allows dextrose solution of ≥15%. Intralipid (fats and essential fatty acids) solutions are commercially available in 10% and 20% concentrations with 20% preferred for children (2 kcal/mL). Protein levels of 1.5-2.0 g/kg per day are common. Vitamins and trace minerals are usually added to meet MDRs. TPN is initiated slowly with infusion rate gradually increasing over 24-48 hours. Because hyperglycemia is a common complication, blood glucose levels should be monitored every 4-6 hours at bedside. Insulin may be ordered (sliding scale) to maintain glucose level <150 mg/dL. Infusion rate should not be changed to manage hyperglycemia or hypoglycemia. TPN should be administered with an infusion pump so that rate of infusion can be precisely managed, and the rate of infusion and amount infused should be checked every 30-60 minutes.

COMPLICATIONS

TPN complications can include the following:

Complication	Signs/Symptoms	Management
Insertion trauma	Pneumothorax, hemothorax: dyspnea, diminished breath sounds Dysrhythmia Air embolism Brachial plexus injury: numbness or weakness in arm	Emergency treatment as indicated, including removal/replacement of catheter
Thrombus	Intraluminal blood clot Occluded catheter	Heparinization of TPN solution
Phlebitis	Inflammation at insertion site (erythema, pain, edema) from infiltration into tissues	Infusion of intralipid solution
Fluid imbalance	Overload or dehydration: change in urinary output, increase or decrease of BUN, creatinine, hematocrit, serum sodium and serum osmolality	Recalculate fluid requirements Evaluate for fluid loss, fever, renal insufficiency, cardiac insufficiency
Hyperglycemia	Increase in serum glucose/urine glucose Increased urinary output	Decrease glucose concentration Slow rate of infusion Administer insulin
Hypoglycemia	Decrease in serum glucose Diaphoresis, pallor, lethargy confusion, weakness, and dizziness	Stop insulin Increase dextrose concentration Slow rate of infusion Evaluate for sepsis

Complication	Signs/Symptoms	Management
Electrolyte imbalance	Varies according to imbalance Maintenance requirements: Na: 2-4 mEq/kg/d K: 2-4 mEq/kg/d Mg: 0.25-1.0 mEq/kg/d Ca: 0.5-3.0 mEq/kg/d P: 0.5-2.0 mmol/kg/d	Frequent laboratory monitoring and adjustment in electrolyte administration
Hyperammonemia	Lethargy, change in mental status Asterixis (flapping, tremors of hands)	Evaluate for hepatic insufficiency Decrease protein concentration in PN formula
Azotemia	Evidence of dehydration: dry mucous membranes, decreased skin turgor, and increased BUN and urinary specific gravity	Decrease amino acids in PN formula or change to NephrAmine
Deficiency of EFAs	Dry skin, flakiness Thrombocytopenia	Increase lipid intake with lipids at least 2x weekly as well as oral fats (if possible) and topical fats
Hyperlipidemia	Triglyceride level increasing Blood specimen cloudy	Decrease lipid administration or stop if triglyceride ≥400 mg/dL Monitor triglycerides every 4 hours initially and then daily

ESOPHAGOGASTRODUODENOSCOPY

Esophagogastroduodenoscopy (EGD), which is performed with a flexible fiberscope equipped with a lighted fiberoptic lens, allows direct inspection of the mucosa of the esophagus, stomach, and duodenum. The scope has a still or video camera attached to a monitor for viewing during the procedure. The scope may be used for biopsies or therapeutically to dilate strictures or treat gastric or esophageal bleeding. The child is positioned on the left side (head supported) to allow saliva drainage. Conscious sedation (midazolam, propofol) is commonly used along with a topical anesthetic spray or gargle to facilitate placing the lubricated tube through the mouth into the esophagus. Atropine reduces secretions. A bite guard in the mouth prevents the older children from biting the scope. The airway must be carefully monitored through the procedure (which usually takes about 30 minutes), including oximeter to measure oxygen saturation. While perforation, bleeding, or infection may occur, most complications are cardiopulmonary in nature and relate to drugs (conscious sedation) used during the procedure, so reversal agents (flumazenil, naloxone) should be available.

FUNDOPLICATION SURGERY

Fundoplication, in which part of the fundus of the stomach (the upper portion) is wrapped either completely or partially around the distal esophagus and then sutured, is the third most common surgery for children. It is done to prevent regurgitation and strengthen the lower esophageal sphincter. When the stomach contracts, this shuts the sphincter, preventing backflow of gastric contents into the esophagus. This procedure is done for children with congenital abnormalities of the esophagus and for those with gastroesophageal reflux, if they do not respond to medical treatment. It is also a common repair after infants have had gastrostomy tubes inserted, damaging the sphincter. There are a number of different procedures, but all are basically variations of the Nissen procedure, which involves a full 360° wrap of the esophagus. In recent years, most procedures have been done with laparoscopy, allowing for small abdominal incisions and less recovery time.

HERNIA REPAIR

Hernia repair (herniorrhaphy) is the most common surgery for infants and children and is done to repair herniation of the peritoneum and a segment of bowel through the abdominal wall. Surgery is necessary to prevent an incarcerated hernia, in which the bowel twists and blood supply is compromised. There are three main types:

- **Inguinal**: Herniation in the inguinal canal. This is common in premature or low birth-weight infants, usually males, and may occur bilaterally.
- **Femoral**: Herniation posterior to the inguinal ligament. This is more common in females.
- **Umbilical**: Herniation in the umbilical ring.

Inguinal and femoral hernias are usually repaired as soon as possible because of the danger of incarceration. Umbilical hernias pose less concern and often heal over time without surgical repair, so surgery for umbilical hernias is rarely done prior to school age. If incarceration has occurred prior to surgery, the affected segment of bowel is resected. Surgery may be done laparoscopically.

HISTAMINE RECEPTOR ANTAGONISTS

Histamine (H) receptor antagonists (actually reverse agonists) are used to treat conditions in which excessive stomach acid causes heartburn and GERD. They block histamine 2 (H_2) (parietal) cell receptors in the stomach, thereby decreasing acid production. These drugs are used less commonly now than proton-pump inhibitors. **Common H_2 antagonists** include:

- **Cimetidine (Tagamet)**: The first H_2 antagonist, it is used less frequently than others because of inhibition of enzymes that results in drug interactions, especially with contraceptive agents and estrogen.
- **Famotidine (Pepcid)**: This may be combined with an antacid to increase the speed of effects as it has a slow onset. It may be used pre-surgically to reduce post-operative nausea.
- **Nizatidine**: The last H_2 antagonist developed, it is used to treat ulcers and GERD. It is about equal in potency and action to ranitidine, which was discontinued due to the presence of NDMA, a cancer-causing contaminant, when stored in high temperatures.

ANTACIDS

Antacids are medications used to reduce stomach acids by raising the pH and neutralizing the acids present. They are commonly used to treat heartburn or indigestion. Adverse reactions are relatively rare unless taken to excess or with renal impairment. Drugs include:

- **Aluminum hydroxide** (Amphojel) may cause constipation and with renal impairment, hypophosphatemia and osteomalacia.
- **Magnesium hydroxide** (Milk of Magnesia) may cause diarrhea and with renal impairment can cause hypermagnesemia.
- **Aluminum hydroxide with magnesium hydroxide** (Maalox, Mylanta) may cause nausea, vomiting and diarrhea, yeast infection (thrush), or hypophosphatemia.
- **Calcium carbonate** (TUMS, Rolaids, Titralac) may cause gastric distention. Excess calcium intake may cause toxic reactions, including kidney stones and renal failure, so excess intake should be avoided.
- **Alka-Seltzer** combines sodium bicarbonate with aspirin and citric acid so this compound may cause gastric irritation, nausea and vomiting, and tarry stools.
- **Bismuth subsalicylate** (Pepto-Bismol). Pepto-Bismol may react with sulfur in the body to create a black tongue and black stools, but this is temporary. Pepto-Bismol has been associated with Reye's syndrome in children with influenza or chickenpox.

PROTON PUMP INHIBITORS

Proton pump inhibitors (PPIs) are now used more frequently than histamine receptor antagonists. PPIs interfere with an acid-producing enzyme in the stomach wall, reducing stomach acid. PPIs are used to treat GERD, stomach ulcers, and *H. pylori* (with antibiotics). PPIs are similar in action and include:

- Esomeprazole (Nexium)
- Lansoprazole (Prevacid)
- Omeprazole (Prilosec)
- Pantoprazole (Protonix)
- Rabeprazole (Aciphex)
- Omeprazole/sodium bicarbonate (Zegerid) (Long-acting form of omeprazole)

Common side effects include gastrointestinal upset (nausea, diarrhea, and constipation), headache, and rash. In rare instances, PPIs may cause severe muscle pain; however, they are usually well-tolerated with few adverse effects. PPIs may interfere with the absorption of some drugs, such as those that are affected by stomach acid. Absorption of ketoconazole is impaired, and absorption of digoxin is increased, sometimes leading to toxicity. Omeprazole impacts the hepatic breakdown of drugs more than other PPIs and may cause increased levels of diazepam, phenytoin, and warfarin.

ANTI-LIPIDS

Anti-lipid medications are frequently used to **lower cholesterol levels** if dietary modifications are unsuccessful in order to decrease coronary artery disease. Four primary **types** of medications include the following:

- **Statins** (3-hydroxy-3-methylglutaryl coenzyme A reductase inhibitors), such as atorvastatin (Lipitor), rosuvastatin (Crestor), fluvastatin (Lescol), lovastatin (Altoprev), pravastatin (Pravachol), and simvastatin (Zocor), inhibit the liver enzyme that produces cholesterol, but different statins vary in the ability to reduce cholesterol and in drug/other interactions (protease inhibitors, erythromycin, grapefruit juice, niacin, and fibric acids). Adverse effects include rhabdomyolysis (which causes severe muscle pain and weakness), headache, rash, weakness, and gastrointestinal disorders.
- **Nicotinic acid** (Niacor, Niaspan) decreases synthesis of lipoprotein, lowers low-density lipoprotein (LDL) and triglycerides, and increases high-density lipoprotein (HDL). It is used for low elevations of cholesterol and may be combined with statins. Adverse effects include flushing, hyperglycemia, gout, upper gastrointestinal disorders, and hepatotoxicity. Liver function must be monitored.
- **Bile acid sequestrants,** such as cholestyramine (Questran, Prevalite), colesevelam (WelChol), and colestipol HCL (Colestid), decrease LDL, increase HDL, and do not affect triglyceride levels. They bind to bile acids in the intestines so that more are excreted in the stool rather than returned to the liver, so the liver has to produce bile acids by converting cholesterol. Adverse effects include gastrointestinal disorders and decrease in absorption of other drugs.

SEROTONIN ANTAGONISTS

Serotonin antagonists block 5-HT$_2$ receptors of serotonin in the central and peripheral nervous systems and gastrointestinal system. An open channel can result in agitation, nausea, and vomiting, but antagonists close the channel and reduce these symptoms. Serotonin antagonists are frequently used to prevent and treat nausea associated with chemotherapy and anesthesia. Medications include:

- **Metoclopramide** (Reglan) is used to reduce nausea and vomiting from a wide range of causes. It is also a prokinetic drug that increases gastrointestinal contractions and promotes faster gastric emptying, so it is used for heartburn, GERD, and diabetic gastroparesis.
- **Ondansetron** (Zofran) reduces vagal stimulation of the medulla oblongata (vomiting center) and is used for nausea related to chemotherapy.
- **Granisetron** (Sancuso) is used to reduce nausea related to chemotherapy, surgery, and radiation.

Serotonin antagonists have fewer side effects than other antiemetics, but they may cause muscle cramping, agitation, diarrhea/constipation, dizziness, and headache.

LAXATIVES

The following are different types of laxatives:

- **Bulk formers** have high fiber content and both soften stool and create more formed stools. These include products such as Metamucil, Citrucel, and FiberCon, which are usually added to liquids because without adequate fluids, they can increase constipation.
- **Lubricants** include both oral mineral oil and glycerin suppositories. They coat the stool, preventing fluid absorption and keeping the stool soft. Mineral oil absorbs fat soluble vitamins and should be used only temporarily
- **Saline**, such as Milk of Magnesia and Epsom Salt, contain ions, such as magnesium phosphate, magnesium hydroxide, and citrate, which are not absorbed through the intestines and draw more fluid into the stool. The magnesium in the preparations also stimulates the bowel. People with impairment of kidney function should avoid magnesium products, and saline laxatives should be used infrequently to avoid dependence. Epsom Salt often has a purging effect and is rarely used.
- **Stool softeners** (emollients, such as Colace, and Philip's Liqui-Gels) use wetting agents, such as docusate sodium, to increase liquid in the stool, thereby softening it. They should not be used with mineral oil because of increased absorption of the oil through the intestines.
- **Hyperosmotics** (available by prescription) contain materials that are not digestible and serve to retain fluid in the stool. Products, such as Kristalose and MiraLAX soften the stool but may result in increased Abdominal distension and flatus, especially initially. There are three types of hyperosmolar laxatives: lactulose, polymer, and saline. Lactulose types use a form of sugar and work similarly to saline laxatives, but more slowly, and may be used for long-term treatment. The salines empty the bowels quickly and are used short-term. The polymers contain polyethylene glycol, which retains fluid in the stool and is used short-term.
- **Combinations** use two or more types, such as stool softener with stimulant, and should be used only short-term.

STIMULANTS

Stimulants increase intestinal motility, moving the stool through the bowel faster and reducing the absorption of fluids so that the stool remains softer. Common ingredients include cascara in Castor oil and senna in Senokot. Stimulants work quickly and are effective but can result in electrolyte imbalance, Abdominal distension, and cramping. Chronic use may cause a cycle of constipation and diarrhea. Stimulant suppositories, such as Dulcolax, are also available.

> **Review Video: Gastroenterological Drugs**
> Visit mometrix.com/academy and enter code: 455152

Genitourinary Acute and Chronic Care

PROCEDURES FOR INSERTION AND REMOVAL OF URINARY CATHETER

Procedure for inserting and removing a urinary catheter:

1. Gather supplies (included in a urinary catheter insertion kit), perform hand hygiene, place a waterproof pad under the patient, and ensure that the light source is adequate to view the urinary meatus.
2. Place females in supine position with knees flexed and males in supine position.
3. Apply gloves and wash the perineal area with facility provided cleanser (sometimes included in the outside of the urinary catheter kit) and allow to dry.
4. Remove gloves and wash hands.
5. Using aseptic technique, place the catheter kit between the patient's legs, open the kit touching only the corners of the drape that wraps around the kit.
6. Apply sterile gloves.
7. Apply sterile drapes to the patient.
8. Following the steps provided with the kit, place the lubricant into the appropriate section of tray, remove the catheter from its plastic and place the tip into the lubricant, and pour iodine over the three cleansing swabs (if they do not come impregnated with iodine already). Attach the 10-cc syringe (filled with sterile water) to the appropriate port of the catheter.
9. Cleanse the urethral meatus with the iodine impregnated swabs.
10. Using the nondominant hand, hold the penis or open the labia to observe the urethral meatus. This hand now becomes "dirty" and cannot be used to touch the catheter.
11. Using the dominant hand, insert catheter with the drainage end attached to the collection bag. Insert until urine flows freely, advancing a little further after that point.
12. Inflate the balloon using the 10-cc sterile water syringe, and ensure the catheter is secure.
13. Secure the catheter to the patient's leg and hang the collection bag below the level of the patient. Secure any tubing to the bed and ensure no kinking is present.

Removal: Straight catheter—remove by pulling out slowly. To remove indwelling catheter, deflate the balloon using the appropriate port and gently pull the catheter out.

REDUCING INFECTION RISKS ASSOCIATED WITH URINARY CATHETERS

Strategies for reducing infection risks associated with urinary catheters include:

- Using **aseptic technique** for both the straight and indwelling catheter insertion
- **Limiting catheter use** by establishing protocols for use, duration, and removal; training staff; issuing reminders to physicians; using straight catheterizations rather than indwelling; using ultrasound to scan the bladder; and using condom catheters
- Utilizing **closed-drainage systems** for indwelling catheters
- **Avoiding irrigation** unless required for diagnosis or treatment
- Using **sampling port** for specimens rather than disconnecting catheter and tubing
- Maintaining **proper urinary flow** by proper positioning, securing of tubing and drainage bag, and keeping the drainage bag below the level of the bladder
- **Changing catheters** only when medically needed
- **Cleansing external meatal area** gently each day, manipulating the catheter as little as possible
- Avoiding placing catheterized patients adjacent to those infected or colonized with antibiotic-resistant bacteria to reduce **cross-contamination**

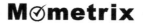

Endocrine Acute and Chronic Care

ORAL HYPOGLYCEMIC AGENTS

Oral hypoglycemic agents are **anti-diabetic treatments** generally used in the treatment of Type II Diabetes. There are five classic categories of oral hypoglycemic agents: sulfonylureas, biguanides, meglitinides, competitive inhibitors of alpha-glucosidases (located in the intestinal brush border), and thiazolidinediones. More recently, two additional novel classes of oral hypoglycemics, DPP-4 inhibitors and SGLT2 inhibitors, were introduced with proven effectiveness when used in conjunction with changes in diet and exercise. Some examples of sulfonylurea oral hypoglycemic agents include the first-generation agents tolbutamide, tolazamide, chlorpropamide, and acetohexamide; and second-generation agents glyburide, glimepiride, and glipizide. The biguanide oral hypoglycemic agent is metformin. Metformin has the distinct advantage of not causing weight gain or hypoglycemic reactions. The meglitinide agent is repaglinide. Examples of alpha-glucosidase inhibitors are acarbose and miglitol. Alpha-glucosidase inhibitors bind tightly to intestinal alpha-glucosidases and decrease the postprandial rise in glucose levels. The only available thiazolidinedione oral hypoglycemic agent is currently pioglitazone; troglitazone was removed from US market in 2000, and rosiglitazone was removed from US market in 2011. Examples of DPP-4 inhibitors include linagliptin, vildagliptin, sitagliptin, and saxagliptin. Examples of SGLT2 inhibitors include canagliflozin, dapagliflozin, and empagliflozin.

INSULIN USED TO TREAT GLYCEMIC DISORDERS

There are a number of different types of **insulin** with varying action times. Insulin is used to metabolize **glucose** for those whose pancreas does not produce insulin. People may need to take a combination of insulins (short- and long-acting) to maintain glucose control. Duration of action may vary according to the individual's metabolism, intake, and level of activity:

- **Humalog** (Lispro H) is a fast-acting, short-acting insulin with onset in 5–15 minutes, peaking at 45–90 minutes and lasting 3–4 hours.
- **Regular** (R) is a relatively fast-acting insulin with onset in 30 minutes, peaks in 2–5 hours, and lasts 5–8 hours.
- **NPH** (N) insulin is intermediate-acting with onset in 1–3 hours, peaking at 6–12 hours, and lasting for 16–24 hours.
- **Insulin Glargine** (Lantus) is a long-acting insulin with onset in 3–6 hours, no peak, and lasting for 24 hours.
- **Combined NPH/Regular** (70/30 or 50/50) has an onset of 30 minutes, peaks at 7–12 hours, and lasts 16–24 hours.

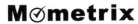

Genitourinary Acute and Chronic Care

RENAL DIALYSIS
PERITONEAL DIALYSIS

Renal dialysis is used primarily for those who have progressed from renal insufficiency to uremia with end-stage renal disease (ESRD). It may also be temporarily for acute conditions. People can be maintained on dialysis, but there are many complications associated with dialysis, so many people are considered for renal transplantation. There are a number of different approaches to **peritoneal dialysis:**

- **Peritoneal dialysis:** An indwelling catheter is inserted surgically into the peritoneal cavity with a subcutaneous tunnel and a Dacron cuff to prevent infection. Sterile dialysate solution is slowly instilled through gravity, remains for a prescribed length of time, and is then drained and discarded.
- **Continuous ambulatory peritoneal dialysis:** a series of exchange cycles is repeated 24 hours a day.
- **Continuous cyclic peritoneal dialysis:** a prolonged period of retaining fluid occurs during the day with drainage at night.

Peritoneal dialysis may be used for those who want to be more independent, don't live near a dialysis center, or want fewer dietary restrictions.

HEMODIALYSIS

Hemodialysis, the most common type of dialysis, is used for both short-term dialysis and long-term for those with ESRD. Treatments are usually done three times weekly for 3-4 hours or daily dialysis with treatment either during the night or in short daily periods. **Hemodialysis** is often done for those who can't manage peritoneal dialysis or who live near a dialysis center, but it does interfere with work or school attendance and requires strict dietary and fluid restrictions between treatments. Short daily dialysis allows more independence, and increased costs may be offset by lower morbidity. A vascular access device, such as a catheter, fistula, or graft, must be established for hemodialysis, and heparin is used to prevent clotting. With hemodialysis, blood is circulated outside of the body through a dialyzer (a synthetic semipermeable membrane), which filters the blood. There are many different types of dialyzers. High flux dialyzers use a highly permeable membrane that shortens the duration of treatment and decreases the need for heparin.

DIALYSIS COMPLICATIONS

There are many complications associated with dialysis, especially when used for long-term treatment:

- **Hemodialysis**: Long-term use promotes atherosclerosis and cardiovascular disease. Anemia and fatigue are common, as are infections related to access devices or contamination of equipment. Some experience hypotension and muscle cramping during treatment. Dysrhythmias may occur. Some may exhibit dialysis disequilibrium from cerebral fluid shifts, causing headaches, nausea and vomiting, and alterations of consciousness.
- **Peritoneal dialysis:** Most complications are minor, but it can lead to peritonitis, which requires removal of the catheter if antibiotic therapy is not successful in clearing the infection within 4 days. There may be leakage of the dialysate around the catheter. Bleeding may occur, especially in females who are menstruating as blood is pulled from the uterus through the fallopian tubes. Abdominal hernias may occur with long use. Some may have anorexia from the feeling of fullness or a sweet taste in the mouth from the absorption of glucose.

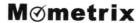

Hematologic Acute and Chronic Care

ANTICOAGULANTS

Common anticoagulants used at home and in the hospital setting are discussed below, including possible complications and the antidotes for each:

- **Antithrombin activators**: Heparin (unfractionated) and derivatives, LWM (Dalteparin, Enoxaparin, tinzaparin), and Fondaparinux.
  - Possible complications: Thrombocytopenia, bleeding/hemorrhage, osteopenia, hypersensitivity.
  - Antidote: Protamine sulfate 1% solution—dosage varies according to drug and drug's dosage. (1 mg protamine neutralizes 100 units of heparin or 1 mg of enoxaparin.)
- **Direct thrombin inhibitors**: Hirudin analogs (bivalirudin, desirudin, lepirudin). Others: Apixaban, Argatroban, and dabigatran.
  - Possible complications: Bleeding/hemorrhage, GI upset, backpain, hypertension, headache.
  - No antidote is available.
- **Direct Xa inhibitor**: Rivaroxaban
  - Possible complications: Bleeding/hemorrhage.
  - No antidote is available.
- **Antithrombin (AT)**: Recombinant human AT, Plasma-derived AT
  - Possible complications: Bleeding/hemorrhage, hypersensitivity.
  - No antidote is available.
- **Warfarin**
  - Possible complications: Bleeding/hemorrhage. Drug interactions may cause thrombosis or increased risk of bleeding.
  - Antidote: Vitamin K_1 usually at 2.5 mg PO or 0.5–1.0 mg IV. If ineffective, FFP or fresh whole blood may be administered.

> **Review Video: <u>Anticoagulants Thrombolytics and Antiplatelets</u>**
> Visit mometrix.com/academy and enter code: 711284

HEPARIN

PHARMACOLOGY

Heparin is an **anticoagulant** derived from the intestinal mucosa of the pig and the lung of the pig. The mechanism of action of heparin is to bind to the surface of the endothelial cell membrane. The activity of heparin depends upon plasma protease inhibitor antithrombin III. Antithrombin III inhibits thrombin and other anti-clotting proteases. In addition, heparin binding causes a change in antithrombin III inhibitor form, resulting in increased antithrombin-protease complex formation activity. After antithrombin-protease complex formation, heparin is subsequently released and is available to bind to more antithrombin molecules.

RISK FACTORS

The major risk factor of heparin use is hemorrhage. Predisposing factors for hemorrhage include advanced age and renal failure. Prolonged use of heparin can result in osteoporosis and fractures. Other risk factors of heparin use include transient thrombocytopenia, severe thrombocytopenia, paradoxical thromboembolism, and heparin-induced aggregation of platelets. These risks can be reduced by careful selection of patients who receive heparin therapy, careful control of the dosage of heparin, and meticulous monitoring of the partial thromboplastin time, or PTT. It is important to remember that thrombocytopenia or the development of a thrombus may be due to heparin itself.

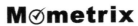

CONTRAINDICATIONS

There are numerous contraindications to the use of heparin, including: hypersensitivity to heparin; diseases of the hematologic system (hemophilia, purpura, or thrombocytopenia); uncontrolled hypertension; intracranial bleed; infectious endocarditis; active tuberculosis; gastrointestinal ulcers; cancer of the gastrointestinal visceral organs; severe liver dysfunction; severe kidney dysfunction; and threatened miscarriage or abortion. Heparin is contraindicated in the following medical procedures: following brain surgery; following spinal cord surgery; following eye surgery; after a lumbar puncture; and after regional anesthesia blocks. The effects of heparin may be reversed by stopping heparin or by the use of a specific antagonist (protamine sulfate).

> **Review Video: Heparin**
> Visit mometrix.com/academy and enter code: 127426

WARFARIN

PHARMACOLOGY

Warfarin causes a deficiency in prothrombin in the plasma and is used as an **anti-thrombotic agent** and to decrease the risk of embolism in humans. This agent causes the liver to manufacture less of the proteins necessary for blood coagulation. Since it is 99% bound to albumin in the plasma, warfarin has a high bio-availability. The mechanism of action of warfarin involves prothrombin, factor VII, factor IX, factor X, and protein C. Warfarin inhibits the g-carboxylation of the glutamate residues in the aforementioned factors. The mechanism of action of warfarin also involves vitamin K. Warfarin has a slow onset of action, usually 24 hours, and a typical duration of 2 to 5 days. Using increased dosages of warfarin as loading dosages will serve to speed up the onset of anti-coagulation. Patients on warfarin must discontinue this medication five days before planned surgery due to its longer duration.

DRUG-DRUG INTERACTIONS

Warfarin has many drug-drug interactions, the most serious of which increases the risk of bleeding. Sulfinpyrazone and phenylbutazone interact with warfarin to cause enhanced decrease in prothrombin, increased inhibition of platelets, and increased risk of peptic ulcer. The following drugs can have adverse effects when co-administered with warfarin: antibiotics such as metronidazole, azithromycin, clarithromycin, dirithromycin, erythromycin, roxithromycin, and telithromycin; broad-spectrum antibiotics such as amoxicillin, imipenem, levofloxacin; antifungal agents such as fluconazole, miconazole, and ketoconazole; barbiturates; and trimethoprim-sulfamethoxazole, amiodarone, cimetidine, and disulfiram. Aspirin inhibits metabolism of the warfarin and nonsteroidal anti-inflammatory drugs (NSAIDs) inhibit the clotting of platelets. The third-generation cephalosporins increase the risk of bleeding with warfarin because these drugs destroy the intestinal bacteria that produce vitamin K. Always check on possible drug-drug interactions when administering warfarin and monitor patients who might be at risk.

> **Review Video: Warfarin**
> Visit mometrix.com/academy and enter code: 844117

THROMBOLYTICS

Thrombolytics are drugs used to dissolve clots in myocardial infarction, ischemic stroke, DVT, and pulmonary embolism. **Thrombolytics** may be given in combination with heparin or low-weight heparin to increase anticoagulation effect. Thrombolytics should be administered within 90 minutes but may be given up to 6 hours after an event. They may increase the danger of hemorrhage and are contraindicated with hemorrhagic strokes, recent surgery, or bleeding. Thrombolytics include:

- **Alteplase tissue-type plasminogen activator** (t-PA) (Activase) is an enzyme that converts plasminogen to plasmin, which is a fibrinolytic enzyme. t-PA is used for ischemic stroke, MI, and pulmonary embolism and must be given IV within 3–4.5 hours or by catheter directly to the site of occlusion within 6 hours.

- **Anistreplase** (Eminase) is used for treatment of acute MI and is given intravenously in a 30-unit dose over 2–5 minutes.
- **Reteplase** (Retavase) is a plasminogen activator used after MI to prevent CHF (contraindicated for ischemic strokes). It is given in 2 doses, a 10-unit bolus over 2 minutes and then repeated in 30 minutes.
- **Streptokinase** (Streptase) is used for pulmonary emboli, acute MI, intracoronary thrombi, DVT, and arterial thromboembolism. It should be given within 4 hours but can be given after up to 24 hours. Intravenous infusion is usually 1,500,000 units in 60 minutes. Intracoronary infusion is done with an initial 20,000-unit bolus and then 2000 units per minute for 60 minutes.
- **Tenecteplase** (TNKase) is used to treat acute MI with large ST elevation. It is administered in a one-time bolus over 5 seconds and should be administered within 30 minutes of the event.

Contraindications to thrombolytic therapy include:

- Evidence of cerebral or subarachnoid hemorrhage or other internal bleeding or history of intracranial hemorrhage, recent stroke, head trauma, or surgery (ruled out by CT scan before administration for ischemic stroke)
- Uncontrolled hypertension, seizures
- Intracranial AVM, neoplasm, or aneurysm
- Current anticoagulation therapy
- Low platelet count (<100,000 mm^3)

Neurological Acute and Chronic Care

ANTICONVULSANTS

Carbamazepine (Tegretol)

Use: Partial, tonic-clonic, and absence seizures; analgesia for trigeminal neuralgia

Side effects: Dizziness, drowsiness, nausea, and vomiting. Toxic reactions include severe skin rash, agranulocytosis, aplastic anemia, and hepatitis

Clonazepam (Klonopin)

Use: Akinetic, absence, and myoclonic seizures; Lennox-Gastaut syndrome

Side effects: Behavioral changes, hirsutism or alopecia, headaches, and drowsiness. Toxic reactions include hepatotoxicity, thrombocytopenia, ataxia, and bone marrow failure.

Ethosuximide (Zarontin)

Use: Absence seizures

Side effects: Headaches and gastrointestinal disorders. Toxic reactions include skin rash, blood dyscrasias (sometimes fatal), hepatitis, and lupus erythematosus.

Felbamate (Felbatol)

Use: Lennox-Gastaut syndrome

Side effects: Headache, fatigue, insomnia, and cognitive impairment. Toxic reactions include aplastic anemia and hepatic failure. It is recommended only if other medications have failed.

Fosphenytoin (Cerebyx)

Use: Status epilepticus prevention and treatment during neurosurgery

Side effects: CNS depression, hypotension, cardiovascular collapse, dizziness, nystagmus, and pruritus.

Gabapentin (Neurontin)

Use: Partial seizures; post-herpetic neuralgia

Side effects: Dizziness, somnolence, drowsiness, ataxia, weight gain, and nausea. Toxic reactions include hepatotoxicity and leukopenia.

Lamotrigine (Lamictal)

Use: Partial and primary generalized tonic-clonic seizures; Lennox-Gastaut syndrome

Side effects: Tremor, ataxia, weight gain, dizziness, headache, and drowsiness. Toxic reactions include severe rash, which may require hospitalization.

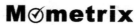

Levetiracetam (Keppra)

Use: Partial onset, myoclonic, and generalized tonic-clonic seizures

Side effects: Idiopathic generalized epilepsy, dizziness, somnolence, irritability, alopecia, double vision, sore throat, and fatigue. Toxic reactions include bone marrow suppression and liver failure.

Oxcarbazepine (Trileptal)

Use: Partial seizures

Side effects: Double or abnormal vision, tremor, abnormal gait, GI disorders, dizziness, and fatigue. A toxic reaction is hepatotoxicity.

Phenobarbital (Luminal)

Use: Tonic-clonic and cortical local seizures; acute convulsive episodes; insomnia

Side effects: Sedation, double vision, agitation, and ataxia. Toxic reactions include anemia and skin rash.

Phenytoin (Dilantin)

Use: Tonic-clonic and complex partial seizures

Side effects: Nystagmus, vision disorders, gingival hyperplasia, hirsutism, dysrhythmias, and dysarthria. Toxic reactions include collapse of cardiovascular system and CNS depression.

Primidone (Mysoline)

Use: Grand mal, psychomotor, and focal seizures

Side effects: Double vision, ataxia, impotence, lethargy, and irritability. Toxic reactions include skin rash.

Tiagabine (Gabitril)

Use: Partial seizures

Side effects: Concentration problems, weak knees, dysarthria, abdominal pain, tremor, dizziness, fatigue, and agitation.

Topiramate (Topamax)

Use: Partial and tonic-clonic seizures; migraines

Side effects: Anorexia, weight loss, somnolence, confusion, ataxia, and confusion. Toxic reactions include kidney stones.

Valproate/Valproic acid (Depakote, Depakene)

Use: Complex partial, simple, and complex absence seizures; bipolar disorder

Side effects: Weight gain, alopecia, tremor, menstrual disorders, nausea, and vomiting. Toxic reactions include hepatotoxicity, severe pancreatitis, rash, blood dyscrasias, and nephritis.

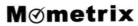

Zonisamide (Zonegran, Excegran)

Use: Partial seizures

Side effects: Anorexia, nausea, agitation, rash, headache, dizziness, and somnolence. Toxic reactions include leukopenia and hepatotoxicity.

HYPERTONIC SALINE SOLUTION

Hypertonic saline solution (HSS) has a sodium concentration higher than 0.9% (NS) and is used to reduce intracranial pressure/cerebral edema and treat traumatic brain injury. Concentrations usually range from 2% to 23.4%. The hypertonic solution draws fluid from the tissue through osmosis. As edema decreases, circulation improves. HSS also expands plasma, increasing CPP, and counteracts hyponatremia that occurs in the brain after injury.

Administration:

- Peripheral lines: HSS <3% only
- Central lines: HSS ≥3%

HSS can be administered continuously at rates varying from 30-150 mL/hr. Rate must be carefully controlled. Fluid status must be monitored to prevent hypovolemia, which increases risk of renal failure. Boluses (typically 30 mL of 23.4%) may be administered over 15 minutes for acute increased ICP or transtentorial herniation.

Laboratory monitoring includes:

- Sodium (every 6 hours): Maintain at 145-155 mmol/L. Higher levels can cause heart/respiratory/renal failure.
- Serum osmolality (every 12 hours): Maintain at 320 mOsm/L. Higher levels can cause renal failure.

MANNITOL

Mannitol is an osmotic diuretic that increases excretion of both sodium and water and reduces intracranial pressure and brain mass, especially after traumatic brain injury. Mannitol may also be used to shrink the cells of the blood-brain barrier in order to help other medications breach this barrier. Mannitol is administered per intravenous infusion:

- 2 g/kg in a 15-25% solution over 30-60 minutes

Cerebral spinal fluid pressure should show decrease within 15 minutes. Fluid and electrolyte balances must be carefully monitored as well as intake and output and body weight. Concentrations of 20-25% require a filter. Crystals may form if the mannitol solution is too cold and the mannitol container may require heating (in 80 °C water) and shaking to dissolve crystals, but the solution should be cooled to below body temperature prior to administration. Mannitol cannot be administered in polyvinylchloride bags as precipitates form. Side effects include fluid and electrolyte imbalance, nausea, vomiting, hypotension, tachycardia, fever, and urticaria.

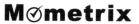

Oncologic/Immunologic Acute and Chronic Care

IMMUNOSUPPRESSANT DRUGS

Drug	Actions	Side Effects
Monoclonal Antibodies	Act to depress particular antigens, such as CD-3, and lower T cell count. Used to treat acute rejection responses.	Marked cell-mediated immune depression increases risk of infection and development of cancer.
Polyclonal Antibodies	(Obtained from animal serum.) Inhibit T cell production and promote destruction of T cells. Used with other immunosuppressant drugs to reduce dosage. Depress cell-mediated immune response and are used to prevent GVHD response.	Allergic/anaphylactic reactions to serum, including serum sickness, fever, arthralgia, urticaria, and erythema.
Azathioprine	Inhibits cell reproduction, especially those that replicate quickly, such as B and T cells. Used with transplantations and autoimmune diseases, such as MS, Crohn's disease and restrictive lung disease.	Bone marrow suppression, increasing risk of infection. Nausea, loss of hair, malaise, and rash. Increased risk of cancer, especially skin tumors, with long-term use.
Methotrexate	Inhibits folic acid, which interferes with RNA/DNA synthesis and cell division. Used for many different cancers and many autoimmune diseases. Also used for elective abortions	Nausea, vomiting, loss of hair, bone marrow suppression with leukopenia, stomatitis. Teratogenic.
Tacrolimus	Used after surgery to prevent rejection of heart, kidney, and liver transplants (usually in combination with azathioprine or MMF). Taken with adrenal corticosteroids. (May interact with grapefruit juice.)	Anaphylaxis, especially with IV infusion, tremor, headache, nausea, diarrhea, hypertension, and kidney dysfunction. Bone marrow suppression may result in increased risk of infection, bleeding, and cancer, especially skin cancer. Increases risk of developing diabetes.

CORTICOSTEROIDS IN CHILDREN

The adrenal cortex, triggered by adrenocorticotropic hormone (ACTH) produced by the pituitary gland, produces three types of steroids from cholesterol: **glucocorticoids** (such as cortisol and hydrocortisone), **mineralocorticoids** (aldosterone), and **androgens** (testosterone). Glucocorticoids, especially cortisol, have a powerful anti-inflammatory effect, inhibiting cell-mediated immune response, and have been synthesized into a number of corticosteroids, which are steroids that resemble cortisol. Replacement therapy for Addison's disease, however, is usually done with natural hydrocortisone and cortisone. **Synthetic corticosteroids** are used to treat many disorders, including arthritis, lupus erythematosus, inflammatory bowel disease, asthma, and cancer, but they have severe side effects, such as increased fatty deposits and weight gain, osteoporosis, sodium retention, adrenal suppression, diabetes mellitus, depression, mood swings, gastric ulcers, acne, thinning of skin, and impaired healing, so use must be carefully monitored.

Corticosteroids include:

- **Betamethasone** is moderately potent and does not cause fluid retention. Topical preparations treat eczema and itching but are not approved for children younger than 13 years old. It may be used IM for treatment of allergic reactions to poison oak/poison ivy. Oral preparations are used for a wide range of disorders, including allergies, dermatologic diseases, endocrine disorders, lymphomas and leukemias, multiple sclerosis (MS), cerebral edema, temporal arteritis, and rheumatoid disorders. It is also used to accelerate maturation of fetal lungs.
- **Budesonide**, with a strong glucocorticoid and mild mineralocorticoid effect, is used to treat mild-moderate Crohn's disease involving the ileum and/or ascending colon for up to 8 weeks with repeated courses if necessary. It is also used to treat the symptoms of asthma in children.
- **Dexamethasone** (Decadron) is used to treat the nausea and vomiting that result from chemotherapy, or in conjunction with other medications to treat nausea and vomiting. It is also used to treat severe croup that does not resolve with other interventions.
- **Hydrocortisone** (Cortef) is frequently used as topical preparations for relief of itching in children older than age 2. Hydrocortisone is used IM and IV (Solu-Cortef) for a wide range of disorders, similar to cortisone, and including MS and trichinosis.
- **Methylprednisolone** has similar uses as hydrocortisone.
- **Prednisolone** has similar uses as hydrocortisone and methylprednisolone.
- **Prednisone** has similar uses as hydrocortisone, methylprednisolone, and methylprednisolone. Prednisone, in oral preparation, is of the most commonly used corticosteroids. It is a common immunosuppressant to treat disease and prevent organ rejection in children.

IMMUNOSUPPRESSANT DRUGS

Drugs	Actions	Side effects
Corticosteroids	Depress cell-mediated immune response, humoral immune response, and inflammation, reducing proliferation of T cells and B cells. Used with transplantations and to prevent GVHD disease.	Weight gain, edema, Cushing syndrome, hyperglycemia, bruising, and osteoporosis. Abruptly stopping drugs may trigger Addisonian crisis.
Ciclosporin	Inhibit activation of T cells. Used to prevent transplantation rejection and to treat autoimmune diseases and nephrotic syndrome.	Tremor, excessive facial hair, gingivitis, bone marrow suppression with increased risk of infection and cancer, especially skin cancer.
Intravenous immuno-globulin G (IVIG)	Used to combat immunosuppression by increasing antibodies to prevent infection or treat acute infection, such as Guillain-Barre. Used off-label for many different disorders and infections.	Dermatitis, headache, renal failure, and venous thrombosis. Infections can occur because IVIG is extracted from pooled plasma.

> **Review Video: Immunomodulators and Immunosuppressors**
> Visit mometrix.com/academy and enter code: 666131

CHEMOTHERAPY

Chemotherapy may be offered during palliative care to enhance patient comfort, wellbeing, and symptom control for **enhanced quality of life**. It is understood that the treatment is not expected to provide a cure and should not be given as a means to maintain a sense of false hope within the patient or family. It should be clear that the expectation of treatment is **prolonged survival** and **control of cancer-related symptoms**. Not all patients will benefit from palliative chemotherapy. The decision to provide chemotherapy is based on the clinical indicators and the patient's wishes. The benefit and cost ratios of treatment need to be considered.

Tumor response to treatment, metastasis, and other disease specific factors will help define chemotherapy's usefulness for an individual patient. Patients also need to be aware that chemotherapy involves a commitment to repeated travel, hospitalizations, invasive procedures, and assessments in order to make an informed decision.

CHEMOTHERAPEUTIC AGENTS

The major chemotherapy agents are alkylating agents, antimetabolites, plant alkaloids, antitumor antibiotics, and steroid hormones.

- **Alkylating agents** work directly by attacking the DNA of cancers such as chronic leukemias, Hodgkin's disease, lymphomas, and lung, breast, prostate, and ovary cancers.
- **Nitrosoureas** inhibit repair in damaged DNA. They are able to cross the blood-brain barrier and are frequently used to treat brain tumors, lymphomas, multiple myeloma, and malignant melanoma.
- **Antimetabolites** block cell growth. This class of chemotherapeutic drugs is used to treat leukemias, choriocarcinoma, and gastrointestinal, breast, and ovary cancers.
- **Antitumor antibiotics** are a broad category of agents that bind to DNA and prevent RNA synthesis and are used with a wide variety of cancers.
- **Plant (vinca) alkaloids** are extracted from plants and block cell division. These are used to treat acute lymphoblastic leukemia, Hodgkin and non-Hodgkin lymphomas, neuroblastomas, Wilms tumor, and lung, breast, and testes cancers.
- **Steroid hormones** have an unclear action but may be useful in treating hormone-dependent cancers such as ovary and breast cancer.

ROUTES OF DELIVERY

Chemotherapy treatments may be provided orally, intramuscularly, intravenously, intra-arterially, intralesionally (directly into the tumor), intraperitoneally, intrathecally, or topically. **Oral chemotherapy** is the easiest and often used in the home. **Intravenous delivery** is the most common chemotherapy route but **intramuscular delivery** may have more lasting effects. The goal of **intra-arterial chemotherapy** is to introduce the agent directly into the blood supply feeding the tumor or affected organ. Ovarian cancer with tumors greater than 2 cm in diameter may be treated with **intraperitoneal therapy**. Acute lymphocytic leukemia is primarily treated with **intrathecal administration**. **Intralesional treatments** are used for melanoma and Kaposi sarcoma. **Topical treatment** is most common with skin cancers.

SIDE EFFECTS

Not every patient will experience every symptom, or in the same degree. **Side effects** can vary greatly; some can be easily controlled with additional medications. Many side effects are due to the effects of the chemotherapy on **cells**, such as bone marrow, hair, and gastrointestinal cells, which have a rapid mitotic rate and rapid turnover. Common side effects can include bone marrow suppression, hair loss (alopecia), mouth ulcers, sore throat and gums, heartburn, nausea, vomiting, loss of appetite, weight loss, anorexia and cachexia, anemia, nerve and muscle problems, dry or discolored skin, kidney and bladder irritation, fatigue, and increased bruising, bleeding, and infection. The patient's sexual function can also be affected, including possible infertility.

RISKS

Infection is a common concern of chemotherapy because of the decreased number of **neutrophils** in the patient's system. **Neutropenia** is silent but dangerous, leaving no neutrophils to fight the threat of infections. Neutropenia can cause a septic situation, which can be life-threatening. Severe **anemia** may result in the need for blood transfusions. **Neurological damage** may include mild alterations in taste or smell, peripheral neuropathy, mental status changes, or seizures. Some anticancer drugs can cause **heart damage** if not monitored closely. Many anticancer drugs cause **kidney damage**, as well as increasing the risk of drug toxicity from decreased renal function. Anticancer drugs can also cause **cataracts** and **retina damage**.

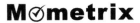

PALLIATIVE SEDATION

Palliative sedation is a treatment method focused on controlling and easing symptoms that have proven otherwise refractory or unendurable in nature. This process was originally named **terminal sedation**. It was changed to palliative sedation to emphasize the differences between symptom management and euthanasia. The purpose of palliative sedation is **symptom control**; it does not hasten or cause death. Through the monitored use of medications such as midazolam or propofol, relief can be provided through varying levels of unconsciousness. Among terminally ill patients, palliative sedation is most often used to calm persistent agitation and restlessness. The second most frequent need is for pain control, followed by confusion, shortness of breath, muscle twitching or seizures, and anguish.

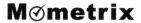

Musculoskeletal Acute and Chronic Care

MONITORING DEVICES FOR EXTREMITY COMPARTMENT SYNDROME

Signs of extremity compartment syndrome include the 5 P's:

- Pain that is severe and out of proportion to injury
- Paresthesia
- Pallor
- Paresis
- Pulse deficit

Pressure is typically measured with a device specially intended for measurement although it can also be measured by attaching a manometer to a needle and syringe. The procedure with the **Stryker intercompartmental pressure monitor device** includes:

- First, the skin is cleansed with antiseptic and a local anesthetic administered.
- The pressure monitor device (or similar) contains a 3 mL syringe, a chamber and needle that connect to the syringe, and a pressure monitor into which the syringe is placed.
- Air is purged from the chamber and needle with the saline.
- The syringe is placed into the pressure monitoring device.
- The device is turned on, zeroed automatically by pressing the "zero" button.
- The needle is inserted into the compartment.
- Once the needle is inserted, about 0.3 mL of NS is injected and the device automatically records the compartment pressure. If the compartment pressure is over 30 mmHg, a fasciotomy is usually needed.

PELVIC STABILIZER

Pelvic stabilizers are used to prevent excessive bleeding associated with pelvic fractures, to maintain the bones in the correct position, and to prevent further damage. Maintaining pressure and reducing the fracture often reduces bleeding. Various methods of stabilizing the pelvis may be employed, including the sheet wrap method in which a sheet is folded, center under the patient, wrapped tightly about the pelvis, and secured. The pneumatic anti-shock garment (PASG) is indicated for hypovolemic shock, and hypotension associated with and for stabilization of pelvic and bilateral femur fractures. PASG is contraindicated with respiratory distress, pulmonary edema, pregnancy (after the first trimester), heart failure, myocardial infarction, stroke, evisceration, abdominal or leg impalement, head injuries, and uncontrolled bleeding above the garment. Another device is the SAM pelvic sling, which has a wide band that fits under and about the pelvis and lateral hips and a belt anteriorly that allows adjustment.

IMMOBILIZATION DEVICES

Immobilization devices include:

- **Cervical collar**: Support the head to prevent spinal cord injury with suspected injury to cervical vertebrae.
- **Cervical extrication splints**: Short board used to immobilize and protect the head and neck during extrication.
- **Backboards**: Used to immobilize the spine to prevent further injury to spinal cord. Both long and short spine boards are available in a number of different shapes and sizes.
- **Full-body splints** (such as vacuum mattress splint): Provide cushioned support to maintain body alignment.
- **Various types of splints for extremities**: Include rigid (should be padded), non-rigid (moldable), traction, and air (pneumatic devices) as well as the use of blankets, rolled towels, sheets, and pillows to maintain position. Traction splints are used for fractured femurs to keep bones in position.

- **Pneumatic anti-shock garment** (PASG): Provides pressure on lower extremities and abdomen and is used to control hemorrhage and shock to prevent pooling of blood in extremities and return blood to general circulation. Often used for pelvic fractures, but may increase risk of internal hemorrhage.

SPINAL IMMOBILIZATION

Spinal immobilization, once a standard for trauma patients, has been shown to have little effect and in some cases may cause harm. Because of these findings, spinal immobilization with backboard is now recommended only for patients with neurological complaints, such as numbness, tingling, weakness, paralysis, pain or tenderness in the spine, spinal deformity, blunt trauma associated with alterations of consciousness, and high energy injuries associated with drugs/alcohol, inability of the patient to communicate, and/or distracting injury. Cervical collars for cervical spine immobilization are to be utilized for trauma based on the NEXUS criteria or Canadian C-spine rules (CCR). According to **NEXUS criteria**, a patient who exhibits all of the following does not require a cervical collar:

- Alert and stable
- No intoxication
- No midline tenderness of the spine
- No distracting injury
- No neurological deficit

Spinal immobilization should be continued for the shortest time possible, so imaging, such as CT, should be carried out upon admission. Cervical collars are applied while the head is supported in neutral position, and the patient is logrolled onto a backboard and strapped in place.

IMMOBILIZATION OF FRACTURES AND DISLOCATIONS

Immobilization techniques for fractures and dislocations include:

- **Cast**: Plaster and fiberglass casts are applied after reduction to ensure that the bone is correctly aligned. Cast should be placed over several layers of padding that extends slightly beyond the cast ends. Cast material, such as plaster, should NOT be immersed in hot water but water slightly above room temperature (70 °F).
- **Splint**: Plaster splints use 12 or more layers of plaster measured to the correct length and then several layers of padding (longer and wider than splint should be measured and cut). The plaster splint is submerged in water to saturate, removed, laid on a flat surface, and massaged to fuse the layers. The padding is laid on top, and the splint is positioned and wrapped with gauze to hold it in place. While setting the splint, position can be maintained by holding it in place with the palm of the hand (not the fingers). After setting, the splint may be wrapped by elastic compression bandages.

TEACHING PATIENTS HOW TO WALK WITH CRUTCHES

Crutches should be properly fitted before a patient attempts ambulation. Correct height is one hand-width below axillae. The handgrips should be adjusted so the patient supports the body weight comfortably with elbows slightly flexed rather than locked in place. The patient should be cautioned not to bear weight under the axillae as this can cause nerve damage but to hold the crutches tightly against the side of the chest wall. The type of gait that the patient uses depends on the type of injury. Typical gaits include:

- **Two-point** in which each crutch is advanced in tandem with the opposite side leg (i.e., the left crutch is advanced at the same time as the right leg, and the right crutch is advanced at the same time as the left leg).
- **Three-point** in which the injured extremity and both crutches are advanced together and then the well leg advances to (or past) the crutches.
- **Four-point** in which the injured side crutch is advanced, followed by the non-injured leg, followed by the non-injured side crutch, followed by the injured leg.

The patient should be advised whether there is partial or no weightbearing and a demonstration should be provided. Stair climbing should be practiced:

- **Ascending**: well foot goes first and then crutches and injured extremity.
- **Descending**: crutches go first and then the well foot.

TRACTION SPLINTING

Traction splints are applied for fractures of long bones, such as midshaft fractures of the femur, in order to reduce pain and prevent further damage to tissue and vasculature. Procedures may vary slightly with different types of traction splints. Two people are usually required.

1. Begin by fitting the splint to the uninjured limb so that it can be adjusted to fit properly.
2. Assess circulation including pedal pulses, toe movement, and sensation while a partner manually stabilizes the femur.
3. Apply manual traction by holding above the ankle and below the knee (only if no lower leg injury is suspected).
4. Slide the splint below the limb.
5. Secure the splint with straps, usually 2 above the knee and two below, being careful to avoid the area of fracture and attaching the ischial strap first.
6. Apply ankle strap.
7. Apply traction hook to ankle strap.
8. Adjust traction until it takes over for manual traction.
9. Reassess pain level, pedal pulses, toe movement, and sensation.

For transport, the patient is placed on a long board with the splint secured to the board.

REDUCTION OF NURSEMAID'S ELBOW

Nursemaid's elbow is a partial dislocation of the elbow (radial head subluxation) that typically occurs when the child is pulled suddenly, lifted by the arm, or falls on the arm. This injury is most common in children between one and four but can occur any time within the first seven years. Typically, the child has pain, will not use the affected arm, and holds it closely to the body. **Reduction procedure**:

1. Calm the child and allow the parents to hold infants and young children securely, facing the practitioner.
2. Grasp the child's forearm or wrist with one hand and the elbow and radial head with the other, placing the thumb against the radial head.
3. Extend (almost to hyperextension) the arm and turn the palm so that it is facing upward (supination) and then flex the elbow rapidly bringing the hand up to the shoulder, using the thumb to guide the radial head into place. A slight click is felt when the radial head pops back into place.
4. The child may still guard the arm for a few more minutes, so wait for 5-10 minutes to determine if the procedure needs to be repeated.

SPINAL FUSION FOR CHILDREN AND ADOLESCENTS

Spinal fusion is done to repair vertebral abnormalities, some resulting in spinal curvature of the spine with disability and deformity that can impair cardiopulmonary function and cause death. While exercises, braces, and electrical stimulation are used to treat mild conditions, **surgical correction** is often required:

- Spinal fusion usually includes spinal realignment and straightening with vertebrae fused together with **bone grafts**, usually from the child's iliac crest or a donor. The grafts may be placed posteriorly or anteriorly, often with the addition of instrumentation (hardware) in the form of rods, screws, wires, hooks, plates, and cages to stabilize and align vertebrae during fusion.
- A **posterior fusion** is done with a vertical incision along the length of the spine to be fused.

317

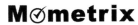

- An **anterior fusion** requires an incision to be back to front on one side of the rib cage (thoracic repair) or across the rib cage and down the abdomen (for thoracic and lumbar repair).
- **Endoscopic surgery** may be done through small incisions.

MUSCULOSKELETAL CONDITIONS THAT MAY REQUIRE SPINAL FUSION FOR CORRECTION

Spinal fusion may be needed for the following conditions:

- **Kyphosis**, a convex angulation of the thoracic spine, may be secondary, such as to arthritis or compression fractures, or may be postural, resulting from skeletal growth faster than muscular. Exercises may help postural kyphosis.
- **Lordosis**, an often-painful concave angulation of the lumbar spine, is frequently associated with obesity, flexion hip contracture, and slipped femoral capital epiphysis. Exercises may give some relief but not a permanent cure.
- **Scoliosis**, a lateral and rotational curvature of the spine, can cause alterations in the structure of the pelvis and chest. It may be nonstructural, related to some other deformity or underlying problem, or structural, with changes in the spine and vertebrae because of congenital or other disorders. It is idiopathic in 70-80% of cases.
- **Spina bifida,** a neural tube defect, results in incomplete closure of the spine with the bones over the defect underdeveloped and unfused.
- A child may have a combination, such as **scoliokyphosis**.

318

Integumentary Acute and Chronic Care

NEGATIVE PRESSURE WOUND THERAPY

Negative pressure wound therapy is used for slow-healing wounds with large volumes of exudate after debridement is completed, leaving the wound tissue exposed. There are a number of different electrical suction NPWT systems, such as the VAC (vacuum-assisted closure) system and the Versatile I (VI). Application steps include:

- Apply nonadherent porous foam cut to fit and completely cover the wound:
  - Polyurethane (hydrophobic, repelling moisture) is used for all wounds EXCEPT those that are painful, have tunneling or sinus tracts, deep trauma wounds, and wounds needing controlled growth of granulation.
  - Polyvinyl (hydrophilic), is used for all wounds EXCEPT deep wounds with moderate granulation, deep pressure ulcers and flaps.
- Secure foam occlusive transparent film.
- Cut opening to accommodate the drainage tube in the dressing and attach drainage tube.
- Attach tube to suction canister, creating closed system.
- Set pressure to 75-125 mmHg, as indicated.
- Change dressings 2-3 times weekly.
- Pediatric patients must be monitored carefully, positions changed at least every 2 hours, and adequate analgesia provided. Patients old enough to understand should be educated about the treatment and the meaning of alarms.

WOUND VACS

Wound vacuum-assisted closure (wound VAC) (AKA negative pressure wound therapy) uses subatmospheric (negative) pressure with a suction unit and a semi-occlusion vapor-permeable dressing. The suction reduces periwound and interstitial edema, decompressing vessels, improving circulation, stimulating production of new cells, and decreasing colonization of bacteria. Wound VAC also increases the rate of granulation and re-epithelialization to hasten healing. The wound must be debrided of necrotic tissue prior to treatment. Wound VAC is used for a variety of difficult-to-heal wounds, especially those that show less than 30% healing in 4 weeks of post-debridement treatment or those with excessive exudate, including chronic stage II and IV pressure ulcers, skin flaps, diabetic ulcer, acute wounds, burns, surgical wound, and those with dehiscence and nonresponsive arterial and venous ulcers. Contraindications include:

- Wound malignancy
- Untreated osteomyelitis
- Exposed blood vessels or organs
- Non-enteric, unexplored fistulas.

Nonadherent porous foam is cut to fit and cover the wound and is secured with occlusive transparent film with an opening cut to accommodate the drainage tube, which is attached to a suction canister in a closed system. The pressure should be set at 75-125 psi and the dressing changed 2-3 times weekly.

PRESSURE REDUCTION SURFACES

Pressure reduction surfaces redistribute pressure to prevent pressure ulcers and reduce shear and friction. There are various types of support surfaces for beds, examining tables, operating tables, and chairs. Functions of pressure reduction surfaces include temperature control, moisture control, and friction/shear control. **General use guidelines** include:

- Pressure redistribution support surfaces should be used for patients with stage II, III, and IV ulcers, as well as for those that are at risk for developing pressure ulcers.
- Chairs should have gel or air support surfaces to redistribute pressure for chair-bound patients, critically ill patients, or those who cannot move independently.
- Support surface material should provide at least an inch of support under areas to be protected when in use to prevent bottoming out. (Check by placing hand palm-up under the overlay below the pressure point.)
- Static support surfaces are appropriate for patients who can change position without increasing pressure to an ulcer.
- Dynamic support surfaces are needed for those who need assistance to move or when static pressure devices provide less than an inch of support.

INCISION AND DRAINAGE

Incision and drainage (I&D) is used to drain localized pockets of purulent material, such as an abscess that is causing pain and inflammation, and has not resolved with other treatment, such as antibiotics. I&D may also be used to drain a hematoma or seroma in some cases. For all I&Ds, position the patient for easy access, use sterile draping and techniques, and cleanse the abscess and 3 inches of surrounding tissue with antiseptic. Procedures:

- **Furuncle/boil**: Apply field block about abscess (1-2% lidocaine with or without epinephrine), make the incision with #11 scalpel and express purulent material. Obtain cultures. Explore cavity with hemostat and then pack with iodoform gauze with wick protruding and cover with dressing.
- **Paronychia**: As above. If under nail, use cautery to bore a small hole or remove part of nail to facilitate drainage.
- **Perianal/ischiorectal abscess**: Place in lithotomy or left lateral position and explore anus/rectum with anoscope or digital exam to determine if there is a fistula present. Freeze the top of the abscess with topical anesthetic (do not use local anesthetic) and incise with a #11 scalpel. Express purulent material and irrigate with NS solution, pack with iodoform gauze with the wick protruding, and cover with dressing.

SUTURE REMOVAL

Prior to suture removal, examine the suture line to determine the type of stitch. If the sutures are crusted, cleanse with a cotton-tipped applicator and hydrogen peroxide, remove hydrogen peroxide with applicator saturated with NS, and then dry with gauze. Procedure:

- **Interrupted stitches**: Lift suture with forceps and slide scissors under the suture and clip. Grasp the knotted end with the forceps and pull suture through skin.
- **Running stitches**: Identify the distal knotted end and lift with forceps if necessary and cut off the knot. Pull the sutures out by grasping the knot at the proximal end with the forceps and gently pulling.
- **Closed and loop sutures or those in awkward anatomic locations**: Lift the suture with forceps and slide a #11 scalpel flat against the skin and under the suture, cutting the suture with the edge of the scalpel. Grasp the knotted end with the forceps and pull the suture through the skin.

Following suture removal, if the suture line appears weak or gaps appear, apply Steri-strips.

STAPLE REMOVAL

Staples should be removed within 7-10 days for staples in the limbs, hands, feet, and trunk, in 3-5 days for the face/neck, and 5-7 days for the ear or scalp as prolonged staple closure may result in scarring and increased risk of infection. Prior to staple removal, examine the staples and wipe with alcohol prep pad if crusted. Procedure for **complete removal**:

1. Using the staple remover, insert the prongs under the most distal staple (to avoid rubbing against other staples during removal) and depress the handle, which will cause both ends of the staple to elevate. Gently rock the remover from side to side if necessary, to loosen the staple, and lift up to remove the staple.
2. Remove all staples in the same manner.
3. Wipe incision line with an alcohol prep pad.

Procedure for **partial removal** (usually reserved for large wounds that are healing poorly or are at risk of dehiscence/evisceration):

1. Proceed as above but remove only every other staple.
2. Apply benzoin to areas where staples were removed and allow to dry until tacky and then apply Steri-strips to those areas.
3. Wipe incision line with an alcohol prep pad.

Infectious Diseases Acute and Chronic Care

ANTIBIOTICS

Antibiotics, produced from microorganisms (such as fungi), are used to combat bacterial infections. Bacteria are critical for human survival and most are benign, but some are pathogenic, leading to infection. Bacteria have simple prokaryote structures, with no membrane-encased nucleus or organelles. Instead, they have a tangle of looped DNA called a nucleoid. Bacteria also have plasmids, which are double strands of DNA outside of the nucleoid that allow for transmission from cell to cell or by attaching to viruses. Essentially, bacteria are able to trade genes, making them very adaptable. The cell membrane of most bacteria, except the Mollicutes (mycoplasmas), is surrounded by a cell wall, the composition of which varies. It is the composition of this cell wall that determines the Gram-staining, either negative or positive. Common side effects include nausea, vomiting, diarrhea, rash, and vaginal yeast infections. Severe reactions include anaphylaxis, super-infection with Clostridium difficile, and bone marrow, liver, and renal impairment.

> **Review Video: Antibiotics: An Overview**
> Visit mometrix.com/academy and enter code: 165628

CLASSIFICATION

Antibiotics may be classified according to their chemical nature, origin, action, or range of effectiveness. There are hundreds of antibiotics. Broad-spectrum antibiotics are useful against both Gram-positive and Gram-negative bacteria. Medium spectrum antibiotics are usually effective against Gram-positive bacteria although some may be effective against Gram-negative as well. Narrow spectrum antibiotics are effective against a small range of bacteria. Depending on the type, antibiotics can kill bacteria by interfering with its biological functions (bacteriocidal) or by preventing reproduction (bacteriostatic). The **main classes of antibiotics** used in children include:

- **Macrolides**: Medium spectrum antibiotics. They prevent protein production by bacteria and are primarily bacteriostatic but may be bactericidal at high doses. They may be irritating to the gastric mucosa, but are less likely to cause allergic responses than penicillins or cephalosporins. Macrolides include erythromycin, clarithromycin, and azithromycin.
- **Sulfonamides**: Sulfonamides are medium spectrum with action against Gram-positive and many Gram-negative organisms as well as Plasmodium and Toxoplasma. Some people are sensitive and may develop an allergic response. Resistance to sulfa drugs is widespread. Sulfa drugs interfere with folate synthesis and prevent cell division, so they are bacteriostatic. Sulfonamides include co-trimoxazole (Bactrim) and trimethoprim (Prismol).
- **Aminoglycosides**: Effective against Gram-negative bacteria. They interfere with protein production in the bacteria and are bacteriocidal. Aminoglycosides cannot be taken orally. They are often given in conjunction with other classes of antibiotics, such as penicillin. Aminoglycosides include gentamicin and tobramycin, neomycin, and streptomycin.
- **Penicillins**: Medium spectrum antibiotics may be combined with β-lactamase inhibitors. They are bacteriocidal and cause breakdown of the bacterial cell wall. They may cause severe allergic reactions in sensitive individuals. Penicillins include ampicillin and amoxicillin.
- **Cephalosporins**: Medium spectrum antibiotics are effective against Gram-negative organisms. They are bacteriocidal and inhibit cell wall synthesis. They are divided into different "generations" according to antimicrobial properties, with succeeding generations having a more powerful effect against resistant strains. First generation includes cephazolin, cephalexin (Keflex), and cefadroxil. Second generation includes cefaclor, cefuroxime, cefotetan (Cefotan), and cefprozil. Third generation includes cefotaxime, cefixime (Suprax), cefpodoxime, ceftazidime (Fortaz), and cefdinir (Omnicef). Fourth generation includes cefepime.
- **Polymyxins**: Narrow spectrum antibiotics are effective against Gram-negative organisms. Interferes with cell membrane of bacteria and are bactericidal. Polymyxins have both neurotoxic and nephrotoxic properties and are not used unless other antibiotics are ineffective. They must be given intravenously.

ANTIFUNGAL AGENTS

Even though antifungal agents are available, systemic fungal infections are difficult to treat. Fungi were originally classified as plants, but they do not produce their own food through photosynthesis and must, like animals, get food from another source. Fungi vary widely, from one-celled microorganisms to multi-celled chains that are miles long. Fungi are used to make antibiotics, but they can also cause infection and disease. Two common classifications of fungi are **molds** (including mushrooms) and **yeast**. Fungi are not motile, but some produce spores, which can be inhaled. Some, such as the yeast Candida albicans, are part of the normal flora of the skin but can overgrow in an opportunistic infection. As microorganisms, fungal infections can invade the sinuses, the mouth, the respiratory system, and the vagina. Antibiotics may affect the balance between bacteria and yeast, causing infection. Fungal infections include histoplasmosis, blastomycosis, and coccidioidomycosis. Fungal infections, such as *Pneumocystis jiroveci* (formerly carinii), pose a serious problem for the immunocompromised.

Fungal infections are common on the skin and mucous membranes, but the use of vascular access devices and other invasive devices has increased the incidence of fungemia in patients. Additionally, powerful antibiotics contribute to fungal infections by altering the balance of organisms. Fungal cells are more difficult to eradicate than bacterial cells because they are more similar to human cells, so treating a fungus can damage other cells and result in serious side effects, such as nausea, diarrhea, anorexia, rash, and itching. Amphotericin B especially has serious side effects, which can cause fever and chills, headache, hypotension, dyspnea, multiple organ damage, and even death. There are a number of different classes of antifungal agents. Below are those most commonly used in the pediatric population:

- **Triazole antifungals** have similar action to imidazole but are newer and less toxic. Fluconazole (Diflucan) may be used for both superficial (skin, mucous membranes) and systemic fungal infections. It is used for both treatment and prophylaxis against candidiasis. It is effective for coccidioidomycosis, cryptococcosis, and histoplasmosis.
- **Polyene antifungals** attack the fungal cell membrane, leading to death of the organism. These antifungals are derived from *Streptomyces* sp. Amphotericin B may be used orally for treatment of thrush, but it is more commonly used intravenously for systemic fungal infections, including aspergillosis and candidiasis.
- **Echinocandin antifungals** also inhibit cell wall synthesis. Anidulafungin (Eraxis) is primarily used for the treatment of systemic candidiasis. It degrades chemically in the presence of normal body pH and is safe to use with liver or kidney impairment. Caspofungin (Cancidas) is used intravenously for treatment of aspergillosis and candidiasis and is often effective when patients have shown resistance to other drugs. Micafungin (Mycamine) is used intravenously to treat a wide variety of candidal infections, including candidiasis, candida peritonitis, and esophageal candidiasis. It is also used as a prophylaxis for those having hematopoietic stem cell transplantation.

ANTIPARASITIC AGENTS

Antiparasitic agents are used for protozoan diseases. **Protozoa** are one-celled organisms from a number of different phyla. Protozoa consume bacteria, so they have a critical role in the cycle of life, but about 10,000 species are parasites that can infect vertebrates. Protozoan infections, especially of the gastrointestinal tract, have become more prevalent in those who are immunocompromised:

- ***Giardia intestinalis*** has become the most common cause of water-borne disease and non-bacterial diarrhea in the United States. Antiparasitic agents include metronidazole (Flagyl), nitazoxanide, and tinidazole.
- ***Dientamoeba fragilis*** occurs worldwide, especially in children, and those who live or travel to areas with poor sanitation. Antiparasitics include iodoquinol, paromomycin, and metronidazole.

- *Entamoeba histolytica* is more prevalent in developing countries, but increasing rates of infection have been found in Hispanics (33%), Asian and Pacific Islanders (17%), recent immigrants, travelers, institutionalized populations, and men having sex with men. Antiparasitics for asymptomatic infections include iodoquinol, paromomycin, and diloxanide furoate. For mild to severe disease, metronidazole and tinidazole.

Antiparasitic agents include **antihelmintic agents** for treatment of parasitic worms:

- **Nematodes** are unsegmented roundworms, including pin worms, hookworms, whipworms, and roundworms. There are over 80,000 varieties. Those that infest humans range from as small as 0.3 mm to as long as 1 m in length. People usually become infected by ingestion of contaminated food or touching contaminated hands to the mouth. Antiparasitic drugs useful against nematodes include albendazole (Albenza), mebendazole (Emverm), pyrantel pamoate (Pin-Away), and ivermectin.
- **Cestodes** are segmented flatworms, also called tapeworms, which live in the intestinal tracts of some animals and fish and infect humans who eat raw or undercooked meat/fish. Antiparasitic drugs include praziquantel (Biltricide), nitazoxanide, and niclosamide.
- **Trematodes** are a type of flatworm called flukes, which can cause diseases in the intestines, blood, liver, and lungs. Fluke infections are caused by ingestion of uncooked meat, plants, or fish from contaminated waters. Antiparasitic drugs include praziquantel and albendazole.
- *Balantidium coli* occur most commonly in the tropics among those in contact with pigs, but outbreaks have occurred in psychiatric hospitals in the United States. Antiparasitics include metronidazole and iodoquinol (topically only).
- *Cryptosporidium parvum* and *Cryptosporidium hominis* have caused a number of outbreaks since first identified in 1976, sometimes related to swimming in pools contaminated with feces or handling dirty diapers. The antiparasitic agent used for treatment is nitazoxanide, which is effective only in those without HIV. Antiretroviral treatment received for HIV infection is, however, affective against cryptosporidia.
- *Isospora belli* occurs worldwide, primarily in tropical areas, but can occur in travelers and those with HIV. The only effective antiparasitic agent is trimethoprim-sulfamethoxazole. There is no alternative for those allergic to sulfa.
- *Cyclospora cayetanensis* occurs worldwide and has been implicated in a number of food-borne outbreaks in the United States since 1996. The antiparasitic agent is trimethoprim-sulfamethoxazole. Those sensitive to sulfa may be treated with nitazoxanide.

Microsporidia are now commonly believed to be basic fungi, closer to fungi than other protozoa, and increasingly recognized worldwide as opportunistic infectious agents, especially in immuno-compromised individuals, such as those with HIV/AIDS, causing microsporidiosis. Fourteen species have been identified as **pathogenic** to humans, some affecting the eyes and muscles. Enterocytozoon bieneusi and Encephalitozoon intestinalis cause most cases of microsporidiosis with gastrointestinal manifestations and are common in HIV/AIDS patients, but there are increasing infections in non-HIV infected travelers and those living in tropical areas. Antiparasitic agents include thalidomide, which is used for chronic diarrhea unresponsive to other medications. Metronidazole is also useful for the treatment of diarrhea. On-going treatment may be needed to prevent recurrence of symptoms. Drugs of choice include:

- *E. Intestinalis*: Albendazole 400 mg daily for children ≥2 years old (200 mg for younger) for 14 days
- *E. Bieneusi*: Fumagillin 60 mg daily for 14 days

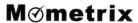

ANTIRETROVIRAL AGENTS FOR HIV AND AIDS

There are four primary classes of antiretroviral agents used for the treatment of HIV/AIDS:

- **Non-nucleoside reverse transcriptase inhibitors** (NNRTIs), such as delavirdine, efavirenz (Sustiva), and nevirapine (Viramune), bind to reverse transcriptase and disable it. Reverse transcriptase is a protein required for HIV replication.
- **Nucleoside reverse transcriptase inhibitors** (NRTIs), such as abacavir (Ziagen), zidovudine (Retrovir), and lamivudine (Epivir), are defective versions of building blocks necessary for replication. When HIV binds to the defective version, it is unable to complete replication.
- **Protease inhibitors** (PIs) disable the protein protease, which HIV requires in order to replicate. PIs include indinavir (Crixivan) and nelfinavir (Viracept).
- **Fusion inhibitors**, such as enfuvirtide (Fuzeon), are entry blockers.

Integumentary Acute and Chronic Care

WART (VERRUCA VULGARIS) REMOVAL

Verruca vulgaris (common warts) are usually self-limiting and will disappear in time, but they can be unsightly and become easily irritated, so requests for removal are common. For all procedures, position the patient so that the lesion is easily accessible. Then cleanse the lesion and 3 inches of surrounding skin with antiseptic, don gloves, and drape the field. Possible procedures for wart removal include the following:

- **Cautery**: Inject 1% lidocaine under the lesion or use a field block for lesions over 4 mm. Use a disposable cautery pen to burn off the lesion. Wipe clean and apply antibiotic ointment and dressing.
- **Duct tape**: Cover the lesion with duct tape and leave in place for 3-6 days. Remove, soak in warm water, and use an emery board or pumice stone to reduce the wart. Wait 10 hours and reapply. Repeat the cycle until the wart disappears.
- **Salicylic acid**: Soak the lesion in warm water for 5-10 minutes, dry, use an emery board or pumice stone to smooth, apply cream to the wart, and let it dry on the skin. Do twice daily for 12 weeks or until the wart is gone.
- **Cryosurgery**: Apply gauze soaked in water to the wart for 5-10 minutes to soften, apply K-Y jelly to the lesion, use a cryoprobe with the appropriately-sized tip to freeze the lesion, and apply antibiotic ointment and dressing.

PHARMACOLOGIC TREATMENT OF WOUND PAIN
TOPICAL ANESTHETICS

There are numerous different types of pain medications that may be used to control pain from wounds, including **topical anesthetics**:

- **Lidocaine 2-4%** is frequently used during debridement or dressing changes. Lidocaine is useful only superficially and may take 15-30 minutes before it is effective.
- **Eutectic Mixture of Local Anesthetics (EMLA Cream)** provides good pain control. The wound is first cleansed and then the cream is applied thickly (1/4 inch) extending about 1/2 inch past the wound to the periwound tissue. The wound is then covered with plastic wrap, which is secured and left in place for about 20 minutes. The wrapped time may be extended to 45-60 minutes if necessary, to completely numb the tissue. The tissue should remain numb for about 1 hour after the plastic wrap is removed, allowing time for the wound to be cleansed, debrided, and/or redressed.

REGIONAL ANESTHESIA

Regional anesthesia (injectable subcutaneous and perineural medications) is administered locally about the wound or as nerve blocks. Medications include lidocaine, bupivacaine, and tetracaine in solution. Epinephrine is sometimes added to increase vasoconstriction and reduce bleeding, although it is avoided in distal areas of the limbs (hands and feet) to prevent ischemia.

- **Field blockade** involves injecting the anesthetic into the periwound tissue or into the wound margins. The effect may be decreased by inflammation. The effects last for limited periods of time.
- **Regional nerve blocks** may involve single injections, the effects of which are limited in duration but can provide pain relief for treatments. Techniques that use continuous catheter infusions are longer lasting and can be controlled more precisely. Blocks may involve nerves proximal to affected areas, such as peripheral nerve blocks, or large nerve blocks near the spinal cord, such as percutaneous lumbar sympathetic blocks (LSB). Long-term blocks may use alcohol-based medications to permanently inactivate the nerves.

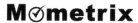

Medication Administration

LIFESPAN CONCERNS

Prescribing drugs across the lifespan requires an understanding of differences in types of medications used and dosages according to age and gender.

Dosage and administration of pediatric medications is **weight and age related**, and only pediatric medications should be prescribed if possible. Adult pills, for example, should not be cut for use for a child, as even small variations in dosage may have adverse effects. Dosage should always be checked. The Broselow tape can be used to measure the child to guide medication dosage.

PHYSIOLOGICAL AND DEVELOPMENTAL CONSIDERATIONS FOR MEDICATION ADMINISTRATION

Absorption of medications can be delayed due to delayed gastric emptying, or delayed or enhanced due to the high pH of the newborn's gastric juices or irregular peristalsis. IM medications can be affected by the small muscle mass and diminished peripheral blood flow of the young child. Topical meds are more rapidly absorbed due to their greater body surface area. The greater body fluid volume can dilute water-soluble medications, and if body fat is increased, a higher dose of a lipid-soluble drug may be needed. An immature liver and temperature fluctuations can affect drug metabolism. Immature kidney function can affect excretion of medications, causing toxicity.

Infants benefit from having the parents assist in medication administration. Toddlers benefit from simple choices, handling any equipment, a positive approach, quick administration and restraint if needed, followed by rewards for positive behavior. Preschoolers need simple explanations, to be able to play with equipment, choices, and parental assistance. School age children benefit from rewards, explanations and play therapy. Adolescents can be treated the same as adults.

SAFE ADMINISTRATION OF ORAL MEDICATIONS

Oral medications can be given by medicine spoon, oral syringe, dropper, nipple, or tube. Suspensions must be shaken. Sometimes tablets need to be crushed or capsules opened if a liquid form is unavailable. Ensure this will not interfere with the action of the drug. Drugs can sometimes be mixed with a pleasant tasting food or flavored. If using a nasogastric, gastrostomy or naso-jejunal tube, ensure proper placement of the tube, and flush the tube before and after administration of medicine.

ADMINISTERING ORAL LIQUID MEDICATIONS

Nurses may have a hard time getting children to take liquid medications and keep them down. There are, however, some methods that may help to make the process a little smoother. Liquid medications can be drawn into a syringe (without a needle) and then the medicine is inserted into the pocket of the child's cheek. Children should not be told that the medicine is candy in order to get them to take it more easily as this can be very confusing. Many medications allow for a drink afterward to wash it down. Having a glass of water on hand to drink after the medication is administered may help. If a medication is very distasteful and the children are old enough, they can drink the liquid through a straw, which may help them taste less of it.

SAFE ADMINISTRATION OF IV MEDICATIONS

IV medication administration permits better control over therapeutic blood levels and is less traumatic for the pediatric patient. The nurse should make sure the drug is given according to pharmacologic guidelines. Check for compatibility with other drugs being given. Check for a patent IV with no complications. The drug should be dissolved completely and be ready for administration prior to entering the patient's room. All ports are cleansed, lines are primed, and rates are set according to protocol. A syringe pump is used for small amounts of fluid. Larger volumes may be administered with a Buretrol or piggyback method (diluted in 50-100 cc bag of saline or dextrose water). The retrograde method can be used for a small amount of medication (injected into the IV line after clamping off close to patient, then the clamp is undone, and medication will dilute and flow with the IV fluid).

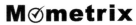

Safe Administration of IM Medications

The safe administration of IM medications is discussed below:

- Infants require a smaller needle and gauge (5/8 inch and 25-27 gauge); toddlers require 1 inch, 22- to 23-gauge needles; and school age children and older require a 1.0-1.5 inch, 22- to 23-gauge needles. Larger gauge needles are used for thicker solutions. Use the smallest gauge needle for the solution and age of the child.
- The preferred site for the infant and toddler is the vastus lateralis; if the child has been walking for at least a year the dorsogluteal muscle can be used. If the child is older than 3 years and has been walking for several years, the ventrogluteal muscle can be used. In children over age 4 or 5, the deltoid can be used.
- The skin is cleaned with alcohol and allowed to dry.
- The needle should be inserted at a 90° angle, aspirated, and then the medicine injected.
- In small infants the needle can be inserted at a 45° angle toward the knee.

Administering Intramuscular Vaccination to Infants

Many types of immunizations are given intramuscularly (IM). In infants, this process typically involves administering the drugs into the large muscles of the thighs. Children from birth until approximately 2 years of age should have IM injections in the anterolateral muscle of the thigh. After preparing the syringe and cleaning the site, the vaccination should be administered at a 90° angle through the skin and subcutaneous fat and into the muscle beneath. Before injecting the medication, aspiration is necessary to avoid giving the drug into the bloodstream. If more than one vaccination is needed, injection sites should be more than 1 inch apart but can be given in the same leg.

Proper Administration of Subcutaneous and Intradermal Medications

Subcutaneous injections are used frequently in children to administer insulin, vaccines, and allergy shots. Intradermal injections are used for tuberculin and allergy testing, and local anesthesia. Subcutaneous injections are given at a 90° angle through skin that has been pinched up to separate the fat from the muscle layer. If you are unable to pinch enough skin, administer subcutaneous injections at a 45° angle. Pain can be minimized by changing the needle to a small gauge after drawing up the medication (provides a sharper, smaller needle) and only injecting small amounts. Sites for subcutaneous injections include the abdomen, the outside of the upper arm and the front center of the thigh. Refer to protocol concerning aspiration before injection. Intradermal injections are given in the inside of the forearm.

Administration of Eye Medications

For eye medication, the child can be supine or sitting. The lower lid is pulled downward while the dominant hand rests on the forehead holding the dropper (to stabilize the dropper). The medication is placed into the conjunctival sac. Alternatively, the lower lid can be pulled down and outward to form a cup, where the medication can be placed. Wipe away excess medication after allowing the child to close his eyes gently. To prevent the medication flowing to the nasopharynx where the child can taste it, apply gentle pressure to the inside corner of the eye for one minute. In infants, place the medication in the corner of the eye with the child supine; when the infant opens their eyes, the medication will flow into the eye. Game-playing with young children may help with administration. Sometimes medication can be administered while the child is sleeping.

Rectal Administration of Medications

The rectal route is sometimes used when the child is vomiting and cannot take oral medications. Acetaminophen, aspirin, antiemetics, sedatives and analgesics are available in suppository form. The absorption of rectal medications is unpredictable due to the presence or absence of stool in the rectum. Using gloves, the suppository is lubricated and inserted into the rectum, beyond the rectal sphincter. The buttocks are held together for 5 to 10 minutes to allow the urge to defecate to pass. Altering the dose of a suppository

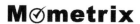

requires cutting it, which doesn't provide an accurate dose. A retention enema is administered in the same manner.

ADMINISTRATION OF MEDICATIONS IN THE EAR AND NOSE

For the administration of ear medication, the child should be supine and turned with the ear up. Under the age of 3, the pinna is pulled downward and then straight back. Over 3 years of age, the pinna is pulled upward and straight back. Administer the medication (for cleanliness use a disposable ear speculum). Loosely placed cotton may be used to prevent the medication from flowing out of the ear canal. The child should be placed on the opposite side for a few minutes.

For nose drops, the child should be supine with the head extended. This prevents the medication flowing into the sinuses and throat where the child can taste it. Keep the child in this position for one minute after administration.

CRUSHING MEDICATIONS FOR ADMINISTRATION TO CHILDREN

Some children cannot tolerate swallowing pills and may benefit from having the pills crushed and mixed with another substance. Permission from the physician is necessary before crushing medications to ensure it will not destroy the activity of the medicine. Pills that are enteric coated, extended release, slow release, or that may irritate the gastrointestinal lining may not be crushed. Pills may be crushed between two spoons or by using a pill-crusher after verifying the correct dose. Crushed medications may be added to applesauce or pudding to assist with administration of the drugs.

GIVING MEDICATION THROUGH A GASTROSTOMY TUBE

Some children use feeding tubes for nutrition, including gastrostomy tubes, also called G-tubes. These tubes are also used for medication administration if the child cannot take medicine by mouth. Many medications are administered in liquid form through tubes; however, some may need to be crushed and diluted with water. The G-tube may have only a button at the site; if this is the case, an extension tube is attached to administer the medications. After drawing up the medicine, the tube is flushed with a small amount of water to clear the tube without adding air. Following the flush, the medication is administered into the tube using a syringe. If more than one type of medication is needed, the tube is flushed between doses with approximately 5 mL of water. Following the last medication dose, the tube is flushed with a small amount of water to ensure that the medicine clears the tube, the extension tubing is removed, and the button is closed.

PATIENT'S AND PARENT'S WILLINGNESS TO ADHERE TO MEDICATION REGIMENS

A patient's willingness to adhere to medication regimens is often critical to the medications' effectiveness. Noncompliance may result in inadequate relief of symptoms, disease complications, super infections, adverse drug effects, and even death. A patient's willingness to adhere to medication regimens depends on a number of variables. The pediatric population's adherence largely depends on parental/guardian support and understanding:

- **Knowledge base**: The patient/parents must be knowledgeable about the administration (time and dosage) of medications and should be aware of uses and adverse effects in order to understand the importance of adhering to a regimen.
- **Relief of symptoms**: Patients/parents who do not see relief of symptoms immediately may believe medications are ineffective.
- **Financial status**: Parents may not be able to afford medications.
- **Ease of administration**: Patients/parents are more likely to comply with medications that are administered orally.
- **Trust**: Patients/parents must trust healthcare providers to provide appropriate treatment.
- **Cultural values/beliefs**: A patient's and their parents' cultural attitudes may influence compliance.

Pharmacologic Pain Management

EQUIANALGESIA

Equianalgesia is a comparison of doses of different analgesics that provide equivalent analgesia/sedation. Children may vary in their ability to metabolize drugs, so they must be monitored carefully with all analgesics. Intravenous analgesics usually take effect within 15 to 30 minutes while oral medications take twice as long. Dosage must be calculated according to age and weight:

Drug	Parenteral	Oral
Morphine sulfate	0.025–0.03 mg/kg/dose	0.08–0.1 mg/kg/dose (comes in 2 mg/mL or 4 mg/mL)
Dilaudid	0.015 mg/kg/dose	0.03–0.08 mg/kg/dose
Fentanyl	1-2 mcg/kg/dose	Varies (patches)
Codeine	Not recommended for children	0.5–1 mg/kg/dose (max dose 60 mg)
Vicodin	Not available parenterally	0.1–0.2 mg/kg/dose

ACETAMINOPHEN AND NSAID PEDIATRIC DOSING AND SIDE EFFECTS

Drug	Dosage	Side Effects
Acetaminophen	Dosages may be repeated every 4 hours to the <u>maximum of 5 doses</u> in 24 hours. Dosage is based on 10-15 mg/kg with adult dosing at 12 years: • 0-3 months: 40 mg • 4-11 months: 80 mg • 1-2 years: 120 mg • 2-3 years: 160 mg • 4-5 years: 240 mg • 6-8 years: 320 mg • 9-10 years: 325–400 mg • 11 years: 480 mg	Allergic response with itching, rash, and edema. Liver toxicity with overdose.
Choline Magnesium Trisalicylate	• <37 kg (81.5 lb): 50 mg/kg/day divided in 2 doses • >37 kg (81.5 lb): 2250 mg/day divided in 2 doses	Tinnitus. GI irritation with nausea, vomiting, diarrhea, constipation, and epigastric discomfort.
Ibuprofen	• <6 months to 12 years: 5-10 mg/kg every 6-8 hours to maximum of 40 mg/kg/day • 12-18 years: 200 to 400 mg every 4 to 6 hours to maximum of 2400 mg/day	Nausea, vomiting, and diarrhea. Gastrointestinal irritation with ulcerations and bleeding. Bleeding nephritis. Retention of fluid.
Naproxen	• >2 years: 20 mg/kg/day divided in 2 doses	Same as ibuprofen
Tolmetin	• >2 years: 15–30 mg/kg/day divided in 3-4 doses	Same as ibuprofen

> **Review Video: <u>NSAIDs and Their Side Effects</u>**
> Visit mometrix.com/academy and enter code: 569064

COX Inhibitors

Cyclooxygenase (COX) inhibitors are NSAIDs that block COX enzymes that develop with inflammation and with precancerous/cancerous tissues. COX enzymes form prostanoids:

- **Prostaglandins**: Cell growth, inflammatory reactions, sensitivity to pain, platelet aggregation/disaggregation, and hormone and calcium regulation
- **Prostacyclin**: Platelet aggregation and vasodilation
- **Thromboxane**: Platelet aggregation and vasoconstriction

COX inhibitors are used as anti-inflammatory analgesics and antiplatelet drugs. Some drugs, such as ibuprofen and aspirin, block both COX-1 and COX-2 enzymes (non-selective inhibitors). Non-selective NSAIDs are associated with irritation of gastric mucosa because of inhibition of COX-1, which has a protective effect on gastrointestinal mucosa. Other drugs, such as celecoxib, block only COX-2 enzymes (selective inhibitors) and these tend to have fewer gastrointestinal adverse effects, but they have been implicated in increased risk for cardiovascular disease and thrombus formation. COX-2 NSAIDs specifically target inflammation. A third COX enzyme, COX-3, has been identified, and some speculate acetaminophen (which has no anti-inflammatory properties) may target this enzyme, but research is inconclusive.

Patient-Controlled Analgesia

Patient-controlled analgesia (PCA) allows the child to control administration of pain medication by pressing a button on an intravenous delivery system with a computerized pump. The device is filled with opioid (as prescribed) and must be programmed correctly and checked regularly to ensure that it is functioning properly and that controls are set. The most-commonly administered medications include morphine, meperidine, fentanyl, and sufentanil. Most devices can be set to deliver a continuous infusion of opioid as well as patient-controlled bolus. Each element must be set:

- **Bolus**: Determines the amount of medication received when the patient delivers a dose
- **Lockout interval**: Time required between administrations of boluses
- **Continuous infusion**: Rate at which opioid is delivered per hour for continuous analgesia
- **Limit** (usually set at 4 hours): Total amount of opioid that can be delivered in the preset time limit

With Authorized Agent Controlled Analgesia (AACA), people who are trained and authorized (such as a nurse, family member, and caregiver) may administer the medication as well as the child.

Non-Pharmacologic Treatments

COMPLEMENTARY THERAPY

Complementary therapies are often used, either alone or in conjunction with conventional medical treatment. These methods should be included if this is what the patient/family chooses, empowering the family to take control of their plan of care. Complementary therapies vary widely and most can easily be incorporated. The **National Center for Complementary and Alternative Medicine** recognizes the following:

- **Whole medical systems**: Chinese medicine (acupressure, acupuncture), naturopathic and homeopathic medicines, and Ayurveda
- **Mind-body medicine**: Prayer, artistic creation, music and dance therapy, biofeedback, focused relaxation, and visualization
- **Biological medicine**: Aromatherapy, herbs, plants, trees, vitamins and minerals, and dietary supplements
- **Manipulation**: Massage and spinal manipulation
- **Energy medicines**: Magnets, electric current, pulsed fields, Reiki, qi gong, and laying-on of the hands

PRECAUTIONS

The use of alternative and complementary therapies should be thoroughly discussed by patients and their physician. Patients should be encouraged to use therapies that are shown to have a beneficial, complementary effect on conventional medical treatment. These therapies include the use of massage, superficial stimulation, relaxation, distraction, hypnosis, and guided imagery.

- Encourage patients to practice the techniques until they are proficient in their use to give them a chance to prove their value.
- Teach the patient how the therapies work to encourage the patient to believe in them to contribute to the placebo effect.
- Caution the patient against abandoning current medical treatment.
- Inform the patient of the high cost of alternate therapies that can divert needed funds and result in little or no benefit.
- Provide the patient with resources in the form of books, pamphlets, and informative websites that prove the results of scientific research so that they can evaluate alternative therapies for themselves.

WHOLE MEDICAL SYSTEMS

Whole medical systems are different philosophies and methods of explaining and treating health and illness. Some systems include:

- **Homeopathic medicine**: This European system uses small amounts of diluted herbs and supplements to help the body to recover from disease by stimulating an immune response.
- **Naturopathic medicine**: This is a European system that uses various natural means (herbs, massage, acupuncture) to support the natural healing forces of the body.
- **Chinese medicine**: Centers on restoring the proper flow of life forces within the body to cure disease by using herbs, acupressure and acupuncture, and meditation.
- **Ayurveda**: This is an Indian system that tries to bring the spirit into harmony with the mind and body to treat disease via yoga, herbs, and massage.

ESSENTIAL OILS AND CUPPING

Essential oils (concentrated oils from plants) are either inhaled (aromatherapy) or diluted and applied to the skin. Essential oils are believed to reduce stress, aid sleep, improve dermatitis, and aid digestion. Commonly used essential oils include eucalyptus, lavender, lemon, peppermint, rosemary, rose, and tea tree. Oils may cause skin irritation when applied to the skin.

Cupping is an ancient practice still used in Southeast Asia and the Middle East to reduce pain, promote healing, and improve circulation. With dry cupping, cups are heated by placing something flammable (such as paper or herbs) inside the cup and setting it on fire to heat the cup, which is then immediately placed on the back along the meridians (generally on both sides of the spine) to form a vacuum that draws blood to the skin and causes circular bruises believed to heal that part of the body. Wet cupping includes leaving the heated cup in place for three minutes, removing it, making small cuts in the skin, and then applying suction cups again to withdraw blood. Cupping should be avoided in children under 4 and limited to short periods in older children.

ACUPUNCTURE

Alternative systems of medical practice include acupuncture, homeopathy, and naturopathy. **Acupuncture**, an ancient Oriental practice, uses stainless steel or copper needles inserted into superficial skin layers at points where energy or life force called *qi* is believed to occur. The needles are supposed to restore balance and the flow of *qi*. The NIH has recognized the effectiveness of acupuncture for certain side effects of other cancer treatments, such as nausea, vomiting, and pain. However, there is no documented scientific evidence to support the principles expounded. Acupuncturists are certified through either formal coursework or apprenticeships, and there is also board certification in this area for physicians. The needles used are classified as class II, which means they have manufacturing and labeling requirements.

HERBAL REMEDIES AND REGULATIONS

In the United States, most **herbal preparations** are classified as dietary supplements. That means that they are not subject to the same rigorous manufacturing, safety, efficacy, and control practices as pharmaceutical drugs. Herbal supplements are only governed by the Dietary Supplement and Health Education Act (DSHEA). As long as no specific disease treatment or curative claims are made, the supplement can be marketed without limitation and safety concerns must be pursued by the FDA after the fact. Nevertheless, some herbal remedies have been undergoing clinical trials in the US to substantiate their health-enhancing or traditional/historical or international use claims. However, the focal point of these studies is still only on the effectiveness of the specific supplement. In Europe, there has been some movement toward greater regulation and licensing of herbal products, but not to the extent of formal drug regulations.

TOXICITIES ASSOCIATED WITH HERBAL REMEDIES

Use of herbal preparations has been associated with a variety of **toxicities**, primarily in categories such as cardiovascular problems, hypersensitivity reactions, disorientation, gastrointestinal problems, and liver malfunction. Because quality control measures are relatively lax for these remedies, contamination from infectious agents and toxic metals can potentially cause other side effects. Many of these herbal medicines **interact with conventional drugs**, thus altering their pharmacodynamics. For example, St. John's wort, which is primarily used for depressive disorders or as a sedative, interacts with a wide range of traditional pharmacologic agents and suppresses their levels in the bloodstream. Kava kava, made from dried roots of a type of pepper bush, is used as a sedative, but it also has been associated with hepatic failure and via interactions with several other drugs can actually induce a comatose state. Ginseng is an Asian remedy touted for its curative properties in a number of diseases. However, it can react with steroidal drugs and induce shaking and manic episodes. These are just a few examples of potential dangers.

NON-PHARMACEUTICAL PAIN RELIEF

Non-pharmaceutical methods to relieve pain that can be used exclusively or combined with medications include massage, heat, cold, electrical stimulation, distraction, relaxation, imagery, visualization, and music. Other **alternatives or adjuncts to pain medication** include hypnosis, magnets, acupuncture, acupressure, and therapeutic touch. Herbs, aromatherapy, reflexology, homeopathic medicine, and prayer may also be accepted by the patient. Any method that the patient feels may help that isn't harmful should be used to help get relief.

MIND-BODY MEDICINE FOR PAIN AND DISEASE

Mind-body medicine (prayer, artistic creation, music and dance, biofeedback, relaxation, and visualization) can help distract people from pain or other symptoms if they are able to concentrate on the method. This can result in the transfer of less painful stimuli to the brain by stimulating the **descending control system**. These methods work if the patient can use them to create alternate sensations in the brain, but will not work if the patient is unable to concentrate due to intense pain.

Relaxation that occurs as a result of using these methods helps to reduce muscular tension that can make pain worse and reduces fatigue caused by chronic pain. Relaxation has been proven to be the most helpful after surgery. Postoperative patients report a greater feeling of control over their pain and tend to request fewer opioids to control pain. Biofeedback can help patients to recognize the feelings of both tension and relaxation and provide a way to indicate their success in managing muscle tension.

USE OF VISUALIZATION

There are a number of methods used for **visualization** to reduce anxiety and promote healing. Some include audiotapes with guided imagery, such as self-hypnosis tapes, but the patient can be taught basic **techniques** that include:

- Sit or lie comfortably in a **quiet place** away from distractions.
- Concentrate on **breathing** while taking long slow breaths.
- **Close the eyes** to shut out distractions and create an image in the mind of the place or situation desired.
- Concentrate on that **image**, engaging as many senses as possible and imaging details.
- If the mind wanders, breathe deeply and **bring consciousness back** to the image or concentrate on breathing for a few moments and then return to the imagery.
- End with positive imagery.

Sometimes, patients are resistive at first or have a hard time maintaining focus, so **guiding** them through visualization for the first few times can be helpful.

STIMULATION OF THE SKIN TO REDUCE PAIN

Skin, muscles, fascia, tendons, and the cornea contain **nociceptors** that are nerve endings that respond to painful stimuli. Massage, transcutaneous electrical nerve stimulation (TENS), heat and cold provide stimulation to other nerves that transfer only sensation, not pain. These signals block some of the transfer of the nociceptor impulses:

- **Massage** not only sends alternate sensation to the brain, but also results in relaxation that decreases the muscular tension that contributes to pain.
- **TENS** works well on incisional and neuromuscular pain by providing a gentle electrical stimulation that overrides the painful impulses from the area and may stimulate endorphins.
- **Heat therapy** increases blood flow and oxygen to promote healing and stimulates neural receptors, decreasing pain. Heat also helps loosen tense muscles that may be contributing to pain.
- **Cold therapy** decreases circulation and reduces production of chemicals related to inflammation, thereby reducing pain.

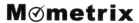

TEMPERATURE-CONTROLLED THERAPIES

METHODS OF HEATING AND COOLING

There are a number of different ways to **heat** (thermotherapy) or **cool** (cryotherapy) for **healing**:

- **Conduction**: Conveyance of heat, cold, or electricity through direct contact with the skin, such as with hot baths, ice packs, and electrical stimulation.
- **Convection**: Indirect transmission of heat in a liquid or gas by circulation of heated particles, such as with whirlpools and paraffin soaks.
- **Conversion**: Heating that results from converting a form of energy into heat, such as with diathermy and ultrasound.
- **Evaporation**: Cooling caused by liquids that evaporate into gases on the skin with a resultant cooling effect, such as with perspiration or vapo-coolant sprays.
- **Radiation**: Heating that results from transfer of heat through light waves or rays, such as with infrared or ultraviolet light.

SUPERFICIAL HEAT

Superficial heat with externally applied heat sources penetrates only the superficial layers of the skin (1-2 cm after about 30 minutes), but it is believed to relax deeper muscles by reflex, decrease pain, and increase metabolisms (2-3 times for every 10 °C increase in skin temperature). Therapeutic temperature range is 40-45 °C. **Superficial heat modalities** include:

- **Moist heat packs** placed on the skin and secured by several layers of towels to provide insulation, applied for 15-30 minutes.
- **Paraffin baths** (52-54 °C) with the hand, foot, or elbow dipped 7 times, cooling between dippings, and then wrapping with plastic and towels for 20 minutes.
- **Fluidotherapy** uses hot-air warmed (38.8-47.8 °C) cellulose particles into which a hand or foot is submerged for 20-30 minutes.

Passive and active range of motion exercises are done after superficial heat treatment. Contraindications include cardiac disease, peripheral vascular disease, malignant tumor, bleeding, and acute inflammation.

Deep heat differs from superficial heat in that the heat is generated internally using ultrasound, short wave, and microwave diathermy rather than applied to the surface of the skin. Deep heating has penetrance to 3-5 cm.

SHORTWAVE DIATHERMY

Shortwave diathermy uses radio waves (27.12 megahertz) to **increase the temperature in subcutaneous tissue** and is used along with passive and active range of motion exercises to **improve range** in painful conditions such as inflammation of the muscles, tendons, and bursae. The radio waves (eddy currents) are transmitted through a capacitor or inductor in a continuous or pulse waveform. Temperatures increase about 15 °C in fatty tissue and 4-6 °C in muscular tissue. Shortwave diathermy should not be used over any organs containing fluid, including the eyes, heart, head, or over pacemakers as the diathermy may disrupt the settings. Because this treatment may increase cardiac demand, it should be avoided in those with preexisting cardiac conditions and should not be used over malignancies. Additionally, it is contraindicated in areas of inflammation because heating the tissue increases inflammation. It cannot be used over prostheses as the metal may heat and damage tissue. Shortwave diathermy should avoid the epiphyses in children, as it may stimulate abnormal growth.

MICROWAVE DIATHERMY

Microwave diathermy is used similarly to shortwave diathermy but has a lower rate of heat increase and penetrance so it is used for muscles and joints near the surface rather than deep muscles, such as the hip. Heat is created by **electromagnetic radiation** (9.15-14.50 MHz) and raises temperature in fatty tissues by about

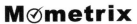

10-12 °C and in muscular tissue by 3-4 °C. **Treatment** is usually given for 15-30 minutes per session and is followed by range of motion exercises (passive and active) to increase flexibility. Contraindications are similar to those of shortwave diathermy in that this treatment should not be used where increase in temperature may be detrimental, such as over organs containing fluid, areas of inflammation, and epiphyses of children. Additionally, it should not be used over prostheses or pacemakers and should be avoided in those with cardiac disease.

CRYOTHERAPY

Cryotherapy uses therapeutic cold treatment to cool the surface of the skin and underlying subcutaneous tissues in order to decrease blood flow, pain, and metabolism. Initially response to cold therapy causes **vasoconstriction** to occur within the first 15 minutes but if the tissues are cooled to -10 °C, then the body responds with **vasodilation**. Cryotherapy affects sensory response so the person will at first feel cold, which progresses to burning, aching, and finally to numbness and tingling. Treatment is usually given for 15-30 minutes. **Treatment modalities** include:

- **Ice packs** such as refrigerated gel packs (-5 °C) or plastic bags filled with water and ice chips are applied directly to the skin for 10-15 minutes for superficial cooling and 15-20 minutes for greater penetrance.
- A **towel dipped in ice and water slurry** is wrapped around limb to provide cold therapy, but this is best used only for emergency situations when ice packs are unavailable, as the towel must be changed frequently as the skin warms the towel rapidly.
- **Ice massage** is applied directly to the affected area for 5-10 minutes, usually rubbing the ice in circular motions on the skin surface. An ice massager is easily made by filled a paper cup with water and freezing it with a tongue depressor or Popsicle stick (to use as a handle) inserted into the center as the water starts to freeze. Then, the paper can be torn away from the bottom and sides when the ice is solid. Ice massage is often followed by friction massage.
- **Ice baths** (13-18 °C) are used for limbs, such as the lower leg, foot, or hand. The body part is immersed for 20 minutes.

Cryotherapy is usually followed by **active and passive exercises**. Contraindications include impaired circulation or sensation, cardiac disease, Raynaud's disease, and nerve trauma.

WHIRLPOOL BATHS

Whirlpool baths are used to increase **circulation** and promote **healing**. They are tubs with a turbine that mixes air with water, which is pressurized and flows into the tub water to create turbulence. Tubs are usually large enough to accommodate the full body although smaller limb-sized whirlpool tubs are available. Water temperature is 95-104 °F (adjusted for the individual) and should be deep enough to completely submerge the affected part. The body part should be cleaned with soap and water before immersion or a shower taken. If the full body is treated, then the patient should wear a swimming suit. During the whirlpool treatment, the muscles relax from the heat and **range of motion exercises** can be done while in the water. Typically, treatments last about 20 minutes, but the patient should be monitored, especially for the first 5 minutes, as some people become lightheaded and can lose consciousness.

CONTRAST BATHS

Contrast baths (alternating hot and cold) are used in the sub-acute phase of healing (after edema begins to subside) for **strains and sprains**. It is believed that contrast baths increase the circulation and help to further decrease edema by a pumping action as the **vasoconstriction and vasodilation** alternate. Two containers are filled with water, one with hot and the other with cold. The hot water should be maintained at about 100-110 °F and the cold at 55-65 °F. The cycle begins and ends with immersion in cold water. Cold water immersions usually last about 1 minute and hot water immersions 4 minutes. Typically, the affected limb is immersed in the cold water for 1 minute, removed, and immediately immersed in hot water for 4 minutes. This cycle is repeated about 3-4 times.

THERAPEUTIC ULTRASOUND

Ultrasound treats soft-tissue injuries (such as myositis, bursitis, and tendinitis) with sound waves (frequency 0.8-3 MHz). Ultrasound utilizes a **piezoelectric crystal** that vibrates, producing sound waveforms, which are transmitted from the transducer through a gel substance into the tissue. The sound waves bounce off of the bone in an irregular pattern that causes an increase in temperature in the connective tissue, such as collagen fibers. Temperatures of the tissue may increase up to 43.5 °C, increasing metabolism in the area, neural conduction, as well as blood flow. Ultrasound is used to **decrease both contractures and scarring**. During treatment, the transducer passes in a circular motion about the skin surface, staying in contact with the gel medium. If a distal limb is submerged in water, the treatment is given with the head of the transducer 0.5-1.0 in from the skin surface. Treatment is followed by range of motion exercises, passive and active. Contraindications are similar to other heat-producing modalities and include peripheral vascular disease, but ultrasound may be used over metal prostheses.

TENS

Transcutaneous electrical nerve stimulation (TENS) uses electrical stimulation to stimulate **peripheral sensory nerve fibers** to reduce acute or recurrent pain. TENS machines may be 2-lead or 4-lead and have adjustments for both frequency (1-20 Hz) and pulse width (50-300 μs, 10-50 mA). Stimulation can be intermittent or continuous. TENS units are small and battery-powered with wires and adhesive electrodes attached so that they can be worn while the person goes about usual activities. The positioning of the electrodes and the settings depend upon the site and type of injury, following guidelines provided by the manufacturer. The TENS machine can be used for a number of hours, but if used for days at a time, it will be less effective. TENS treatment is contraindicated with demand pacemakers and should not be used on the head or neck or over irritated skin.

REHABILITATION
SAID PRINCIPLE OF REHABILITATION AND RECONDITIONING

The Specific Adaptation to Imposed Demands (SAID) principle suggests that when a person is injured or stressed, that person attempts to overcome the problem by **adapting** to the demands of the situation. This is based on **Wolff's law** (systems adapt to demands). For example, if one hand is not usable, the person adapts and uses the other hand. Unfortunately, this adaptation can lead to increasing disability, so when the SAID principle is applied to rehabilitation, it means that the person must do exercises that specifically aim to correct the problem. Thus, the functional needs of the person should always be considered when designing a specific exercise program for that individual (such as treadmill running for soccer players). The exercise activities should as closely mirror the functional activities as possible. For example, if the goal is increased strength rather than endurance, then the exercise program should rely more heavily on strengthening exercises.

MASSAGE FOR REHABILITATION AND RECONDITIONING

Massage therapy is commonly used in sports and may be employed before activities, at breaks during activities, and after the activity is completed. Many types of massage are used in sports, and some massage therapists specialize in sports massage, but all nurses who work with athletes of any age should know the basic techniques of **sports massage** as it is used to both treat and prevent injuries. Sports massage is based primarily on Swedish massage although the massage may be deeper and targeted toward a particular injury, and other types of massage may be incorporated into a sports massage program. Massage of an injured area is delayed for the first **48-72 hours** to prevent further injury to tissues. Different techniques include:

- **Compression**: Deep rhythmical compressions of the muscles are done to increase circulation and temperature and make muscles more pliable. It may be used prior to deeper massage techniques.
- **Effleurage**: This is usually the beginning massage and begins softly and increases in intensity with the hands gliding over the tissue, so it is done with some type of oil or emollient. Massage is done in rhythmical broad strokes with the palms of the hands. This massage helps to relax the athlete and identify areas of tightness or pain that may require additional attention.

- **Friction**: These are massages either in line with muscle fibers or across the muscle fibers to create stretching and to reduce adhesions and scarring during healing. The tissue is pressed firmly against the underlying tissue and then pressure moves the underlying tissue until resistance is felt. Friction massage may be done deeply, and this can be uncomfortable. Usually, the thumb or fingers are used for this type of massage.
- **Petrissage**: This is kneading massage and is usually used on large muscle areas, such as the calf or thigh. It increases circulation, so it is useful to relax and to improve circulation and drainage as well as to stretch muscles. The full hand is used for this massage with the heel and thumb stabilizing the tissue while the fingers squeeze the tissue.
- **Tapotement**: This type of massage uses quick rhythmic tapping, usually with the edge of the palm and little finger or the heel of the hand with the fingers elevated. It is done to increase circulation or relieve cramped muscles.
- **Vibration**: Vibratory massage is used for deep muscle relaxation and reduction of pain. Usually, the entire hand is placed against the skin, compressing the muscle and then vibrating the hand to cause movement.
- **Trigger point**: Pressure is applied with a finger or thumb to areas of point tenderness to reduce spasticity and pain.

PROGRESSION IN STRENGTHENING EXERCISES

Strengthening exercise progression includes the following exercises:

- **Isometric exercises** are done with the muscle and limb in static position with no movement of the joint or lengthening of the muscle. The muscle is contracted against resistance.
- **Isotonic exercises** include movement of the joint during exercise (such as running, weight lifting) and both shortening and lengthening of the muscles through eccentric or concentric contractions. Isotonic refers to tension, so the tension is constant during shortening and lengthening of the muscle.
- **Isokinetic exercises** utilize machines (such as stationary bicycles that can be set with various parameters) to control the rate and extent of contraction as well as the range of motion. Both speed and resistance can be set so the athlete is limited by the settings of the machine.
- **Plyometrics** is a particular type of exercise program that uses activities to allow a muscle to achieve maximal force as quickly as possible, and the sequence is a fast, eccentric movement (to stretch) followed quickly by a strong concentric movement (to contract).

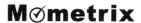

Psychosocial and Child/Family-Centered Care

FAMILY TYPES

A table of the different family types is provided below:

Family Type	Description
Nuclear	This husband-wife-children model was once the most common family type but is no longer the norm. In this model, the husband is the provider, and the mother stays home to care for the children. This makes up only about 7% of current American families.
Dual career/ dual earner	This model, where both parents work, is the most common in American society, affecting about 66% of two-parent families. One parent may work more than another, or both may work fulltime. There may be disparities in income that affect family dynamics.
Childless	10-15% of couples have no children because of infertility or choice.
Extended	These may include multigenerational families or shared households with friends, parents, or other relatives. Childcare responsibilities may be shared or primarily assumed by an extended family member, such as a grandparent.
Extended kin network	Two or more nuclear families live close together, share goods and services, and support each other, including sharing childcare. This model is common in the Hispanic community.
Single-parent	This is one of the fastest growing family models. Typically, the mother is the single parent, but in some cases, it is the father. The single parent may be widowed, divorced, or separated but more commonly has never married. In cases of divorce or abandonment, the child may have minimal or no contact with one parent, often the father. Single parents often face difficulties in trying to support and care for a child and may suffer economic hardship.
Stepparent	Because of the high rate of divorce, stepparent families are common. This can result in stress and conflict when a new child enters the picture. There may be jealousy and resentment on the part of siblings and estranged family members. In some cases, families can work together to achieve harmony and provide added support to children.
Binuclear/co-parenting	In this model, children share time between two primarily nuclear families because of joint custody agreements. While this may at times result in conflict, the child benefits from having a continued relationship with both parents.
Cohabiting	This model refers to unmarried heterosexual couples living together. The relationships within this model may vary, with some similar to the nuclear family. In some cases, people are in committed relationships and may avoid marriage because of economic or personal reasons. A planned child may strengthen the relationship, but an unplanned child may cause conflict.
Same sex	Whether those in same sex relationships marry or cohabit, they have the opportunity to create families using sperm donors, adoption, or surrogacy.

FAMILY THEORY

FAMILY DEVELOPMENTAL THEORY

According to the family developmental theory, families move through different developmental stages, which are accompanied by certain tasks:

- **Marriage**: Get to know significant other, establish good relationships with new kin, and discuss parenthood.
- **Birth of first child**: Adjust to and bond with new baby, maintain spousal relationship.

- **Preschool children**: Provide for different children's needs while family grows, teach socialization skills, maintain healthy relationships between immediate family and extended family, cope with decreased energy and privacy.
- **School-age children**: Encourage academic achievement and good relationships with peers and teachers.
- **Teenagers**: Help teens balance freedom and responsibility, maintain good communication between parents and teens, renewed focus on career and marital relations.
- **Launching adult children**: Allow children to start their own life, jobs, etc., welcome new family members by marriage, help with aging parents' needs, and work on marital relationship.
- **Empty nest**: Maintain relationships with children and aging parents, establish stronger marital relationship.
- **Aging family**: Adjust to health issues, reduced income and loss of spouse/family members/friends.

Limitation: The theory assumes a traditional, nuclear, middle-class family.

STRUCTURAL-FUNCTIONAL THEORY

According to the structural-functional theory, the family, a social system, serves society by performing functions needed for survival:

- **Affective**, or providing love and acceptance to each member
- **Socialization and social placement**, or teaching the children how to get along with others and fit into society as adults
- **Reproductive**, or producing of offspring to continue the family line
- **Economic**, or providing and distributing the necessary resources to the family members
- **Health care**, or providing basic necessities (food, clothing, shelter) and health care, as well as teaching basic hygiene to maintain good health

Limitation: The theory assumes the traditional definition of family and doesn't address the changes that a family encounters.

FAMILY SYSTEMS THEORY

According to the family systems theory, the family is a system where members can only be understood in relationship to other family members. They are interdependent, so that as one member experiences a change, other family members will change to maintain equilibrium. Each member has specific roles, with certain rules governing them.

Limitation: The theory is vague and therefore difficult to apply.

FAMILY STRESS THEORY

The stress theory has several different models. Most assume a stressor (sometimes more than one stressor can occur at the same time, termed **stressor pileup**), resources that are available to the family in coping with the stressor, and how the family perceives the stressor. These factors together will determine whether the family experiences stress or a crisis. Stress causes changes within the family, but it is usually short-lived. A crisis occurs when the family cannot recover from a stress using the resources at hand or the stress is too large for the family to handle.

RESILIENCY MODEL

The resiliency model assumes that some families develop strength over time by facing changes common to all families. These strengths, as well as strong resources and relationships, help protect against crises when uncommon stressors are present. Families respond to stressful events in two phases. The **adjustment phase** occurs when the family makes minor changes to its roles and routines. When the family moves into the **adaptation phase**, it makes major changes to its structure and functions.

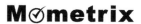

FAMILY ASSESSMENT AND FACTORS THAT INFLUENCE RELATIONSHIPS AND PARENTING

Family assessment is the collection of data concerning the structure of the family and how family members relate to each other and society. It is an ongoing process, using assessment tools, such as a genogram (a map of a three generational family tree, including relationships and health histories), an ecomap (a chart depicting the relationships within and outside of the family and the support networks available to the family), interviews, questionnaires, and observations.

There are many factors that influence family relationships and parenting. These include: the type of family unit (nuclear, blended, single parent, gay, or lesbian), parental culture, parenting a foster child, adolescent parenting, parenting an adopted child, parenting by grandparents.

FAMILY FUNCTIONING AND DYNAMICS

Cultural/lifestyle factors that affect family integration include the following:

- **Values**: Values based on attitudes, ideas, and beliefs often connect family members to common goals. However, these values may be influenced by many external factors, such as education, social norms, and attitudes of peers, extended family, and coworkers, so values may change, which may affect family integration.
- **Roles**: In some families, roles are clearly defined by gender and task (homemaker and breadwinner), but the roles blur or are shared in many families, and in some cases the father becomes the primary caregiver while the mother works. Other common roles include peacemaker, nurturer, and social planner. How these roles are perceived and actualized affects the manner in which a child is integrated into the family and cared for.
- **Decision making**: Family power structures vary widely, but in many families, power rests with one person who makes ultimate decisions and whose opinions affect other family members. In many traditional cultures (Hispanic, Asian, Middle Eastern) power lies with the father, grandfather, or other male family member. However, in American society, this may vary because of diversity. Power may be shared or rest with the mother or the father.
- **Socioeconomic**: Employment trends, marriage rates, and economic trends all affect family integration. Many people have become unemployed and are unable to support their families, resulting in severe stress, which may be exacerbated by the arrival of a new child or illness. The divorce rate is high, leaving many parents with inadequate funds to support a child. Even if both parents are employed, the cost of living continues to escalate, including the cost of caring for a child.

IDENTIFYING PRIMARY CAREGIVER

Identifying the primary caregiver is especially important in the emergency care of infants and children, as their ability to report is limited and may not be reliable, depending on age. With the diversity of family models, one cannot assume that the mother, father, or person accompanying the child is the primary caregiver. In some cases, custodial arrangements designate one parent as custodial and the other as non-custodial, and they may or may not share legal rights over medical care for the child. Therefore, the nurse should ask who is the primary caregiver in order to glean information about the child and ask who has the legal right to make medical decisions to determine who should sign consent forms and make decisions.

IMPACT AND COMPLICATIONS WHEN PATIENT HAS MULTIPLE CAREGIVERS

Continuity of care is especially important for infants and young children, and the lack of stability in caregivers can lead to various problems. Even when children must have **multiple caregivers**, a primary care giver should be identified and should oversee care and ease the transitions whenever possible by introducing other caregivers and coordinating care activities. The greater the number of changes, the greater the impact on the child. The impacts/complications involved when a patient has multiple caregivers, either at the same time or sequentially, include:

- Inadequate communication of the patient's needs and condition
- Different approaches to caregiving, leading to confusion or discord
- Inability of the patient to adequately bond and form attachment with the caregivers
- Patient insecurity and impaired sociopsychological development
- Increased stress and anxiety
- Behavioral problems

Some children are able to adapt to multiple changes over time and can better handle the demands of change than others.

FUNCTIONAL COPING STRATEGIES OF FAMILIES

Some families utilize a number of functional coping strategies to deal with stress. These families exhibit resilience in difficult situations. Strategies include:

- The family gathers information, increases organization, discusses issues, and tries to jointly solve problems.
- Family members draw together as a strengthened family unit to deal with stressful situations.
- The family attempts to carry on as normal a routine as possible while making accommodations as needed for a child who is ill. This provides the child with a sense of security.
- The family accepts those things that cannot be changed rather than wasting energy trying to deny or alter reality.
- The family communicates openly and directly, avoiding family secrets and including the child in discussions as appropriate to the child's age.
- The family uses humor to deflect stress.
- The family uses resources outside of the immediate family for support, such as extended family, spiritual advisors, and community agencies.

DYSFUNCTIONAL COPING STRATEGIES OF FAMILIES

Some families are not resilient when dealing with stressful situations and exhibit dysfunctional coping strategies, which include:

- Family members may resort to substance abuse, such as alcohol and/or drugs, rather than facing problems. This adds to the family dysfunction and negatively affects all members.
- The family may take out frustrations through domestic violence, aimed at the child or other family members. This can include physical, sexual, or mental abuse and can create an environment of fear within the family.
- The family denies problems and refuses to acknowledge that family dynamics have changed, attempting to carry on as usual.
- The family uses threats, aggression, and/or withholding of affection to retain control and maintain the family unit.
- The family may blame vulnerable members, such as the child, for the stressful situation, often scapegoating the member that they "blame" rather than dealing with the real problems.

METHODS TO GET PARENTS MORE INVOLVED IN THEIR CHILD'S HEALTH AT SCHOOL

Most children spend a great deal of time at school, and children with health conditions are often monitored and supported by school health staff, such as the school nurse, health aide, psychologist, or counselor. Parents can be involved with their child's health at school by maintaining communication with these professionals to provide the most comprehensive care for their child. This may mean partnering with school officials to develop a care plan to use at school, signing documents approving medication administration at school, and attending meetings to discuss the effects of their child's health on the classroom experience. Parents provide the health care providers in the school system with much of the information needed for their child to have a sufficient school experience without health issues standing in the way. School nurses can reinforce this behavior by keeping in frequent contact with parents about their child's health, communicating when the child receives health services at school, and keeping records updated and accurate.

FACTORS THAT INFLUENCE THE RELATIONSHIP BETWEEN THE CHILD AND PARENTS

Factors influencing parent-child relationships are cultural (some children consider themselves a part of the American culture, while their parents still hold true to the cultural practices of their home country), religious (some youth rebel against their religious upbringing, especially in the teen years), parenting style, and family structure (nuclear, extended, blended, gay/lesbian, single parent, adolescent parent, adoptive parenting, grandparents raising the children, and foster parenting).

APPROPRIATE DISCIPLINARY PRACTICES FOR FAMILIES TO USE

Appropriate discipline practices should be discussed with parents. These include:

- Make rules clear and appropriate for the age of the child.
- Set the consequences before the rule has been broken, making sure they are appropriate for the broken rule and age of the child. The consequence should be administered directly after the rule has been broken, with a calm attitude.
- Use lots of praise when the child behaves appropriately.

TEMPERAMENT

Temperament is the way a person relates or responds to his environment and the people around him. Temperament is inborn, but it can be affected by how parents relate to the child/adolescent.

ATTRIBUTES

The nine attributes of temperament are:

- **Activity**: How active is the child is during normal activities?
- **Rhythmicity**: How regular are the child's normal physiological activities, such as bowel movements, sleep cycle, and eating patterns?
- **Approach-withdrawal**: How does the child respond to different stimuli, such as being drawn readily to a new stuffed animal or withdrawing from the noise of fireworks?
- **Adaptability**: How does the child adapt to new circumstances?
- **Intensity of reaction**: How forcefully does the child respond to new circumstances?
- **Threshold of responsiveness**: How much stimulus is needed before the child responds?
- **Mood**: How much positive vs. negative behavior is exhibited in different situations?
- **Distractibility**: How easily can the child be distracted and the behavior changed?
- **Attention span and persistence**: How long will the child continue an activity and how much distraction is needed to pull the child away from the activity (persistence)?

TYPES

Types of temperament include:

- **Easy**: Easily adapts to new situations, gets along with others well, easy going behaviors
- **Difficult**: Responds negatively to new situations, behaviors are unpredictable, does well in highly structured environment
- **Slow-to-warm-up**: Moody, shy, slow to adapt to new situations, low activity level

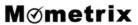

EFFECTS OF PARENTING STYLES ON TEMPERAMENT OF CHILDREN

Although children are born with their own temperament, the parenting style they grow up with can influence how this temperament manifests over time.

- **Authoritarian (autocratic)** parents desire obedience without question. They tend toward harsh punishments, using their power to make their children obey. They are emotionally withdrawn from their children and enforce strict rules without discussing why the rules exist. These children tend to have low self-esteem, be more dependent, and are introverted with poor social skills.
- **Authoritative (democratic)** parents provide boundaries and expect obedience, but use love when they discipline. They involve their children in deciding rules and consequences, discussing reasons for their decisions, but will enforce the rules consistently. They encourage independence and take each child's unique position seriously. These children tend to have higher self-esteem, good social skills, and confidence in themselves.
- **Indulgent (permissive)** parents stay involved with their children, but have few rules in place to give the children boundaries. These children have a difficult time setting their own limits and are not responsible. They disrespect others and have trouble with authority figures.
- **Indifferent (uninvolved)** parents spend as little time as possible with their children. They are self-involved, with no time or patience for taking care of their children's needs. Guidance and discipline are lacking and inconsistent. These children tend toward delinquency, with a lack of respect for others.

METHODS TO ASSIST CAREGIVERS

Caregivers for children are most often the parents, with the greatest burden of care often falling on the mother. Caregiving can be extremely stressful, especially if the child suffers from a chronic or serious disease. Part of caring practices is to recognize that the caregivers need care as well.

- **Conflict resolution** brings people with conflict together with a neutral person or group in order to attempt to negotiate or reach agreement. Nurses are in a unique position to assist with conflict resolution because they see people at their most vulnerable, when they are dealing with stress.
- **Debriefing** allows the caregiver to talk about experiences that have caused trauma or stress.
- **Crisis intervention** takes place when an individual is overwhelmed by a situation and is not able to function adequately. It involves intervening during the crisis in order to help the person stabilize and to help him or her to function and to facilitate problem solving.

EFFECTS OF DEVELOPMENTAL STAGE OF THE LEARNER ON TEACHING

Many children have chronic conditions, such as those receiving insulin or managing colostomies, and the nurse must **guide the child** and family in helping the child become independent in care based on the **development stage** of the child and the learner:

- **Infant/toddler**: Caregivers provide care; instruction encourages bonding and acceptance.
- **Early childhood**: Children learn by participation, such as role-playing, simple explanation, and teaching dolls. Children should be independent in emptying colostomy pouch by kindergarten.
- **Childhood**: By age 6, children should be independent in care at school. They should have supplies at school, and the school nurse should know about care so the nurse can provide assistance. Child should be completely independent in care by 6th grade. Parents and child should be taught together.
- **Adolescence/young adulthood**: The adolescent may be angry and resistive. Extra time and guidance, including visits with other young patients facing the same or similar challenges may help. Parents should allow adolescents to be independent in care.

INCREASING KNOWLEDGE BASE OF HEALTHCARE COMMUNITY

There are numerous ways to contribute to and advance the **knowledge base** of the healthcare community:

- **Research** may be a review of literature and compilation of findings on a given subject or may be clinical research in which different treatment approaches are used and evaluated.
- **Presentations** may include any variety of informal or formal presentations in meetings, workshops, or classes.
- **Publications** may include research results or nurse-related educational courses, such as continuing education courses related to a field of expertise. Publications may be in journals, online, or intended for in-house use only.
- **Involvement in professional organizations** is especially important in the field of nursing because changes occur rapidly, not only in medical treatments but also in regulations. Professional organizations provide up-to-date information and provide a means to lobby legislators about issues related to nursing practice, such as nurse-patient ratios.

INTELLECTUAL DISABILITY

Intellectual disability is usually diagnosed <18. Individuals may have difficulty adapting to changing environments, need guidance in decision-making, and have self-care or communication deficits. Behaviors range from shy and passive to hyperactive or aggressive. Those with associated physical characteristics (Down syndrome) or problems are often diagnosed early. Intellectual disability may be inherited (Tay-Sachs), toxin-related (maternal alcohol consumption), perinatal (hypoxia), environmental (lack of stimulation/neglect), or acquired (encephalitis, brain injury). Diagnosis involves performance results from standardized tests along with behavior analysis. **Intellectual disability classifications** are divided into mild, moderate, severe, and profound with criteria broken down across three domains: conceptual, social, and practical.

- **Mild (85% of cases)**: Educable to about 6th grade level. May not be diagnosed until adolescence. Usually able to learn skills and be self-supporting but may need assistance and supervision.
- **Moderate (10% of cases)**: Trainable and may be able to work and live in sheltered environments or with supervision.
- **Severe (3-4% of cases)**: Language usually delayed and can learn only basic academic skills and perform simple tasks.
- **Profound (1-2% of cases)**: Usually associated with neurological disorder with sensorimotor dysfunction. Require constant care and supervision.

ATTENTION-DEFICIT HYPERACTIVITY DISORDER

A child with attention-deficit hyperactivity disorder (ADHD) may display some or all of the following symptoms:

- Inattention (short attention span, distractible)
- Hyperactivity (can't sit still, moves constantly)
- Impulsivity (impatience, acts before thinking)

Inattention and hyperactivity/impulsivity can be present separately or in combination. A diagnosis of ADHD is based on several criteria. The most important criteria are that symptoms of impulsivity/hyperactivity and/or inattention be present for at least 6 months and that some symptoms were present before the age of 12.

TREATMENT

Treatment for ADHD is aimed at controlling the behavior (pharmacotherapy and behavior management), controlling the environment (educational interventions) and educating the family. Medications used include stimulants (Ritalin, Dexedrine, and Adderall), antihypertensives (Catapres, Tenex), antidepressants (Wellbutrin), or Strattera, a nonstimulant. Stimulants are addictive and the side effects include weight loss, insomnia, headache, palpitations, and high blood pressure. Behavior therapy involves using positive reinforcement to help the child follow rules, stay on task, and have more self-control. ADHD is a developmental disorder, meaning that the school system must provide accommodations for these children in mainstreamed classrooms if at all possible. Families should be educated as to the nature of ADHD and coping skills. Some controversial treatments are used, although they are part of the standard of care. These can include vitamins, mineral and herbal supplements, biofeedback, dietary changes, and chiropractic care.

AUTISM SPECTRUM DISORDERS

Autism spectrum disorders (ASD) affect approximately 3.4 per 1000 children in the United States and present with a wide range of symptoms, including impairment in thinking and expressions of emotion, using language, and communicating and relating with others. Some children are profoundly impaired and are diagnosed early, but more high functioning children, such as those with Asperger's, may go undiagnosed. All exhibit some degree of impairment in 3 areas:

- Social interaction
- Communication (verbal and nonverbal)
- Repetitive behavior

Because they may lack social skills, children with ASD are often isolated and bullied. They may do well in school or have some degree of intellectual disability. About 25% suffer from seizure disorders as well. ASD may be identified through developmental screening, and/or specific screening instruments for autism. Intervention includes referrals to special education programs, including early intervention programs for children under the age of 3 and may include behavioral and speech therapy. Early diagnosis helps maximize the child's potential and may allow the child to live independently as an adult.

EARLY INDICATORS OF AUTISM

Although there is no specific test that defines a diagnosis of autism, there are many indications that can point to autistic development that caregivers should be aware of. Further testing may be indicated with a child who does not make sounds such as babbling or giggling; fails to show positive facial expressions or mimic smiles or laughter; lacks the ability to repeat activities, words, or sounds when another person initiates these; fails to utter speech sounds at all by 16 months of age; fails to initiate gestures, such as waving, pointing to objects, or reaching for items; and appears to turn backwards in development, such as a sudden loss of speech, words, or social skills.

MOOD DISORDERS

Mood disorders can be broken down into two types: **bipolar** (depression alternating with mania) and **depressive** (chronic or episodic). The major symptom of mood disorders is depression, usually lasting 7–9 months. Other symptoms to watch for are disinterest in activities the child used to enjoy, changes in eating or sleeping patterns, agitation or anxiety, low self-esteem, being more tired than usual, problems with concentration, and suicidal thoughts. They may also exhibit physical complaints, such as stomach aches, diarrhea, and headaches.

BIPOLAR DISORDER

In children with bipolar disorder, the hallmark symptom is intense rage. They may experience rage episodes lasting for 2–3 hours. Many parents do not seek treatment for younger children for several years until the child becomes older and the behavior becomes more disruptive. For many younger children, the first symptom exhibited is depression. Symptoms in children under the age of nine usually include labile emotions and irritability rather than more classic manic symptoms. However, as the child becomes older and enters adolescence, the symptoms become more classic-like and include abnormally elevated mood and delusions of grandeur. They may exhibit racing thoughts and pressured speech. Bipolar disease may occur with ADHD, depression, reactive attachment disorder, conduct disorder, and oppositional defiant disorder, so diagnosis and treatment may be complicated. Children often experience academic and behavioral problems as well as

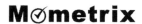

suicidal ideation. Initial treatment is monotherapy with a mood stabilizer, such as lithium, carbamazepine, divalproex, or atypical antipsychotics.

DEPRESSION

Depression is increasingly recognized as a risk factor for children, manifesting in young children as feigning illness or refusal to go to school and in older children as behavioral problems, negativity, and difficulties at school rather than the more common withdrawal and overt depression of some adults. However, children may feel persistent anxiety and sadness, and they often have profound fears that something will happen to a parent. Usually changes in behavior become apparent. One study showed that 29% of children with depression had suicidal thoughts, making early diagnosis and intervention very important. While there is some concern about antidepressants and children, suicide is a leading cause of death in teenagers, so medications with careful monitoring along with psychotherapy, such as cognitive behavioral therapy, seem to provide the best form of treatment, providing >70% with clinical improvement.

EATING DISORDERS

ANOREXIA NERVOSA

Eating disorders are a profound health risk and can lead to death, especially for adolescent girls, although boys also have eating disorders, often presenting as excessive exercise. Anorexia nervosa is characterized by profound fear of weight gain and severe restriction of food intake, often accompanied by abuse of diuretics and laxatives, which can cause electrolyte imbalances, kidney and bowel disorders, and delay or cessation of menses.

- **Symptoms** include growth retardation, amenorrhea (missing 3 consecutive periods), unexplained and sometimes precipitous weight loss (at least 15% below normal weight), dehydration, loss of appetite, hypoglycemia, hypercholesterolemia, or carotenemia with yellowing of skin, emaciated appearance, osteoporosis, bradycardia, and food obsessions and rituals.
- **Diagnosis** includes complete history, physical, and psychological exam with CBC and chemical panels to rule out other disorders.
- **Treatment** includes volume and electrolyte replacement initially with referral to psychiatric care for long-term management of the disorder and nutritional plans.

BULIMIA NERVOSA

Bulimia nervosa includes binge eating followed by vomiting (at least once a week for at least 3 months), often along with diuretics, enemas, and laxatives. Some may engage in periods of fasting or excessive exercise rather than vomiting to offset the effects of binging. Gastric acids from purging can damage the throat and teeth. While bulimics may maintain a normal weight, they are at risk for severe electrolyte imbalances that can be life-threatening. Binge eating affects 2-5% of females and includes grossly overeating, often resulting in obesity, depression, and shame. Symptoms include hypokalemia, metabolic acidosis, fluctuations of weight, dental caries and loss of enamel, knuckle scars (from contact with teeth while inducing vomiting), parotid and submandibular gland enlargement, and insulin-dependent diabetes. Diagnosis includes complete history, physical, and psychological exam with CBC and chemical panels to rule out other disorders. Treatment includes volume and electrolyte replacement initially with referral to psychiatric care for long-term management of the disorder and nutritional plans, as well as SSRIs, naltrexone, and ondansetron.

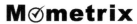

ANXIETY DISORDERS IN CHILDREN

Some anxiety is normal and assists the child in adjusting to new situations. Overwhelming anxiety to unspecific events can produce psychological and physical symptoms. Classifications of anxiety disorders in children include the following:

- **Social anxiety disorder** occurs when the child feels embarrassed, judged, or humiliated in the social environment.
- **Specific phobia** involves extreme fear/anxiety when exposed to a specific object/scenario, which may present as crying/screaming or freezing in the child.
- **Separation anxiety disorder** occurs when the child becomes stressed upon being separated from familiar surroundings or people.
- **Generalized anxiety disorder** presents as excessive worry over future events or day-to-day situations. Symptoms of anxiety may include stomachaches, nausea, vomiting, headaches, dizziness, palpitations, slight fever, tiredness, crying, irritability, and sleeping and eating difficulties.

TREATMENT AND NURSING MANAGEMENT

Treatment for anxiety disorders focuses on relieving symptoms and normalizing the child's daily activities. Education of the child and family, cognitive behavioral, family, and individual therapy, and medication are some treatment modalities. School teachers should be involved in the plan of care. To return the child to school, cognitive therapies such as desensitization and conditioning can be used. Medication is used in combination with therapy; antidepressants or anti-anxiety drugs are commonly used.

Assess for physical symptoms of anxiety (stomachaches or headaches that go away later in the day) and excessive absences from school. Diagnoses can include fear of separation, fear of interacting with others outside the home, and poor coping skills. A good outcome might include being able to be away from home for extended periods of time with little anxiety, attending school with little anxiety, good coping skills, and good social skills. The family should be included in the implementation of therapy. They can be taught signs of anxiety and ways to help the child gain independence and increase self-confidence.

PHYSIOLOGICAL EFFECTS OF CHRONIC STRESS ON A CHILD'S BODY

Children experience and struggle with stress, even at a very young age. Stressful situations can cause potential harm when a child lives in a chronic state of stress. Physiologically, a child who experiences continuous life stress may secrete increased levels of cortisol from the adrenal glands. This can contribute to a decreased immune response, resulting in increased illnesses and diminished protection from diseases. Increased levels of cortisol also damage the part of the brain that promotes memory and learning, which can lead to learning disabilities and difficulties in school. **Chronic stress** can alter brain growth, and when begun at a very early age, it can result in a smaller brain. Finally, continuous levels of stress may make a child less likely to tolerate stressful situations in life, leading to a decreased threshold for tolerating demanding activities.

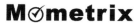

SUICIDAL IDEATION/SUICIDE ATTEMPTS

Suicide is the third leading cause of death among adolescents, with about 1 million attempting suicide in the US each year. Additionally, antidepressants and atypical antipsychotics may increase suicidal ideation and depression.

Suicidal Ideation Indications	High Risk for Repeated Suicide Attempt
<ul><li>Depression or dysphoria</li><li>Hostility to others</li><li>Problems with peer relationships, and lack of close friends</li><li>Post-crisis stress (divorce, death in family, graduation, college)</li><li>Withdrawn personality</li><li>Quiet, lonely appearance, behavior</li><li>Change in behavior (drop in grades, wearing black clothes, unkempt appearance, sleeping excessively, or not sleeping)</li><li>Co-morbid psychiatric problems (bipolar, schizophrenia)</li><li>Drug abuse</li></ul>	Children who actually attempt suicide should be hospitalized and assessed for repeated suicide risk after initial treatment: <ul><li>Violent suicide attempt (knives, gunshots)</li><li>Suicide attempt with low chance of rescue</li><li>Ongoing psychosis or disordered thinking</li><li>Ongoing severe depression and feeling of helplessness</li><li>History of previous suicide attempts</li><li>Lack of social support system</li></ul>

HOMICIDAL IDEATION/ATTEMPTS

Homicidal ideation or attempts are rare in young children but can occur during adolescence for a variety of reasons.

- **Sociopathy/psychopathy**: These children usually appear quite normal and may even seem charming, but they can be very dangerous because they lack empathy for others. Some are involved in gangs in which violent behavior is expected and valued.
- **Psychosis**: Uncontrolled schizophrenia and paranoia may result in a child behaving in a homicidal manner.
- **Medications**: Medications such as antidepressants, SSRIs, and antipsychotics as well as interferon have been associated with homicidal ideation in some patients. Children on multiple medications may experience involuntary intoxication that results in rage reactions and sometimes even the death of others.

Children who express homicidal ideation or who have attempted homicide require immediate psychiatric referral and may require restraint. The nurse should conduct a complete review of medications and notify security personnel if the child poses a danger.

TREATMENTS FOR CHILDREN AND FAMILIES WITH PSYCHOSOCIAL DISORDERS

Treatments for children and families with psychosocial disorders includes a variety of approaches:

- **Individual therapy** involves the child and therapist working together on the psychosocial and developmental problems.
- **Family therapy** involves the whole family working with the therapist. The focus is on family relationships, communication, and assisting each family member in individual development within the family.
- **Group therapy** involves a group of children or teens working on socialization skills.

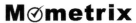

- **Play therapy** uses play to allow the child to explore and bring out his feelings. The therapist helps the child understand these emotions and use them in positive ways. The child learns to control his actions and emotions, thereby increasing his self-esteem.
- **Art therapy** uses the child's own art projects to bring out emotions and deal positively with them.

TYPES OF PHYSICAL RESTRAINTS FOR PEDIATRIC PATIENTS
There are a number of different types of physical restraints to ensure child safety:

- **Swaddling**: Used for infants and small children for treatments and examinations of the head, neck, and throat, venipuncture, and gavage feedings to prevent movement. A papoose board with straps or a mummy wrap is used.
- **Jacket**: Used to prevent children from falling out of chairs/beds or to maintain horizontal position. A jacket is applied with ties in the back and long ties secured out of reach in the back of the wheelchair or underside of the crib.
- **Limb**: Used to prevent arm or leg movement that might cause injury or to protect IV access. Commercial restraints are sized, so they should fit properly and should be padded to prevent pressure.
- **Elbow**: This restraint is used to prevent the child from reaching the head or face, usually after surgery, or to prevent scratching. The most common restraint is a muslin wrap with pockets for tongue depressors for infants. Commercial restraints are available for older children.

SSRIS FOR CHILDREN
Escitalopram (Lexapro) and fluoxetine (Prozac for children ages 8 and older) are the only two SSRIs approved by the FDA for children. They are the first-line pharmacologic treatment in pediatric depression. All SSRIs have similar action but may have different chemical properties that cause various side effects, so some people tolerate one better than others. Side effects include nausea, weight gain, sexual dysfunction, excitation and agitation, and insomnia, drowsiness, increased perspiration, headache, and diarrhea. In rare cases, **serotonin syndrome** may occur from high levels of serotonin from overdose or combination with monoamine oxidase (MAO) inhibitors, so SSRIs must not be taken within two weeks of each other. Symptoms include severe anxiety and agitation, hallucinations, confusion, blood pressure swings, fever, tachycardia, seizures, and coma. SSRIs are not addictive but abrupt cessation may trigger discontinuation syndrome (flu-like symptoms).

SECOND-GENERATION/ATYPICAL ANTIPSYCHOTICS FOR CHILDREN
Second-generation antipsychotics (SGAs), also called atypical antipsychotics, are used for bipolar disorders, schizophrenia, and psychosis in children. Children may also receive atypical antipsychotics for a wide range of non-psychotic disorders, such as mood disorders (most common), eating disorders, developmental disorders (autism spectrum), and tic disorders. Use is most common during adolescence. Children should receive the lowest effective dose of medication.

LITHIUM
Lithium carbonate (Lithobid) is used to control the manic episodes associated with bipolar disorder. While it is FDA-approved only for children over age 12, it is increasingly used for younger children. Children should be started on ≤30 mg/kg/day with blood levels monitored every other day initially. Lithium has a very narrow therapeutic window, and toxicity is a medical emergency that can lead to death. Target serum levels are 0.6-1.2 mEq/L. Increased blood levels can cause **toxicity**:

- 1.5-2.5 mEq/L: Severe vomiting and diarrhea, increased muscle tremors and twitching, lethargy, body aches, ataxia, ringing in the ears, blurry vision, vertigo, or hyperactive deep tendon reflexes.
- >2.5 mEq/L: Elevated temperature, low urine output, hypotension, ECG abnormalities, decreased level of consciousness, seizures, coma, or death.

Plasma levels will usually decrease to an acceptable level within 48 hours after discontinuation of the medication; however, in severe cases involving acute renal failure, dialysis may be necessary.

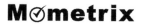

SHIFT REPORTING

Shift reporting should include bedside handoff when possible with oncoming staff members. The nurse handing off the patient should follow a specific format for handoff (such as I PASS the BATON) so that handoff is done in the same manner every time, as this reduces the chance of omitting important information. The shift report should include introduction of the oncoming staff to the patient, the triage category or acuity level of the patient, diagnosis (potential or confirmed), current status, laboratory and imaging (completed or pending) and results if available, and medications or treatments administered and pending. Any monitoring equipment (pulse oximetry, telemetry) should be examined. Any invasive treatments (Foley catheter, IV) should be discussed and equipment examined. The nurse should report any plans for admission, transfer, or discharge. It is essential that all staff be trained in shift reporting and the importance of consistency.

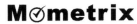

Palliative/End-of-Life Care

INFANT RESPONSE TO ILLNESS AND HOSPITALIZATION

Infants respond to illness and pain with crying, grimacing, and withdrawal from the stimulus. Infants up to 4 months tolerate hospitalization fairly well, if their needs are met. They may exhibit separation anxiety from 4 months on, when their parents are not close by.

Nursing Interventions: Let parents participate in the care of the infant as much as possible. Keep the infant's schedule the same as the home schedule. Meet basic needs quickly and gently. Provide age-appropriate toys. Interact often with the infant (holding, talking to her). The key is to make the hospital environment match the home environment as closely as possible. This will encourage the infant to continue to trust her environment and the people in it.

TODDLER RESPONSE TO ILLNESS AND HOSPITALIZATION

Toddlers tend to experience a great deal of stress when dealing with an invasive procedure. Pain produces crying, pulling away, and resistance if they've experienced painful procedures before. Toddlers regress when hospitalized. Their usual control of their environment is lost and they will exhibit separation anxiety if their caregiver is absent.

Nursing Interventions: Encourage the parents to stay in the room. Ask them to bring items from home that remind the child of the parents. Discourage the parents from leaving the room while the child is sleeping. Keep routines the same as at home. Use terms that the child is used to. Provide age-appropriate toys and activities. Allow the child to do as much as he can for himself. Allow him some control over his environment and schedule.

PRESCHOOLER RESPONSE TO ILLNESS AND HOSPITALIZATION

Preschoolers think illness is caused by something they can see or experience and may blame their illness on something totally unrelated. They may also think the illness or hospitalization is a punishment. They fear body mutilation, and will therefore be very afraid of any invasive procedure. An IV can bring on a fear of body contents leaking out. Preschoolers, like toddlers, will exhibit regression as a defense mechanism. They experience a loss of control over their environment and fear their parents do not love them if they are separated from them.

Nursing Interventions: Keep invasive procedures to a minimum. Use dolls/puppets to show how procedures will be done. Use band-aids after giving injections. Use terms understood by the child. Give rewards. Stay with the child for procedures. Keep the routine as close to the home routine as possible. Encourage parents to stay. Provide appropriate toys and activities. Assure the child that she did not cause the illness.

SCHOOL AGE CHILDREN RESPONSE TO ILLNESS AND HOSPITALIZATION

The school age child fears being mutilated, being held down, and having to take clothes off for exams. They have a basic understanding of the severity of different illnesses and think illness is caused by something outside themselves. These children take a brave stance when they are truly scared (reaction formation). They become depressed and withdrawn when separated from family. School age children are stressed by the loss of control experienced in the hospital and by their fear of pain, injury, and death.

Nursing Interventions: Allow parents to stay. Allow the child to do things for himself. Encourage him to talk about what is happening. Let him know it's ok to be scared and cry. Be honest and use models to explain procedures. Provide appropriate play activities. Keep the routine as normal as possible, allowing the child to read, play games, and do homework. Let the child assist in his care by letting him help with charting and keeping track of procedures and medication times.

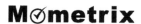

ADOLESCENT RESPONSE TO ILLNESS AND HOSPITALIZATION

Adolescents who are hospitalized experience stress due to changes in body image, loss of peer interaction, dependence on others, and fear that illness is a punishment. They use denial to deal with these feelings and tend to become angry and withdraw. Their world often revolves around peer interactions, so losing control over this part of their lives can result in many negative behaviors.

Nursing Interventions: Allow her to have as much control over her environment as possible (wear own clothes, decorate room, have telephone, have privacy). Set limits and provide appropriate activities as diversions. Allow a routine that she is comfortable with, including schoolwork, peer interactions, and self-care. Involve her in the management of her care, along with the parents.

FEELINGS AND RESPONSE OF CHILDREN TO CHRONIC ILLNESS

The most stressful aspect of having a **chronic illness** is how much the symptoms and treatment tend to embarrass children and make them feel different. Young children tend to focus on pain, while school age children are concerned with aspects of their illness that interfere with their activities. School age children are more apt to refuse treatments because they have a limited understanding of why those treatments are necessary. As the school age child matures, he takes more responsibility for the care of his illness. In adolescence, difficulties arise when the youth seeks independence and control over his environment, which is difficult to do with a chronic illness. He may either become very controlling and preoccupied with his illness or rebel against treatments, resorting to risky behaviors. Near the end of adolescence, maturity brings a more responsible outlook on his disease, when he will want to work with his illness to fit it in around his life.

IMPACT OF CHRONIC ILLNESS ON THE CHILD

Chronic illnesses/disorders may interfere with the normal development of the child. Adjustments need to be made, as much as possible, to facilitate normal development. For example, allowing a wheelchair-bound adolescent to participate in sports designed for handicapped individuals. Schools are required by law to provide a free education for all children, regardless of handicaps. This includes any modifications that need to be made to the school environment. Most children are able to be mainstreamed into regular classrooms. Dealing with the general public's reactions to a child who looks different is difficult for most kids. The nurse and caregivers can role-play with the child to practice what to say to people who stare or make comments. School nurses should educate classmates about the child's illness and assure them that she is just like them on the inside. Most school age children adjust well to a classmate's disorder and become protective of her.

ASSISTING CHILDREN IN DEALING POSITIVELY WITH ILLNESS

Children generally want to be defined by who they are on the inside, not by the illness that changes their appearance and affects their daily life. They need help in creating a sense of normalcy in their life. Treatments may need to be modified for their situation, and they should have control over how much information is told to family and peers. A thorough assessment using open-ended questions to elicit as much information as possible on what the child wants and needs is essential. All treatment plans should involve the child's input. Assessment should include the coping strategies being used, such as social support from family, peers, and school and health officials, problem solving techniques, managing emotions (using humor, relaxation, talk therapy, distraction), and spiritual help (prayer, time with church family). If coping strategies are not working, different ones can be suggested, including support groups. Negative coping strategies might include using risky behaviors, regression, withdrawal, blaming, and antisocial behaviors.

REACTIONS OF FAMILY TO CHILD'S ILLNESS OR HOSPITALIZATION

Families may not have the coping skills in place to deal with a serious illness, increasing their levels of fear and anxiety, which in turn makes it hard for the family to help the child cope with his illness. They may regress to helplessness and display many signs of stress, such as physical ailments, guilt, anger, depression, and denial.

The nurse needs to assess the family's coping skills, support system, parenting style, present stressors, cultural and religious beliefs, education and how each parent was raised by their own parents. Identify areas that need support and allow the parents to ask questions, bring in support systems from outside and participate in support groups. Provide information on the child's treatment, progress and anticipated needs. The outcomes identified should focus on strengthening the parents and enabling them to assist the child in coping.

CHALLENGES FACED BY PARENTS OF CHRONICALLY ILL CHILDREN

Families with chronically ill children experience stress, lack of social contacts, and worry about the other family member's psychosocial health. They may cope in the following ways: educating themselves, making sure they are experts at their child's care, gaining social support, including church contacts, being positive, and recognizing that there are other's whose illnesses are worse. Parents do tend to become overwhelmed at times. They may work through the grieving process several times during their child's life, especially at milestones. Families attempt to normalize their lives as much as possible, incorporating family rituals and activities that the whole family participates in. The more the family works together and remains cohesive, the better their coping strategies will work to decrease everyone's stress and the healthier the ill child will remain. The family will be strengthened by working together and networking with other caregivers.

Parents first need to work through the emotions that come with the diagnosis of a chronic illness. Then they need to learn how to operate any equipment, troubleshoot any problems, anticipate any changes in the child's health, and recognize dangerous conditions. The caregivers need support, encouragement and assistance in setting short term goals during this time. Eventually they take over as CEO of the illness and treatments. Over time the parent will gradually give control over the disease to the child. When this will happen depends on the developmental level and readiness of the child. The **nurse plays a vital role** in this transition as a teacher and coach. Time management is another challenge, especially finding time to spend with the parent's other children and spouse. Other caregiver stressors include lack of sleep, managing conflict in the family, and roles of other family members. Nurses can help by arranging respite care for short- or long-term periods.

STRESSORS FACED BY SIBLINGS OF CHRONICALLY ILL CHILDREN

Siblings are exposed to the emotions and stress of the caretakers. They usually receive less attention and take on more responsibilities earlier. They respond better when taught about the condition and the need for treatments. Efforts need to be made for the siblings to have their own activities. They also need role-playing to learn to deal with peers' reactions to the ill child, which may transfer to themselves. They would like to be involved in the ill child's care, but need their own time also. The parents and nurse need to be aware that they do worry about what will happen to their ill sibling, as well as about their own future if they should ever be expected to take on his or her care.

NURSING MANAGEMENT OF FAMILY OF CHILD WITH CHRONIC ILLNESS

Educate the family about the condition, its expected progression, and the available treatments. Teach the family to care for the child and any equipment needed. Provide education about psychosocial aspects of caring for a chronically ill child, including normal feelings of grief, denial, anger, etc. Encourage parents to talk to siblings about the illness and to take time for them. Refer them to support groups for siblings. Make sure the family meets with the healthcare team on a regular basis and that the parent's and child's wants and needs take primary consideration. Refer them to support groups. Talk with school officials about any needed modifications and continuing education when the child cannot be at school. Encourage participation in school and community activities. Teach school personnel about any equipment to be used. Arrange any home health care that is needed.

GRIEF

Grief is an emotional response to a **loss** that begins at the time a loss is anticipated and continues on an individual timetable. While there are identifiable stages or tasks, it is not an orderly and predictable process. It involves overcoming anger, disbelief, guilt, and a myriad of related emotions. The grieving individual may move back and forth between stages or experience several emotions at any given time. Each person's grief response is unique to their own coping patterns, stress levels, age, gender, belief system, and previous experiences with loss.

KUBLER-ROSS'S FIVE STAGES OF GRIEF

Kubler-Ross taught the medical community that the dying patient and family welcomes open, honest discussion of the dying process and felt that there were certain **stages** that patients and family go through. The stages may not occur in order, but may vary or some may be skipped. Stages include:

- **Denial:** The person denies the diagnosis and tries to pretend it isn't true. During this time, the person may seek a second opinion or alternative therapies. They may use denial until they are better able to emotionally cope with the reality of the disease or changes that need to be made. Patients may also wish to save family and friends from pain and worry. Both patients and family may use denial as a coping mechanism when they feel overwhelmed by the reality of the disease and threatened losses.
- **Anger:** The person is angry about the situation and may focus that rage on anyone.
- **Bargaining:** The person attempts to make deals with a higher power to secure a better outcome to their situation.
- **Depression:** The person anticipates the loss and the changes it will bring with a sense of sadness and grief.
- **Acceptance:** The person accepts the impending death and is ready to face it as it approaches. The patient may begin to withdraw from interests and family.

> **Review Video: <u>Patient Treatment and Grief</u>**
> Visit mometrix.com/academy and enter code: 648794

ANTICIPATORY GRIEF

Anticipatory grief is the mental, social, and somatic reactions of an individual as they prepare themselves for a **perceived future loss**. The individual experiences a process of intellectual, emotional, and behavioral responses in order to modify their self-concept, based on their perception of what the potential loss will mean in their life. This process often takes place ahead of the actual loss, from the time the loss is first perceived until it is resolved as a reality for the individual. This process can also blend with past loss experiences. It is associated with the individual's perception of how life will be affected by the particular diagnosis as well as the impending death. Acknowledging this anticipatory grief allows family members to begin looking toward a changed future. Suppressing this anticipatory process may inhibit relationships with the ill individual and contribute to a more difficult grieving process at a later time. However, appropriate anticipatory grieving does not take the place of grief during the actual time of death.

DISENFRANCHISED GRIEF

Disenfranchised grief occurs when the loss being experienced cannot be openly acknowledged, publicly mourned, or socially supported. Society and culture are partly responsible for an individual's response to a loss. There is a **social context** to grief; if a person incurring the loss will be putting himself or herself at risk if grief is expressed, disenfranchised grief occurs. The risk for disenfranchised grief is greatest among those whose relationship with the individual they lost was not known or regarded as significant. This is also the situation found among bereaved persons who are not recognized by society as capable of grief, such as young children, or needing to mourn, such as an ex-spouse or secret lover.

GRIEF VS. DEPRESSION

Normal grief is preoccupied with self-limiting to the loss itself. Emotional responses will vary and may include open expressions of anger. The individual may experience difficulty sleeping or vivid dreams, a lack of energy, and weight loss. Crying is evident and provides some relief of extreme emotions. The individual remains socially responsive and seeks reassurance from others.

Depression is marked by extensive periods of sadness and preoccupation often extending beyond 2 months. It is not limited to the single event. There is an absence of pleasure or anger and isolation from previous social support systems. The individual can experience extreme lethargy, weight loss, insomnia, or hypersomnia, and has no recollection of dreaming. Crying is absent or persistent and provides no relief of emotions. Professional intervention is required to relieve depression.

Loss

Loss is the blanket term used to denote the absence of a valued object, position, ability, attribute, or individual. The aspect of **loss** as it is associated with the death of an animal or person is a relatively new definition. Loss is an individualized and subjective experience depending on the **perceived attachment** between the individual and the missing aspect. This can range from little or no value of attachment to significant value. Loss also can be represented by the **withdrawal of a valued relationship** one had or would have had in the future. Depending on the unique and individual responses to the perception of loss and its significance, reactions to the loss will vary. Robinson and McKenna summarize the aspects of loss in three main attributes:

- Something has been removed.
- The item removed had value to that person.
- The response is individualized.

Mourning

Mourning is a public grief response for the death of a loved one. The various aspects of the mourning process are partially determined by **personal and cultural belief systems**. Kagawa-Singer defines mourning as "the social customs and cultural practices that follow a death." Durkheim expands this to include the following: "mourning is not a natural movement of private feelings wounded by a cruel loss; it is a duty imposed by the group." Mourning involves participation in religious and culturally appropriate customs and rituals designed to publicly acknowledge the loss. These rituals signify they are adjusting to the change in their relationships created by the loss, as well as mark the beginning of the reorganization and forward movement of their lives.

Bereavement

Bereavement is the emotional and mental state associated with having suffered a **personal loss**. It is the reactions of grief and sadness initiated by the loss of a loved one. Bereavement is a normal process of feeling deprived of something of value. The word bereave comes from the root "reave" meaning to plunder, spoil, or rob. It is recognized that the lost individual had value and a defining role in the surviving individual's life. Bereavement encompasses all the acts and emotions surrounding the feeling of loss for the individual. During this grieving period, there is an increased mortality risk. A **positive bereavement experience** means being able to recognize the significance of the loss while still recognizing the resilience and value of life.

Risk Factors Complicating Bereavement

The caregiver should assess for multiple **life crises** that take energy away from the grieving process. An important factor is the grieving individual's history with past grieving experiences. Assess for other recent, unresolved, or difficult losses that may need to be addressed before the individual can move toward resolution of the current loss. Age, mental health, substance abuse, extreme anger, anxiety, or dependence on the individual facing the end of life can add additional stressors and handicap natural coping mechanisms. Income strains, community support, outside and personal responsibilities, the absence of cultural and religious beliefs, the difficulty of the disease process, and age of the loved one lost can also present additional risk factors.

Counseling and Providing Emotional Support Regarding Grief and Loss to Children

The approach to counseling and providing emotional support regarding grief and loss to children is dependent on the age of the child. When available, children and family should be provided information about **peer support groups** (especially adolescents) and **bereavement art therapy groups** as these may be especially helpful. Healthcare professionals should use appropriate words (death, died) instead of euphemisms (passed on) when talking about the deceased and should encourage the child to ask questions. Children are often reluctant to express feelings directly, so it may be beneficial to encourage them to keep a journal about their feelings or draw pictures to express them. Parents should be encouraged to share their feelings of grief with their children rather than trying to hide their emotions and should be aware that children express grief in different ways and may regress or complain of physical ailments (stomach ache, headache) in response to grief. Children should be prepared for changes in routines or living situations, such as a stay-at-home parent having to take a job, which may occur as a result of a death or serious illness.

SIGNS OF A CHILD HAVING ISSUES MANAGING GRIEF

Management of **grief** comes in stages for children as well as for adults. Grief may be complicated for a child who does not understand the significance of the situation, such as in the case of a parent's death, or for someone who does not have the necessary support systems in place, as in the case of a child who has a grieving parent who consequently becomes unavailable. **Signs that a child is not coping well with grief** include extended periods of sadness, lack of interest in regular activities, sleep disturbances, loss of appetite, statements of wishing for death or joining a person who has died, difficulties with concentration, problems taking direction at school, poor school performance, and fear of being alone.

INTERVENTIONS FOR PATIENTS AND FAMILY EXPERIENCING LOSS AND GRIEF

Loss is painful and frightening. Loss can occur through death or loss of health, self-esteem, or relationships. Loss can also occur from threats, such as fire, flood, theft, or severe weather. The severity of the loss, preparation for it, and the maturity, stability, and coping mechanisms of the person all affect the grieving process. Multiple losses and substance abuse can complicate grief and recovery. Previous life experience and cultural and religious beliefs can help in resolution of grief. Many emotions are triggered, and if the loss is not acknowledged, the person may become depressed or develop health problems. **Interventions** for those experiencing grief and loss include:

- Teach patients to recognize symptoms, such as SOB, empty feelings in the chest or abdomen, deep sighing, lethargy, and weakness as signs of grief.
- Assist the patient and family to heal themselves by accepting the loss, recognizing the pain from it, making changes to adapt to and assimilate the loss, and moving toward new relationships and activity.
- Refer to groups or counseling for more intense support if needed.

SUPPORTING FAMILIES AND PATIENTS AS THEY RECEIVE BAD NEWS

It is often best if the patient can **receive bad news** while being **supported** by family, friends, physicians, nurses, support staff, social workers, and clergy if they so desire. However, the patient may not want family members or others to be present, and this too should be respected.

- Provide privacy and ensure that there will be no interruptions.
- Provide seating for all participants.
- Do not provide too much information at once, as the opening statement may be all that the patient can comprehend at one time.
- Allow time for reactions before providing more information.
- Wait for the patient to signal the need for more information and then provide an honest answer in layman's terms. Information may not be absorbed and may need to be repeated as the patient and family are ready for it later after the initial conference.
- Use techniques of therapeutic communication. People may need others to sit and listen and provide comforting empathy many times before having a conversation about problem solving.

SPIRITUALITY

Spirituality provides a connection of the self to a higher power and a way of finding meaning in life experiences. It provides guidance for behavior and can help to clarify one's purpose in life. It can offer hope to those who are ill or facing loss and grief and can give comfort, support, and guidance. **Spirituality** is not always connected to a religion and is highly individualized. A person may lose faith and confidence in his/her spiritual beliefs during trying times:

- Ask patients about their spiritual beliefs.
- Listen attentively and do not offer opinions about their beliefs or share your own unless invited.
- Show respect for their views and offer to obtain spiritual support by calling a spiritual leader or setting up a spiritual ritual that has meaning for them.

This support can help them to regain their beliefs and endure illness by helping them to rise above their suffering and find meaning in this experience.

PALLIATIVE AND HOSPICE CARE

Palliative care attempts to make the rest of the patient's life as comfortable as possible by treating distressing symptoms to keep them controlled. It does not attempt to cure but only to control discomfort caused by the disease. Palliative care does not require terminal illness/prognosis and can be implemented for any patient with chronic disease and suffering.

Hospice care uses palliative care as it supports the patient and family through the dying process. Hospice teams support the daily needs of the patient and family and provide needed equipment, medical expertise, and medications to control symptoms. They offer spiritual, psychological, and social support to the patient and family as needed and desired. Assistance with end-of-life planning is given to help the patient and family accomplish goals important to them. Bereavement support is also given. The team consists of the attending physician, hospice physician advisor, nurses, social worker, clergy, hospice aides, and volunteers. Hospice care is given in the home when the patient has family who are willing to assume care with the assistance of the hospice team. Hospice care also occurs in hospice facilities, hospitals, and extended care facilities. To qualify for Hospice care, the patient must be deemed terminal and given a 6-month or less life expectancy by two separate physicians. Should the patient survive 6 months in hospice, they can be extended for two 90-day periods, and then an unlimited number of 60-day periods per physician order.

THERAPEUTIC COMMUNICATION

FACILITATING COMMUNICATION

Therapeutic communication begins with respect for the patient/family and the assumption that all communication, verbal and nonverbal, has meaning. Listening must be done empathetically. The following are some techniques that facilitate communication.

Introduction:

- Make a personal introduction and use the patient's name: "Mrs. Brown, I am Susan Williams, your nurse."

Encouragement:

- Use an open-ended opening statement: "Is there anything you'd like to discuss?"
- Acknowledge comments: "Yes," and "I understand."
- Allow silence and observe nonverbal behavior rather than trying to force conversation. Ask for clarification if statements are unclear.
- Reflect statements back (use sparingly): Patient: "I hate this hospital." Nurse: "You hate this hospital?"

Empathy:

- Make observations: "You are shaking," and "You seem worried."
- Recognize feelings:
  - Patient: "I want to go home."
  - Nurse: "It must be hard to be away from your home and family."
- Provide information as honestly and completely as possible about condition, treatment, and procedures and respond to the patient's questions and concerns.

Exploration:

- Verbally express implied messages:
  - Patient: "This treatment is too much trouble."
  - Nurse: "You think the treatment isn't helping you?"
- Explore a topic but allow the patient to terminate the discussion without further probing: "I'd like to hear how you feel about that."

Orientation:

- Indicate reality:
  - Patient: "Someone is screaming."
  - Nurse: "That sound was an ambulance siren."
- Comment on distortions without directly agreeing or disagreeing:
  - Patient: "That nurse promised I didn't have to walk again."
  - Nurse: "Really? That's surprising because the doctor ordered physical therapy twice a day."

Collaboration:

- Work together to achieve better results: "Maybe if we talk about this, we can figure out a way to make the treatment easier for you."

Validation:

- Seek validation: "Do you feel better now?" or "Did the medication help you breathe better?"

AVOIDING NON-THERAPEUTIC COMMUNICATION

While using therapeutic communication is important, it is equally important to avoid interjecting **non-therapeutic communication**, which can block effective communication. *Avoid the following:*

- Meaningless clichés: "Don't worry. Everything will be fine." "Isn't it a nice day?"
- Providing advice: "You should…" or "The best thing to do is…." It's better when patients ask for advice to provide facts and encourage the patient to reach a decision.
- Inappropriate approval that prevents the patient from expressing true feeling or concerns:
  - Patient: "I shouldn't cry about this."
  - Nurse: "That's right! You're an adult!"
- Asking for an explanation of behavior that is not directly related to patient care and requires analysis and explanation of feelings: "Why are you so upset?"
- Agreeing with rather than accepting and responding to patient's statements can make it difficult for the patient to change his or her statement or opinion later: "I agree with you," or "You are right."
- Making negative judgments: "You should stop arguing with the nurses."
- Devaluing the patient's feelings: "Everyone gets upset at times."

- Disagreeing directly: "That can't be true," or "I think you are wrong."
- Defending against criticism: "The doctor is not being rude; he's just very busy today."
- Changing the subject to avoid dealing with uncomfortable topics;
  - o Patient: "I'm never going to get well."
  - o Nurse: "Your family will be here in just a few minutes."
- Making inappropriate literal responses, even as a joke, especially if the patient is at all confused or having difficulty expressing ideas:
  - o Patient: "There are bugs crawling under my skin."
  - o Nurse: "I'll get some bug spray,"
- Challenging the patient to establish reality often just increases confusion and frustration:
  - o "If you were dying, you wouldn't be able to yell and kick!"

COMMUNICATING WITH PATIENTS WITH DISABILITIES

Guidelines for communicating with individuals with disabilities:

- Do not assume that the person with disabilities also has impaired cognition.
- Always treat the person with respect and dignity.
- Use first names with the patient if asked to do so, but start out formally as with any patient.
- Offer to shake hands even when a prosthesis is present.
- Be patient if communication is impaired.
- Offer assistance, but allow the patient to tell you what is helpful; otherwise don't assist.
- When a wheelchair is used, sit down so the patient does not have to strain their neck to speak with you.
- If providing directions, consider the obstacles that may be in the way and assist the person to find an appropriate way around them.

COMMUNICATION WITH PATIENTS WITH COGNITIVE DISABILITIES

The person with cognitive disabilities may be easily distracted, so verbal communication should be attempted in a quiet area:

- Address people with dignity and respect.
- Do not try to discuss abstract ideas but stick with concrete topics.
- Keep words and sentences very simple and try rephrasing when necessary. People may have difficulty in distinguishing your spoken words and deriving the meaning from them.
- Be very patient with people's attempts to speak to you since they may have difficulty in processing thoughts and changing them into spoken words.
- Use objects around you and gestures to illustrate your words since the patient may also use pointing and gesturing when unable to find the words to communicate with you. The person may prefer written communication, although some may be unable to read.
- Use touch to convey your regard during communication, as this is recognized by the patient as reassurance of your care and concern for them.
- Give a few instructions at a time as to not overwhelm them.

COMMUNICATING WITH DEAF OR HEARING-IMPAIRED PATIENTS

Communicating with a person with deafness or hearing impairment:

- Try to communicate in a quiet environment if possible.
- Wave or touch the person to let him or her know you are trying to communicate.
- Determine the method the person uses to communicate: sign language, lip reading, hearing devices, or writing.
- Fingerspell or use some signs if able to do so.
- Address the person directly when you speak even though the person may be looking at an interpreter or your lips.
- Look at the person as the interpreter tells you what was said.
- Speak slowly so the interpreter can keep up with you.
- If the person reads lips, face the person and speak clearly and normally, using normal volume.
- If writing a communication, do not speak while writing.
- Do not be afraid to check that the person understands you, and ask questions if you do not understand the person.

COMMUNICATION WITH PEOPLE WITH LOW VISION OR BLINDNESS

Communicating with a person with low vision or blindness:

- Greet the person with low vision or blindness, identifying yourself and others present.
- Always say goodbye when you are leaving.
- Alert the person to written communications, such as warning signs or printed notices.
- Face the person and touch briefly on the arm to let the person know you are speaking to him or her if you are in a group.
- Speak at normal loudness.
- Make any directions given specific in terms of the length of walk and obstacles, such as stairs.
- Use the position of hands on a clock face to give directions (potatoes at 3 o'clock) as well as using *right* or *left*.
- Mention sounds that the person may hear in transit or on arrival at a destination.
- Do not be afraid to use the word *see*, as the person will probably use it as well.

COMMUNICATING WITH A PATIENT ON A VENTILATOR

When a patient on a ventilator is conscious, he or she may still be able to communicate by blinking, nodding, shaking the head, or pointing to a picture or word board:

- If the person is able to write, try to reposition the IV line to leave the dominant hand free to communicate.
- Discuss the need for communication with the physician and ask if a valve or an electric larynx can be used to permit speech.
- Help the patient practice lip reading of single words.
- Remember the patient's glasses or hearing aids when attempting to communicate.
- Enlist the aid of a speech therapist if there is frustration on the part of the patient and family due to communication difficulty.

COMMUNICATING WITH PERSONS WITH SPEECH PROBLEMS DUE TO A STROKE

Methods to communicate with stroke patients with speech problems:

- **Dysarthria**: Patients have problems forming the words to speak them aloud. Give them time to communicate, offer them a picture board or other means of communicating, and give encouragement to family members who are frustrated with the difficulty of trying to communicate.

- **Expressive aphasia**: The patients' efforts at speech come out garbled when they try to say sentences, but single words may be clear. Encourage the patients to try to write and to practice the sounds of the alphabet. Resist the urge to finish sentences for the patients.
- **Receptive aphasia**: The patients have a problem comprehending the speech they hear. Communicate in simple terms and speak slowly. Test comprehension of the written word as an alternative method of communication.
- **Global aphasia**: The patient has both receptive and expressive aphasia. Use simple, clear, slow speech augmented by pictures and gestures.

COMMUNICATION PROBLEMS OF PATIENTS WITH PARKINSON'S DISEASE

Parkinson's disease causes problems with speaking in the majority (75-90%) of patients. The reason for this is not clear but may relate to increasing rigidity and changes in movement. Speech is often very low-pitched or hoarse, given in a monotone and with a soft voice. Speech production may decrease because of the effort required to speak. **Speech therapy** can develop exercises for the patient that can assist them in remembering to speak slowly and carefully, as patients are not always aware that their **communication** is impaired:

- Allow time for the patient to communicate, asking for repetition if you do not understand the message.
- Help family by teaching ways to facilitate communication with the patient and encouraging them to assist the patient to do the exercises provided by the therapist.
- If speech volume is very low, suggest amplification devices that can be obtained through speech therapy.

COMMUNICATION WITH PATIENTS WITH PSYCHIATRIC PROBLEMS

Persons with psychiatric disorders appreciate being addressed with respect, dignity, and honesty:

- Speak simply and clearly, repeating as necessary.
- Encourage patients to discuss their concerns regarding treatment and medications to improve compliance.
- Use good eye contact and be attentive to your body language messages.
- Be alert, but unless the person is known to be violent, try to relax and listen to them.
- Don't try to avoid words or phrases pertaining to psychiatric problems, but if you do say something inappropriate, apologize honestly to the patient.
- Offer patients outlets for their thoughts and feelings.
- Learn more about their disorder and ways to use therapeutic communication to help them with their problem, such as re-orienting them as needed.

CULTURAL COMPETENCE

Different cultures view health and illness from very different perspectives, and patients often come from a mix of many cultures, so the nurse must be not only accepting of cultural differences but must be sensitive and aware. There are a number of characteristics that are important for a nurse to have **cultural competence**:

- **Appreciating diversity**: This must be grounded in information about other cultures and understanding of their value systems.
- **Assessing own cultural perspectives**: Self-awareness is essential to understanding potential biases.
- **Understanding intercultural dynamics**: This must include understanding ways in which cultures cooperate, differ, communicate, and reach understanding.
- **Recognizing institutional culture**: Each institutional unit (hospital, clinic, office) has an inherent set of values that may be unwritten but is accepted by the staff.
- **Adapting patient service to diversity**: This is the culmination of cultural competence as it is the point of contact between cultures.

CULTURAL CHARACTERISTICS
HISPANIC PATIENTS

Many areas of the country have large populations of Hispanics and Hispanic Americans. As always, it's important to recognize that cultural generalizations don't always apply to individuals. Recent immigrants, especially, have cultural needs that the nurse must understand:

- Many Hispanics are Catholic and may like the nurse to make arrangements for a priest to visit.
- Large extended families may come to visit to support the patient and family, so patients should receive clear explanations about how many visitors are allowed, but some flexibility may be required.
- Language barriers may exist as some may have limited or no English skills, so translation services should be available around the clock.
- Hispanic culture encourages outward expressions of emotions, so family may react strongly to news about a patient's condition, and people who are ill may expect some degree of pampering, so extra attention to the patient/family members may alleviate some of their anxiety.

Caring for Hispanic and Hispanic American patients requires understanding of cultural differences:

- Some immigrant Hispanics have very little formal education, so medical information may seem very complex and confusing, and they may not understand the implications or need for follow-up care.
- Hispanic culture perceives time with more flexibility than American culture, so if parents need to be present at a particular time, the nurse should specify the exact time (1:30 PM) and explain the reason rather than saying something more vague, such as "after lunch."
- People may appear to be unassertive or unable to make decisions when they are simply showing respect to the nurse by being deferent.
- In traditional families, the males make decisions, so a woman waits for the father or other males in the family to make decisions about treatment or care.
- Families may choose to use folk medicines instead of Western medical care or may combine the two.
- Children and young women are often sheltered and are taught to be respectful to adults, so they may not express their needs openly.

MIDDLE EASTERN PATIENTS

There are considerable cultural differences among Middle Easterners, but religious beliefs about the segregation of males and females are common. It's important to remember that segregating the female is meant to protect her virtue. Female nurses have low status in many countries because they violate this segregation by touching male bodies, so parents may not trust or show respect for the nurse who is caring for their family member. Additionally, male patients may not want to be cared for by female nurses or doctors, and families may be very upset at a female being cared for by a male nurse or physician. When possible, these cultural traditions should be accommodated:

- In Middle Eastern countries, males make decisions, so issues for discussion or decision should be directed to males, such as the father or spouse, and males may be direct in stating what they want, sometimes appearing demanding.
- If a male nurse must care for a female patient, then the family should be advised that *personal care* (such as bathing) will be done by a female while the medical treatments will be done by the male nurse.

Caring for Middle Eastern patients requires understanding of cultural differences:

- Families may practice strict dietary restrictions, such as avoiding pork and requiring that animals be killed in a ritual manner, so vegetarian or kosher meals may be required.
- People may have language difficulties requiring a translator, and same-sex translators should be used if at all possible.

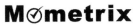

- Families may be accompanied by large extended families that want to be kept informed and whom patients consult before decisions are made.
- Most medical care is provided by female relatives, so educating the family about patient care should be directed at females (with female translators if necessary).
- Outward expressions of grief are considered as showing respect for the dead.
- Middle Eastern families often offer gifts to caregivers. Small gifts (candy) that can be shared should be accepted graciously, but for other gifts, the families should be advised graciously that accepting gifts is against hospital policy.
- Middle Easterners often require less personal space and may stand very close.

ASIAN PATIENTS

There are considerable differences among different Asian populations, so cultural generalizations may not apply to all, but nurses caring for Asian patients should be aware of common cultural attitudes and behaviors:

- Nurses and doctors are viewed with respect, so traditional Asian families may expect the nurse to remain authoritative and to give directions and may not question, so the nurse should ensure that they understand by having them review material or give demonstrations and should provide explanations clearly, anticipating questions that the family might have but may not articulate.
- Disagreeing is considered impolite. "Yes" may only mean that the person is heard, not that they agree with the person. When asked if they understand, they may indicate that they do even when they clearly do not so as not to offend the nurse.
- Asians may avoid eye contact as an indication of respect. This is especially true of children in relation to adults and of younger adults in relation to elders.

Caring for Asian patients requires understanding of cultural differences:

- Patients/families may not show outward expressions of feelings/grief, sometimes appearing passive. They also avoid public displays of affection. This does not mean that they don't feel, just that they don't show their feelings.
- Families often hide illness and disabilities from others and may feel ashamed about illness.
- Terminal illness is often hidden from the patient, so families may not want patients to know they are dying or seriously ill.
- Families may use cupping, pinching, or applying pressure to injured areas, and this can leave bruises that may appear as abuse, so when bruises are found, the family should be questioned about alternative therapy before assumptions are made.
- Patients may be treated with traditional herbs.
- Families may need translators because of poor or no English skills.
- In traditional Asian families, males are authoritative and make the decisions.

RELIGIOUS OBJECTIONS TO TREATMENT

JEHOVAH'S WITNESSES

Jehovah's Witnesses have traditionally shunned transfusions and blood products as part of their religious beliefs. In 2004, the *Watchtower*, a Jehovah's Witness publication, presented a guide for members. When medical care indicates the need for blood transfusion or blood products and the patient and/or family members are practicing Jehovah's Witnesses, this may present a conflict. It's important to approach the patient/family with full information and reasons for the transfusion or blood components without being judgmental, allowing them to express their feelings. In fact, studies show that while adults often refuse transfusions for themselves, they frequently allow their children to receive blood products, so one should never assume that an individual would refuse blood products based on the religion alone. Jehovah's Witnesses can receive fractionated blood cells, thus allowing hemoglobin-based blood substitutes. The following guidelines are provided to church members:

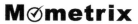

Basic **blood standards for Jehovah's Witnesses**:

- **Not acceptable**: Whole blood: red cells, white cells, platelets, plasma.
- **Acceptable**: Fractions from red cells, white cells, platelets, and plasma.

CHRISTIAN SCIENTISTS

Christian Science, a religion developed by Mary Baker Eddy in 1879, promotes the belief that sickness is most effectively treated through prayer alone. While Christian Scientists do not avoid all medical interventions, their beliefs are conservative regarding medical treatment. Most notably, Christian Scientists, for the most part, do not believe in vaccinations and may only agree to such if required by law, as they do acknowledge the importance of community health. They have widely appreciated the use of exemptions from mandatory vaccines, but as these exemptions have become more limited, religious leaders have given their members the right to decide upon vaccinations.

IMPACT OF CULTURE AND RELIGION ON DIETARY PREFERENCES

When performing a dietary assessment, the nurse should remember that culture and religion might dictate which foods and spices are used. The manner in which food is prepared, cooked, and served may also be specified. The utensils used at the meal as well as the persons who may eat together may be important. Mealtimes and required fasts should be determined. Holidays may be accompanied by particular foods. Alcohol (including extracts made with alcohol) and caffeine may be prohibited. The culture may also consider obesity a sign of affluence and success. The nurse should evaluate the foods that are eaten in light of the patient's medical condition. The patient may not wish to eat the usual hospital fare and may need to have a special diet prepared or food brought from home. The nurse can guide the patient and family to foods that are acceptable and within the patient's requirements for health.

Professional Role and Responsibilities

Standards of Practice

COLLEGIALITY

Collegiality is a term used to describe the relationship between people who work together. Within nursing, collegiality is a standard of practice to promote the profession of nursing, improve work situations, and educate peers about care issues. Examples within nursing practice are as follows: promoting some nurses to clinical educators or resource personnel; establishing a mentoring program; providing preceptors to nurses who are new to staff; supporting membership in professional organizations and work groups; and providing professional workshops or seminars that support team-building, leadership, or direction.

PERSONAL RESPONSIBILITIES NECESSARY TO SUPPORT COMPETENT CAREGIVING

Nurses who care for themselves are better able to handle the pressures that come with caring for others. While professional accountability and conduct are important to give adequate patient care, **personal responsibility** is necessary to support nurses outside of work and to provide balance between work and personal life. Personal responsibilities of nurses include caring for themselves physically and mentally by practicing healthy habits and doing restful activities while not at work. Nurses can also examine their own personal beliefs and practices to provide a solid foundation to guide them through decisions they must make while at work.

PEER REVIEW PROCESS

The Joint Commission focuses on the process of peer review in both design and function. Peer review should be a review by a like nurse with similar training, experience, and expertise. In some cases, the pool of nurses within one organization may be too small, so external peer reviews may be required. Peer review is often triggered by root cause analysis that indicates the need to focus on an individual, sometimes related to utilization review:

- The **design** should include definitions of peer, methods in which peer review panels are selected, triggering events, and timeframes. It should also outline the participation of the person being reviewed.
- The **function** must be consistently applied to all individuals, balanced and fair, adherent to timelines, ongoing, and valuable to the organization. Decisions should be based on solid reason and literature review and must be defensible.

ROLES OF LEADERS
MENTOR

The experienced pediatric nurse is in an ideal position to serve as a mentor, both informally and formally. There are a number of elements that enhance mentoring:

- **Nurturing**: Being supportive and interested in furthering the skills and education of the staff.
- **Providing clinical expertise**: Guiding the staff by demonstrating a personal commitment to excellence in provision of care.
- **Motivating others**: Encouraging others and supporting them throughout their careers.
- **Providing an example**: Teaching others by being a good example.
- **Listening**: Being non-judgmental in discussions with others and listening to determine different perspectives and needs.

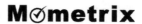

- **Providing feedback**: Being honest in evaluation and assisting others to improve care, providing feedback about how their practices affect patient outcomes.
- **Role modeling**: Providing assistance to others in gaining certification and understanding the role of the pediatric nurse.

PRECEPTOR

The nurse is often in the position of having many roles in clinical practice, including educating others and serving as a preceptor for graduate students who are studying to enter the field. While mentoring may entail a long-term relationship, preceptoring is usually a time-limited arrangement related to a term of study, such as a semester, orientation period, or a clinical rotation. The pediatric nurse must balance responsibilities and ensure that he or she is able to provide adequate clinical supervision and guidance to the student on a daily basis. This may require coordinating schedules and planning carefully to ensure all responsibilities can be met. The nurse preceptor helps the student to understand his or her impact on the spheres of influence (patient/client, nurse and nurse practice, and organization/system) by including the student in all nursing activities. The preceptor may engage in shared care as well as direct supervision in order to improve the student's skills.

RESOURCE USE

Resource use is a standard of care for nurses, involving the use of resources in a cost-effective manner. Resources can be equipment used for patient treatments or the analysis of budget data to determine where reductions can be made. Examples of resource use as part of nursing standards of care include determining the safest, most cost-effective option when presented with a choice of treatment plans; using health care assistive personnel, such as nursing assistants or medication aides and delegating tasks to them; and assisting families with finding the resources necessary to provide adequate, cost-effective care for their child.

SPECIFIC EVIDENCE-BASED INTERVENTIONS IN PEDIATRICS

KANGAROO CARE

Kangaroo care involves holding an infant with skin-to-skin contact to promote warmth and bonding between a mother and child. Ideally, kangaroo care occurs naturally, with a mother carrying her infant in this position as often as possible. However, in the neonatal intensive care unit, many infants are connected to tubing and wires and may be too medically unstable to be held in this manner. Instead, parents may perform kangaroo care during times when the infant is hemodynamically stable and for short intervals to promote bonding and breastfeeding. In this method, the infant is undressed down to a diaper and held against the mother or father's bare chest.

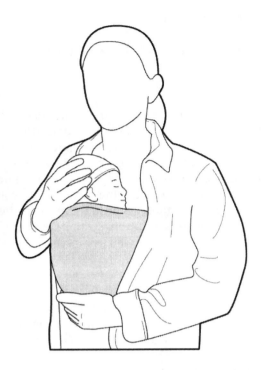

SUCTIONING A HIGH-RISK NEWBORN AND A CHILD WITH A TRACHEOSTOMY

Suctioning should not be considered a routine procedure. It is only performed when necessary, as determined by lung sounds, oximeter reading, or restlessness. Suctioning can cause bradycardia, bronchospasm, hypoxia, and increased ICP (may lead to IVH). Always use aseptic technique. The suction catheter is premeasured so that it is not inserted past the end of the endotracheal tube. The catheter should be inserted quickly and withdrawn using intermittent suction; a suctioning episode should last no more than 5 seconds. A pulse oximeter should be used before, during, and after suctioning to ascertain oxygen status, and the results should be documented. An in-line suction device can be used for very ill infants. This will ensure an adequate oxygen supply during suctioning and is more aseptic. The infant should be placed supine with the head in the sniffing position or on the side with the head in alignment. When suctioning a tracheostomy, make sure the catheter's diameter is half that of the tracheostomy tube.

CHLORHEXIDINE (CHG) BATHS AND ORAL SUCROSE

Chlorhexidine (CHG) baths and oral sucrose are evidence-based interventions on the pediatric unit:

- **Chlorhexidine (CHG) baths**: Chlorhexidine gluconate has been used to prevent hospital acquired infections across hospital units for decades. From CHG baths, to CHG soaked dressings and skin preparation solutions, this method of infection prevention has proven effective, particularly on units with patients who are ventilated or have central lines. For that reason, many pediatric inpatient units implement daily CHG baths as part of the HAI prevention protocol.
- **Oral sucrose**: Oral sucrose, a simple sugar solution, is used as a non-pharmacologic pain reliever for infants less than 28 days old during short procedures that may induce pain or distress. The sucrose is administered orally to the infant's tongue, and its analgesic effect lasts for about five to eight minutes. This is most commonly used prior to the following procedures: heel pricks, circumcision, IV-line insertion, injections, eye examination, lumbar puncture, amongst other brief pain-inducing procedures.

ADHD INTERVENTIONS

Because of research studies, interventions, surveys, and collaboration with parents and teachers, health care workers have access to evidence-based practice information about how to help children diagnosed with **attention-deficit/hyperactivity disorder (ADHD)**. Continued work with children with this condition and follow-up with practice guidelines can be successful because evidence through previous outcomes is available. Nurses can use evidence-based practices to treat as well as educate parents about their child with ADHD by performing interventions to help with decreased impulse control, short attention spans, hyperactivity, decreased concentration, and memory problems. These interventions can be implemented in any situation in which the child is having difficulty, such as at home, in the classroom, with peers, or in other group settings.

PREVENTION OF HOSPITAL-ACQUIRED INFECTIONS

Hospital-acquired infections can occur in several ways among children in health care facilities, such as after surgery or invasive procedures and after exposure to infectious organisms from other patients in the hospital or from central lines or endotracheal tubes. Nurses can perform research to determine the effectiveness of interventions aimed at preventing infections. Because of the large number of studies related to infection control, many evidence-based practices are well recognized and accepted in the health care environment. Some interventions that may be used to prevent hospital-based infections include regular and appropriate hand washing between patients, use of waterless hand sanitizer, sterile technique when performing invasive procedures, proper cleaning and disinfection of reusable equipment, reducing the number of breaks in central lines, and using isolation precautions for infectious patients.

CASES OF CHILD ABUSE OR NEGLECT

Evidence-based practices are in use for health care workers and social service workers who treat **victims of child abuse**. Evidence-based practices can be used to find case studies about treatment protocols, long-term effects of child abuse, and policies related to reporting incidents. Evidence-based practices can be used to change practices for reporting cases and prosecuting offenders; to train practitioners to recognize child abuse and methods by which to collect evidence; and to educate families about domestic violence, anger management, respite opportunities, and the negative outcomes of child abuse.

POSITIVE BEHAVIOR ANALYSIS

Positive behavior analysis is a treatment method that involves using certain types of techniques to affirm positive behaviors with the hope of the child repeating the positive behavior. For example, positive behavior analysis might involve giving a child a sticker when he makes a positive choice. The child may be more likely to make the same choice in a future situation if he or she remembers a positive outcome from the last time. Applied behavioral analysis, when used with children with autism, may teach them social skills and more positive interactions. This is done by setting up a situation that will teach the children something new and then help them to succeed at learning so that they associate positive outcomes with change.

Patient and Nurse Safety

CONTINUOUS QUALITY IMPROVEMENT

Continuous quality improvement is a multidisciplinary management philosophy that can be applied to all aspects of an organization, whether related to such varied areas as the cardiac unit, purchasing, or human resources. The skills used for epidemiologic research (data collection, analysis, outcomes, action plans) are all applicable to the analysis of multiple types of events, because they are based on solid scientific methods. Multi-disciplinary planning can bring valuable insights from various perspectives, and strategies used in one context can often be applied to another. All staff, from housekeeping to supervising, must be alert to not only problems but also opportunities for improvement. Increasingly, departments must be concerned with cost-effectiveness as the costs of medical care continue to rise, so the quality professional in the cardiovascular unit is not in an isolated position in an institution but is just one part of the whole, facing similar concerns as those in other disciplines. Disciplines are often interrelated in their functions.

JURAN'S QUALITY IMPROVEMENT PROCESS

Joseph Juran's quality improvement process (QIP) is a 4-step method of change (focusing on quality control) which is based on a trilogy of concepts that includes quality planning, control, and improvement. The steps to the QIP process include the following:

1. **Defining** the project and organizing includes listing and prioritizing problems and identifying a team.
2. **Diagnosing** includes analyzing problems and then formulating theories related to cause by root cause analysis and test theories.
3. **Remediating** includes considering various alternative solutions and then designing and implementing specific solutions and controls while addressing institutional resistance to change. As causes of problems are identified and remediation instituted to remove the problems, the processes should improve.
4. **Holding** involves evaluating performance and monitoring the control system in order to maintain gains.

FOCUS PERFORMANCE IMPROVEMENT MODEL

Find, organize, clarify, uncover, start (FOCUS) is a performance improvement model used to facilitate change:

- **Find**: Identifying a problem by looking at the organization and attempting to determine what isn't working well or what is wrong.
- **Organize**: Identifying those people who have an understanding of the problem or process and creating a team to work on improving performance.
- **Clarify**: Determining what is involved in solving the problem by utilizing brainstorming techniques, such as the Ishikawa diagram.
- **Uncover**: Analyzing the situation to determine the reason the problem has arisen or that a process is unsuccessful.
- **Start**: Determining where to begin in the change process.

FOCUS, by itself, is an incomplete process and is primarily used as a means to identify a problem rather than a means to find the solution. FOCUS is usually combined with PDCA (FOCUS-PDCA), so it becomes a 9-step process; however, beginning with FOCUS helps to narrow the focus, resulting in better outcomes.

NURSE'S INVOLVEMENT IN QUALITY IMPROVEMENT

The following are ways in which nurses can be involved in quality improvement in their facility:

- **Identify situations** in the nursing unit that require improvement and might benefit patient outcomes (cost containment, incident reporting, etc.) if changed.
- **Identify potential items** that can be measured to be able to test the problem or to be able to monitor patient outcomes.
- **Collect data** on those measurements and determine current patient outcomes.
- **Analyze the data** and identify procedures, methods, etc., that can be utilized to potentially make positive changes in patient outcomes, doing research if necessary.
- **Make recommendations for changes** to be implemented to determine the effect on patient outcomes.
- **Implement recommendations** after approval from administrative personnel.
- **Collect data** using the same measurements and determine if the changes improved patient outcomes or not.

RISK MANAGEMENT

Risk management attempts to prevent harm and legal liability by being proactive and by identifying a patient's **risk factors**. The patient is educated about these factors and ways that they can modify their behavior to decrease their risk. Treatments and interventions must be considered in terms of risk to the patient, and the patient must always know these risks in order to make healthcare decisions. Much can be done to avoid mistakes that put patients at risk. Patients should note medications and other aspects of their care so that they can help prevent mistakes. They should feel free to question care and to have their concerns heard and addressed. When mistakes are made, the actions taken to remedy the situation are very important. The physician should be made aware of the error immediately, and the patient notified according to hospital policy. Errors must be evaluated to determine how the process failed. Honesty and caring can help mitigate many errors.

NURSING MALPRACTICE, NEGLIGENCE, UNINTENTIONAL TORTS, AND INTENTIONAL TORTS

- **Malpractice** is unethical or improper actions or lack of proper action by the nurse that may or may not be related to a lack of skills that nurses should possess.
- **Negligence** is the failure to act as any other diligent nurse would have acted in the same situation.
- Negligence can lead to an **unintentional tort**. In this case, the patient must prove that the nurse had a duty to act, a duty proven via standards of care, and that the nurse failed in this duty and harm occurred to the patient as a result of this failure.
- **Intentional torts** differ in that the duty is assumed and the nurse breached this duty via assault and battery, invasion of privacy, slander, or false imprisonment of the patient.

> **Review Video: Medical Negligence**
> Visit mometrix.com/academy and enter code: 928405

PROTOCOL FOR NEEDLESTICK INJURY AND POSTEXPOSURE PROPHYLAXIS

If the healthcare provider experiences a **needlestick injury**, the individual's initial response should be to irrigate the wound with soap and water. As soon as possible, the incident must be reported to a supervisor and steps taken according to established protocol. This may include testing and/or prophylaxis, depending on the patient's health history. In some cases, the patient may also be tested for communicable diseases, such as HIV, in order to determine the risk to the healthcare provider. PEP (post-exposure prophylaxis) is available for exposure to HIV (human immunodeficiency virus) and hepatitis B virus (hepatis B immune globulin). However, no PEP is available for HCV (hepatitis C virus) although the CDC does provide a plan for management. PEP should be initiated within 72 hours of exposure. All testing and treatments associated with the needlestick injury must be provided free of cost at a hospital or medical facility.

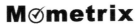

Legal and Ethical Issues

REGULATION OF NURSING BY STATES' NURSE PRACTICE ACT

Each state's **nurse practice act** seeks to regulate nursing within the state. It specifies the amount and type of education required to become an RN or LPN/LVN. It defines the nurse's role and responsibilities in healthcare settings. It lists actions that the nurse may take and defines advanced practice education, experience, responsibilities, and limitations. It gives nurses the authorization to perform as required. It also regulates delegation and supervision responsibilities of the nurse. Nurse practice acts are administrated by the state board of nursing, which is responsible for issuing and renewing nurse licenses as well as discipline and censure of nurses. Most state boards of nursing now have a website that provides state-specific information about licensure and nursing rights and responsibilities.

NURSE'S ACCOUNTABILITY FOR NURSING CARE

Nurses are part of an interdisciplinary team responsible for patient outcomes. Nurses have the responsibility for the outcomes of nursing care as a professional group. This responsibility is outlined in each state's nurse practice act, the American Nurses Association (ANA) practice guidelines, and the nurse's job description. Tools, such as the nursing care plan that includes standardized nursing diagnoses, interventions, and expected outcomes, enable the nurse to fulfill this responsibility. Empowerment to act as the patient advocate allows the nurse to point out factors in the patient's individual situation that can be addressed to further improve outcome. Critical thinking during decision-making and detailed documentation are also important. The nurse is held accountable for delegation as well as supervising care by others and evaluation of the outcomes of that care as well. The nurse has personal **accountability** in terms of ethical and moral conduct. Since clinical knowledge is crucial to critical thinking, the nurse must strive to increase knowledge continuously through professional development throughout his or her career.

ADVANCE DIRECTIVES

In accordance to Federal and state laws, individuals have the right to self-determination in health care, including the right to make decisions about end of life care through **advance directives** such as living wills and the right to assign a surrogate person to make decisions through a durable power of attorney. Patients should routinely be questioned about an advanced directive as they may present at a healthcare provider without the document. Patients who have indicated that they desire a do-not-resuscitate (DNR) order should not receive resuscitative treatments for terminal illness or conditions in which meaningful recovery cannot occur. Patients and families of those with terminal illnesses should be questioned as to whether the patients are Hospice patients. For those with DNR requests or those withdrawing life support, staff should provide the patient palliative rather than curative measures, such as pain control and/or oxygen, and emotional support to the patient and family. Religious traditions and beliefs about death should be treated with respect.

HIPAA

The Health Insurance Portability and Accountability Act (HIPAA) and state laws govern **who may receive healthcare information** about a person, how permission is to be obtained, how the information may be shared, and patients' rights concerning personal information. HIPAA strives to protect the **privacy** of an individual's healthcare information. Facilities must prevent this information from being accessed by unauthorized personnel. Healthcare information is required to be protected on the **administrative**, **physical**, and **technical** levels. The patient must sign a release form to allow any sharing of patient information. There are stiff penalties for violation of these laws, ranging from $100 for an unintentional violation to $50,000 for a willful violation. Facilities that violate HIPAA may also be subject to corrective actions. Penalties are governed by the Department of Health and Human Services' Office for Civil Right and the state attorneys general.

APPLICATION OF HIPAA TO PRACTICE

As an integral member of the health care team, the nurse must always be aware of HIPAA regulations and apply this knowledge to practice. The nurse is responsible for the following efforts to protect and maintain patient privacy:

- The nurse must read and follow facility policies regarding the transfer of patient data.
- Communication between health care personnel about a patient should always be in a private place so that this information is not overheard by those who do not have the right to share the information.
- Access to charts must be restricted to only those health care team members involved in that patient's care.
- Patient care information for unlicensed workers cannot be posted at the bedside, but must be on a care plan or the patient chart in a protected area.
- The nurse must not give information casually to anyone (e.g., visitors or family members) unless it is confirmed that they have the right to have that information.
- Family members must not be relied upon to interpret for the patient; an interpreter must be obtained to protect patient privacy.
- Computers with patient information must have passwords and safeguards to prevent unauthorized access of patient information.
- The nurse should not leave voicemail messages containing protected healthcare information for a patient but should instead ask the patient to call back.

> **Review Video: What is HIPAA?**
> Visit mometrix.com/academy and enter code: 412009

OSHA

The **Occupational Safety and Health Act (OSHA)** seeks to keep workers safe and healthy while on the job. OSHA mandates that employers maintain a safe environment, workers are made fully aware of any hazards, and that access to personal protective gear is made available to workers who come into contact with hazardous materials. By following these regulations, an employer keeps injury and illness of workers to an absolute minimum. This fosters productivity, since workers are not absent due to illness or injury, employee health costs are contained, and the turnover rate is decreased, saving money spent on hiring and training new employees. OSHA is concerned about healthcare employee exposure to radiation, as well as chemical and biological agents, when caring for patients. Information is available to help hospitals and other facilities write plans that comply with best practices to deal with this and other threats to employees. Cleaning procedures, decontamination, and hazardous waste disposal are all covered by OSHA and apply to everyday hospital operation as well as disaster situations.

> **Review Video: What is OSHA (Occupational Safety and Health Administration)**
> Visit mometrix.com/academy and enter code: 913559

CMS

The **Centers for Medicare and Medicaid (CMS)**, part of the US Department of Health and Human Service department, see to it that healthcare regulations are observed by healthcare facilities that receive federal reimbursement. They reimburse facilities for care given to Medicare, Medicaid, and the state Children's Health Insurance Program (CHIP) recipients. They also monitor adherence to HIPAA regulations concerning healthcare information portability and confidentiality. CMS examines documentation of patient care when deciding to reimburse for care given. CMS has regulations for all types of medical facilities, and these regulations have profoundly impacted nursing practice because nurses must ensure that they comply with regulations related to the quality of patient care and concerns regarding cost-containment. Each facility should provide guidelines to assist nursing staff in meeting the specific documentation requirements of CMS.

AHRQ

The **Agency for Healthcare Research and Quality (AHRQ)** is part of the US Department of Health and Human Services. This agency is concerned about health care and primarily promotes scientific research into the safety, effectiveness, and quality of healthcare. It encourages evidence-based healthcare that produces the best possible outcome while containing healthcare costs. It makes contracts with institutions to review any published evidence on healthcare in order to produce reports used by other organizations to write guidelines. The agency operates the National Guideline Clearinghouse, which is available online. It is a repository of evidence-based guidelines that address various health conditions and diseases. These guidelines are written by many different health-related professional organizations and are used by primary healthcare providers, nurses, and healthcare facilities to guide patient treatment and care.

PATIENT RIGHTS AND RESPONSIBILITIES

Empowering patients and families to act as their own advocates requires that they have a clear understanding of their **rights and responsibilities.** These should be given (in print form) and/or presented (audio/video) to patients and families on admission or as soon as possible:

- **Rights** include competent, non-discriminatory medical care that respects privacy and allows participation in decisions about care and the right to refuse care. They should have clear understandable explanations of treatments, options, and conditions, including outcomes. They should be apprised of transfers, changes in care plan, and advance directives. They should have access to medical records and billing information.
- **Responsibilities** include providing honest and thorough information about health issues and medical history. They should ask for clarification if they don't understand information that is provided to them, and they should follow the plan of care that is outlined or explain why that is not possible. They should treat staff and other patients with respect.

> **Review Video: Patient Advocacy**
> Visit mometrix.com/academy and enter code: 202160

INFORMED CONSENT

The patient or their legal guardian must provide informed consent for all treatment the patient receives. This includes a thorough explanation of all procedures and treatment and associated risks. Patients/guardians should be apprised of all options and allowed to have input on the decision-making process. They should be apprised of all reasonable risks and any complications that might be life threatening or increase morbidity. The American Medical Association has established **guidelines for obtaining informed consent:**

- Explanation of the diagnosis
- Nature and reason for the treatment or procedure
- Risks and benefits of the treatment or procedure
- Alternative options (regardless of cost or insurance coverage)
- Risks and benefits of alternative options, including no treatment

Obtaining informed consent is a requirement in all states; however, a patient may waive their right to informed consent. If this is the case, the nurse should document the patient's waiving of this right and proceed with the procedure. Informed consent is not necessary for procedures performed to save life or limb in which the patient or guardian is unable to consent.

CONFIDENTIALITY

Confidentiality is the obligation that is present in a professional-patient relationship. Nurses are under an obligation to protect the information they possess concerning the patient and family. Care should be taken to safeguard that information and provide the privacy that the family deserves. This is accomplished through the use of required passwords when family call for information about the patient and through the limitation of who is allowed to visit. There may be times when confidentiality must be broken to save the life of a patient, but those circumstances are rare. The nurse must make all efforts to safeguard patient records and identification. Computerized record keeping should be done in such a way that the screen is not visible to others, and paper records must be secured.

ETHICAL PRINCIPLES

Autonomy is the ethical principle that the individual has the right to make decisions about his or her own care. In the case of children or patients with dementia who cannot make autonomous decisions, parents or family members may serve as the legal decision maker. The nurse must keep the patient and/or family fully informed so that they can exercise their autonomy in informed decision-making.

Justice is the ethical principle that relates to the distribution of the limited resources of healthcare benefits to the members of society. These resources must be distributed fairly. This issue may arise if there is only one bed left and two sick patients. Justice comes into play in deciding which patient should stay and which should be transported or otherwise cared for. The decision should be made according to what is best or most just for the patients and not colored by personal bias.

Beneficence is an ethical principle that involves performing actions that are for the purpose of benefitting another person. In the care of a patient, any procedure or treatment should be done with the ultimate goal of benefitting the patient, and any actions that are not beneficial should be reconsidered. As conditions change, procedures need to be continually reevaluated to determine if they are still of benefit.

Nonmaleficence is an ethical principle that means healthcare workers should provide care in a manner that does not cause direct intentional harm to the patient:

- The actual act must be good or morally neutral.
- The intent must be only for a good effect.
- A bad effect cannot serve as the means to get to a good effect.
- A good effect must have more benefit than a bad effect has harm.

NURSING CODE OF ETHICS

There is more interest in the **ethics** involved in healthcare due to technological advances that have made the prolongation of life, organ transplants, prenatal manipulation, and saving of premature infants possible, sometimes with poor outcomes. Couple these with healthcare's limited resources, and **ethical dilemmas** abound. Ethics is the study of **morality** as the value that controls actions. The American Nurses Association Code of Ethics contains nine statements defining **principles** the nurse can use when faced with moral and ethical problems. Nurses must be knowledgeable about the many ethical issues in healthcare and about the field of ethics in general. The nurse must help a patient to reveal their values and morals to the health care team so that the patient, family, and team can resolve moral issues pertaining to the patient's care. As part of the healthcare team, the nurse has a right to express personal values and moral concerns about medical issues.

ETHICAL ASSESSMENT

While the terms *ethics* and *morals* are sometimes used interchangeably, ethics is a study of morals and encompasses concepts of right and wrong. When making **ethical assessments,** one must consider not only what people should do but also what they actually do, as these two things are sometimes at odds. Ethical issues can be difficult to assess because of personal bias, which is one of the reasons that sharing concerns with other internal sources and reaching consensus is so valuable. Issues of concern might include options for care, refusal of care, rights to privacy, adequate relief of suffering, and the right to self-determination. Internal sources might include the ethics committee, whose role is to make decisions regarding ethical issues. Risk management can provide guidance related to personal and institutional liability. External agencies might include government agencies, such as the public health department.

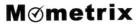

ETHICAL ANALYSIS OF A SITUATION

Assessment of the situation is done to reveal the ethical, legal, and professional **conflicts** that are present. Those who are involved are identified, including the patient, family, and healthcare personnel. The decision maker is determined if it is not the patient. Information about the situation is collected to determine medical facts about the disease and condition of the patient, options for treatment, and nursing diagnoses. Any pertinent legal information is included. The patient and family's cultural, religious, and moral values are determined. Possible courses of action are listed and compared in terms of outcomes for the patient using the utilitarian or deontological theory of ethics. Professional codes of ethics are also applied. A decision is made and evaluated as to whether it is the most morally correct action. Ethical arguments for and against the decision are given and responded to by the decision maker.

PROFESSIONAL BOUNDARIES

GIFTS

Over time, patients may develop a bond with nurses they trust and may feel grateful to the nurse for the care provided and want to express thanks, but the nurse must make sure to maintain professional boundaries. Patients often offer **gifts** to nurses to show their appreciation, but some adults, especially those who are weak and ill or have cognitive impairment, may be taken advantage of easily. Patients may offer valuables and may sometimes be easily manipulated into giving large sums of money. Small tokens of appreciation that can be shared with other staff, such as a box of chocolates, are usually acceptable (depending upon the policy of the institution), but almost any other gifts (jewelry, money, clothes) should be declined: "I'm sorry, that's so kind of you, but nurses are not allowed to accept gifts from patients." Declining may relieve the patient of the feeling of obligation.

SEXUAL RELATIONS

When the boundary between the role of the professional nurse and the vulnerability of the patient is breached, a boundary violation occurs. Because the nurse is in the position of authority, the responsibility to maintain the boundary rests with the nurse; however, the line separating them is a continuum and sometimes not easily defined. It is inappropriate for nurses to engage in **sexual relations** with patients, and if the sexual behavior is coerced or the patient is cognitively impaired, it is **illegal**. However, more common violations with adults, particularly elderly patients, include exposing a patient unnecessarily, using sexually demeaning gestures or language (including off-color jokes), harassment, or inappropriate touching. Touching should be used with care, such as touching a hand or shoulder. Hugging may be misconstrued.

ATTENTION

Nursing is a giving profession, but the nurse must temper giving with recognition of professional boundaries. Patients have many needs. As acts of kindness, nurses (especially those involved in home care) often give certain patients extra attention and may offer to do **favors**, such as cooking or shopping. They may become overly invested in the patients' lives. While this may benefit a patient in the short term, it can establish a relationship of increasing **dependency** and **obligation** that does not resolve the long-term needs of the patient. Making referrals to the appropriate agencies or collaborating with family to find ways to provide services is more effective. Becoming overly invested may be evident by the nurse showing favoritism or spending too much time with the patient while neglecting other duties. On the other end of the spectrum are nurses who are disinterested and fail to provide adequate attention to the patient's detriment. Lack of adequate attention may lead to outright neglect.

COERCION

Power issues are inherent in matters associated with professional boundaries. Physical abuse is both unprofessional and illegal, but behavior can easily border on abusive without the patient being physically injured. Nurses can easily **intimidate** older adults and sick patients into having procedures or treatments they do not want. Regardless of age, patients have the right to choose and the right to refuse treatment. Difficulties arise with cognitive impairment, and in that case, another responsible adult (often the patient's child or

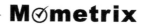

spouse) is designated to make decisions, but every effort should be made to gain patient cooperation. Forcing the patient to do something against his or her will borders on abuse and can sometimes degenerate into actual abuse if physical coercion is involved.

PERSONAL INFORMATION

When pre-existing personal or business relationships exist, other nurses should be assigned care of the patient whenever possible, but this may be difficult in small communities. However, the nurse should strive to maintain a professional role separate from the personal role and respect professional boundaries. The nurse must respect and maintain the confidentiality of the patient and family members, but the nurse must also be very careful about **disclosing personal information** about him or herself because this establishes a social relationship that interferes with the professional role of the nurse and the boundary between the patient and the nurse. The nurse and patient should never share secrets. When the nurse divulges personal information, he or she may become vulnerable to the patient, a reversal of roles.

Pediatric Nurse Practice Test

Want to take this practice test in an online interactive format?
Check out the bonus page, which includes interactive practice questions and much more: **mometrix.com/bonus948/pediatricnurse**

1. A 6-week-old male infant is brought into the ED by his mother. He has a weeklong history of progressively worsening emesis that is projectile in nature. What is his most likely diagnosis?

    a. Intussusception.
    b. Appendicitis.
    c. Pyloric stenosis.
    d. Pancreatitis.

2. An 8-year-old male has contracted chicken pox (varicella virus). With which of the following family members can the child have contact?

    a. 20-year-old aunt on chemotherapy.
    b. 35-year-old uncle with HIV.
    c. 95-year-old grandfather on long-term steroid therapy.
    d. 2-year-old brother who has never had varicella but has had the vaccine.

3. A 5-year-old girl has a fever, headache, and complaints of a stiff neck. The physician suspects bacterial meningitis. What is the best test culture site to detect the bacteria?

    a. Lumbar puncture.
    b. Clean catch urine.
    c. Blood culture.
    d. Nasal swab.

4. A 2-year-old child has severe dental caries in the upper and lower front teeth, posterior aspects. What is the most likely cause for this type of caries?

    a. Lack of fluoridation in the water.
    b. Sleeping with water in a nighttime bottle.
    c. Low carbohydrate diet.
    d. Sleeping with sugared liquid in nighttime bottle.

5. Which of the following patients will likely need surgical correction of his/her fracture?

    a. 10-year-old with humeral head fracture.
    b. 5-year-old with tuft fracture of the distal phalanx.
    c. 4-year-old with tuft fracture of the toe.
    d. 16-year-old with radial head fracture.

6. An infant with a chronic respiratory condition should be offered all of the following vaccines EXCEPT:

    a. Hepatitis A.
    b. Hepatitis B.
    c. Hepatitis C.
    d. influenza.

7. A 14-year-old boy with leukemia is receiving an IV infusion of packed red blood cells. The client reports that he is feeling anxious and short of breath even though his respiratory rate is 24. What should the nurse do in this situation?

    a. Give a dose of ibuprofen (Motrin).
    b. Give a dose of acetaminophen (Tylenol).
    c. Give a dose of diphenhydramine (Benadryl).
    d. Stop infusion and notify physician.

8. As part of counseling for a 7-year-old child with mild persistent asthma, the nurse tells the client's family that the most reliable indicator of worsening asthma is:

    a. coughing.
    b. fever.
    c. decreased peak flow.
    d. fatigue.

9. A patient is experiencing dizziness, shortness of breath, lightheadedness, and nausea caused by encephalitis. Which of the following descriptions most accurately describes the patient's condition?

    a. Metabolic acidosis.
    b. Respiratory alkalosis.
    c. Metabolic alkalosis.
    d. Respiratory acidosis.

10. 10-year-old male with sickle cell disease comes into the ED complaining of pain in his legs due to a vasoocclusive crisis. In addition to IV fluids, what is the other initial treatment for this client?

    a. Elevate legs.
    b. Ace wrap to legs.
    c. Nitroglycerine paste.
    d. Pain medication.

11. 14-year-old male with renal failure is given an arteriovenous fistula (shunt) for future dialysis. How does the nurse assess the shunt post-operatively for patency?

    a. Assess for bruit and thrill.
    b. Monitor blood pressure on that arm.
    c. Ease of venipuncture at shunt site.
    d. Rate of flow during dialysis.

12. A nurse is admitting a 16-year-old female to the mental health unit with a diagnosis of bulimia and anorexia. What OTC medications should the client's belongings be screened for as they may interfere with treatment?

    a. Imodium.
    b. Acetaminophen (Tylenol).
    c. Laxatives.
    d. Ibuprofen (Motrin).

13. A 10-year-old is accidentally shot in the forearm by a small caliber firearm. The wound enters the dorsum of the forearm and exits on the ventral side. The patient is ambulatory and has minor pain at the site. What test is likely needed for evaluation of the injury?

    a. Arteriogram.
    b. CT of arm.
    c. MRI of arm.
    d. Ultrasound of arm.

14. A 17-year-old female with severe acne wants treatment for her condition. What form of treatment requires the patient use 2 forms of contraception and sign a consent form?

   a. Benzoyl peroxide cream.
   b. Tetracycline (Sumycin) pills.
   c. Isotretinoin (Accutane) pills.
   d. Ultraviolet light treatment.

15. An 8-year-old with suspected appendicitis is evaluated. The physician asks the child to lie on his left side and extend the hip, eliciting pain in the RLQ. What is this test called?

   a. Rovsing's sign.
   b. Psoas sign.
   c. Kernig's sign.
   d. Brudzinski's sign.

16. In order to collect proper blood culture samples, the nurse should do which of the following?

   a. Sterilize site with chlorhexidine gluconate.
   b. Draw sample from femoral site.
   c. Wipe culture bottles with alcohol pad.
   d. Shave collection site.

17. The child of a celebrity client is admitted to a nursing floor, and the nurse taking care of this patient notices a medical assistant not involved in the care of the patient looking at her chart. What would be the most appropriate course of action?

   a. Confront medical assistant and make her apologize.
   b. Notify nursing supervisor of HIPAA violation.
   c. Place chart in locked cabinet.
   d. Place chart at end of client's bed.

18. A 7-year-old female is newly diagnosed with celiac disease. What is the best choice for a carbohydrate food source for this patient?

   a. Baked potato.
   b. Pasta.
   c. Bread.
   d. Saltine crackers.

19. The parents of a newborn male ask you about the benefits of circumcision. It is appropriate to inform them that circumcision seems to decrease the risk of transmission of which of the following sexually transmitted diseases?

   a. Human papillomavirus (HPV).
   b. Syphilis.
   c. HIV.
   d. Hepatitis C.

20. A 15-year-old female is diagnosed with a newly acquired infectious disease. Which of the following is NOT a mandatory reportable disease to the health department?

   a. TB.
   b. Varicella.
   c. Syphilis.
   d. Rabies.

21. Following an exposure to a TB-infected family member, a twelve-year-old male is screened for TB with a PPD (Mantoux) test. After administration of the test, when should he be brought back for reading of the result?

a. 24 to 36 hours.
b. 36 to 48 hours.
c. 48 to 72 hours.
d. 72 to 96 hours.

22. A newborn is scheduled for a chloride sweat test. For which genetic disorder does this test screen?

a. Muscular dystrophy.
b. Cystic Fibrosis.
c. Trisomy 18.
d. Fragile X.

23. A teenage female at a school health clinic asks the nurse what she can do to prevent contracting the human papilloma virus (HPV). All of the following would be considered suitable means of prevention EXCEPT:

a. abstinence.
b. condom use.
c. gardasil vaccine.
d. intrauterine devices.

24. Which of the following children has a fracture most likely caused by abuse?

a. 6-month-old with a spiral fracture of the femur.
b. 5-year-old with a wrist fracture.
c. 8-year-old with a clavicle fracture.
d. 15-year-old with an avulsion fracture of the ankle.

25. Which of the following conditions increases the risk of testicular cancer?

a. Undescended testes.
b. Umbilical hernia.
c. Inguinal hernia.
d. Hiatal hernia.

26. A 2-year-old client with a corneal abrasion needs to be examined. What is the best positioning for this client?

a. Restrained on papoose board.
b. Restrained by parent on gurney.
c. Under sedation in an operative room.
d. Held on a parent's lap

27. Following a diagnosis of cystic fibrosis in their infant child, the parents should be educated in all of the following EXCEPT:

a. genetic counseling.
b. sign language.
c. home chest percussions.
d. dietary modifications.

28. Which of the following medications has been linked to the development of Reye's syndrome when given to febrile children?

    a.   Acetaminophen (Tylenol).
    b.   Naprosyn (Aleve).
    c.   Aspirin.
    d.   Ibuprofen (Motrin).

29. A newborn with jaundice is treated with outpatient ultraviolet light therapy. What blood test is tested to ensure that the jaundice is clearing?

    a.   Bilirubin.
    b.   CBC.
    c.   AST.
    d.   Amylase.

30. A 2-month-old male is being evaluated for gastroesophageal reflux. What is the best test to confirm this diagnosis?

    a.   CT scan.
    b.   Barium enema.
    c.   Upper GI barium series
    d.   Night-time Ph probe

31. A 16-year-old female is undergoing an evaluation for possible juvenile rheumatoid arthritis. What lab test serves as a marker for general inflammation?

    a.   Monospot.
    b.   Erythrocyte sedimentation rate.
    c.   White blood count (WBC).
    d.   Mean corpuscular volume (MCV).

32. A 7-year-old female is evaluated for possible leukemia. She is scheduled for a bone marrow biopsy the next morning. What part of the body should be listed on the consent form for the biopsy?

    a.   Radius.
    b.   Skull.
    c.   Posterior pelvis.
    d.   Calcaneus (heel).

33. While performing trauma resuscitation on a 5-year-old male, neither peripheral nor central IV access can be obtained. The physician orders an intraosseous line. What is the best site on the body for this line?

    a.   Radius.
    b.   Proximal anterior tibia.
    c.   Skull.
    d.   Medial malleolus.

34. A 5-year-old is diagnosed with probable "Fifth's disease" caused by Parvovirus B19 although she does not yet have a rash. Which of the following should the child avoid?

    a.   Contact sports.
    b.   Tylenol.
    c.   Pregnant women.
    d.   Spicy food.

35. A 13-year-old female is diagnosed with *Clostridium difficile* colitis. What is the most probable cause of this infection?

    a.   Recent antibiotic use.
    b.   Travel to Central America.
    c.   Drinking from a stream.
    d.   Eating undercooked pork.

36. A 14-year-old male is suspected of having infectious mononucleosis. What Point of Care Testing (POCT) device can be used to confirm this diagnosis?

    a.   Urine dip.
    b.   Monospot.
    c.   Rapid strep test.
    d.   Rapid influenza test.

37. A 12-year-old female immigrant from the Philippines has a positive PPD (Mantoux) skin test. What vaccine given routinely in her native country can cause false positive PPD tests?

    a.   Varicella.
    b.   Yellow fever.
    c.   Influenza.
    d.   BCG.

38. Which of the following congenital hernias is more commonly seen in African-American children?

    a.   Umbilical hernia.
    b.   Inguinal hernia.
    c.   Hiatal hernia.
    d.   Femoral hernia.

39. A 13-year-old female has the development of breast buds and sparse long, downy pubic hair. What Tanner stage does this development suggest?

    a.   Tanner 1.
    b.   Tanner 2.
    c.   Tanner 3.
    d.   Tanner 4.

40. Apocrine sweat glands develop during onset of puberty. In which part of the body are these glands most commonly located?

    a.   Scalp.
    b.   Feet.
    c.   Hands.
    d.   Axilla.

41. A 16-year-old male has hearing loss at the 4000-Hertz range on audiogram. What is the most common cause for such a hearing deficit?

    a.   Cerumen in the ear canal.
    b.   Prolonged exposure to noises over 100 decibels.
    c.   Medulla oblongata tumor.
    d.   Ruptured tympanic membrane.

42. Which of the following would NOT be considered a pediatric patient at high risk for dehydration?

  a. 4-year-old male with 30% body surface area burn.
  b. 7-year-old female with diabetic ketoacidosis.
  c. 12-year-old male with hyperventilation due to anxiety.
  d. 8-year-old male with cellulitis in the right arm.

43. A 15-year-old female is evaluated for an intentional overdose of aspirin. The excessive ingestion of this medication puts the patient at risk for what acid-base disorder?

  a. Metabolic acidosis.
  b. Metabolic alkalosis.
  c. Respiratory acidosis.
  d. Respiratory alkalosis.

44. Symptoms consistent with a diagnosis of dehydration in children would include all of the following EXCEPT:

  a. thirst.
  b. bradycardia.
  c. dry mucous membranes.
  d. depressed fontanelles.

45. A 6-year-old female with dehydration due to vomiting is evaluated with a complete blood count (CBC). What lab finding is expected?

  a. Decreased mean corpuscular (cell) volume (MCV).
  b. Increased MCV.
  c. Increased hematocrit.
  d. Normal red cell distribution width (RDW).

46. What is the leading cause of death in children in developing countries?

  a. Accidental trauma.
  b. TB.
  c. AIDS.
  d. Infectious diarrhea.

47. What is the most common cause of viral (non-bacterial) diarrhea in pediatric patients?

  a. Rotavirus.
  b. Parainfluenza.
  c. Influenza.
  d. Parvovirus B19.

48. After a camping trip a 14-year-old male develops diarrhea, flatulence, steatorrhea, and abdominal cramping. The other campers who drank water from a stream also have similar symptoms. What is the most likely causative organism?

  a. *E. coli.*
  b. Giardia Lamblia.
  c. Rotavirus.
  d. *Shigella.*

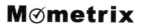

49. A 2-year-old female is undergoing an evaluation for celiac disease (sprue). Which of the following is NOT a risk factor for this disease?

    a. First degree relative with the disease.

    b. Recent travel to Mexico.

    c. Congenital trisomy 21.

    d. History of type 1 diabetes mellitus.

50. A 6-year-old male grabbed a pot of boiling water off of a stove and has a burn on the dorsum of the forearm. The burn area is red with edema and thin-walled blisters. What classification of burn is this?

    a. First-degree burn.

    b. Second-degree burn.

    c. Third-degree burn.

    d. Fourth-degree burn.

51. Antibodies exist in the body to respond to allergens and protect the body against disease. Which antibodies act primarily against parasitic infections?

    a. IgE.

    b. IgM.

    c. IgG.

    d. IgA.

52. A child presents with history of fever for 2 days at 102 degrees F. At what age would the child likely need a spinal tap and full work up for sepsis based on the fever only?

    a. 3 months.

    b. 3 years.

    c. 6 years.

    d. 12 years.

53. In caring for a child with a history of HIV infection, which of the following immunizations should NOT be given to the child?

    a. Hep B.

    b. DTaP.

    c. Influenza.

    d. Varicella.

54. Due to sickle cell disease, a 7-year-old female is considered to be asplenic from repeated splenic sequestration crises. What vaccine should she get to protect her from encapsulated bacteria?

    a. MMR.

    b. Tetanus.

    c. Pneumococcal vaccine (PCV).

    d. Varicella.

55. Which of the following children over the age of 6 months should NOT be given the influenza vaccine?

    a. 2-year-old with chronic renal disease.

    b. 7-year-old with HIV.

    c. 13-year-old with type 1diabetes.

    d. 2-year-old with streptococcal pharyngitis.

56. Which of the following patients would be most at risk from meningitis due to the severity of their current infection?

    a. 7-year-old with leg cellulitis.
    b. 4-year-old with finger cellulitis.
    c. 3-year-old with peri-orbital cellulitis.
    d. 12-year-old with appendicitis.

57. A 5-year-old with suspected meningitis is evaluated with a lumbar puncture. Which of the following lab results would NOT be consistent with a diagnosis of bacterial meningitis?

    a. Decreased WBC.
    b. Elevated protein level.
    c. Decreased glucose level.
    d. Cloudy fluid.

58. Bronchodilators are used to improve respiratory function and relax pulmonary musculature. Which of the following medications is NOT a bronchodilator?

    a. Albuterol (Proventil).
    b. Theophylline.
    c. Prednisolone (Prelone).
    d. Levalbuterol (Xopenex).

59. Cystic fibrosis patients can develop breathing difficulty due to the viscosity of their sputum. Which of the following medications is used as a mucolytic agent to thin out the mucous and help them breathe better?

    a. Acetylcysteine (Mucomyst).
    b. Albuterol (Proventil).
    c. Prednisolone (Prelone).
    d. Theophylline.

60. Acute otitis media is a very common disease in early childhood. Many different bacteria can cause otitis media. Which of the following is NOT a common bacterial pathogen in acute otitis media?

    a. *Haemophilus influenzae.*
    b. *Streptococcus pneumoniae.*
    c. *Clostridium difficile.*
    d. *Moraxella catarrhalis.*

61. Which of the following pediatric upper respiratory infections can lead to respiratory compromise and often requires intubation?

    a. Croup.
    b. Acute otitis media.
    c. Nasopharyngitis.
    d. Epiglottiditis.

62. Cystic fibrosis is an inherited disease that affects the respiratory and digestive systems. What is the genetic etiology of cystic fibrosis?

    a. Autosomal dominant.
    b. Autosomal recessive.
    c. Y chromosome linked.
    d. Spontaneous mutation.

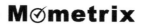

63. Due to insufficiencies in chloride channel function in cells, children with cystic fibrosis often need supplementation for proper digestion. What medication is commonly needed for these patients?

    a. Protein pump inhibitors.
    b. Pancreatic enzymes.
    c. Antacids.
    d. Laxatives.

64. A nurse is advising a new mother on care of her newborn. The newborn has a cleft palate. What should NOT be advised regarding feeding of this infant prior to surgical correction?

    a. The infant should be fed slowly and burped frequently.
    b. Special nipples should be provided for infants unable to suck adequately with a standard nipple.
    c. Sucking should be stimulated by rubbing the nipple on the lower lip.
    d. The infant should be fed in the Trendelenburg (head down) position.

65. A 6-month-old male is diagnosed with an intussusception of the colon. What diagnostic test is often therapeutic in reducing the invagination of one part of the intestine into another?

    a. Barium enema.
    b. Ultrasound.
    c. CT.
    d. MRI.

66. New red blood cells are made by the bone marrow and transport oxygen and carbon dioxide. What is the life span of a red blood cell?

    a. 30 days.
    b. 60 days.
    c. 90 days.
    d. 120 days.

67. Typical symptoms of anemia in a pediatric patient would include all of the following EXCEPT:

    a. fatigue.
    b. easy bruising tendency.
    c. pink oral mucosa.
    d. conjunctival pallor.

68. The red blood cell index that measures the size of the red blood cells and is useful in classifying anemia is:

    a. hemoglobin.
    b. hematocrit.
    c. mean corpuscular volume.
    d. platelets.

69. A 2-year-old female is evaluated for iron deficiency anemia. Which of the following would NOT likely be found?

    a. Larger RBC size.
    b. Decreased hemoglobin level.
    c. Decreased RBC mass.
    d. Decreased oxygen carrying capacity of the blood.

70. An African-American newborn is evaluated for a possible hemoglobinopathy. What is the most common hemoglobinopathy in this population, occurring in 1 in 375 live births?

    a. Thalassemia.
    b. Sickle cell disease.
    c. Babesiosis.
    d. Malaria.

71. Idiopathic thrombocytopenic purpura (ITP) is an acquired disease that causes hemorrhage. What circulating blood component is reduced with ITP?

    a. Platelets.
    b. Red blood cells.
    c. White blood cells.
    d. Iron.

72. Discharge instructions are being given to the parents of a child with iron deficiency anemia. Which of the following food choices would NOT be a good source of iron in the diet?

    a. Lean beef.
    b. Spinach.
    c. Chicken.
    d. Potatoes.

73. At which age would a blood pressure reading of 80/40 be considered normal?

    a. 16 years.
    b. 7 years.
    c. 12 years.
    d. 3 months.

74. In analysis of an ECG, what component of the heart's function does the P-wave represent?

    a. Ventricular repolarization.
    b. Atrial depolarization.
    c. Ventricular depolarization.
    d. Resting period of the heart.

75. Diuretic medications are used to manage edema in pediatric patients with heart failure. Which of the following medications is NOT a diuretic medication?

    a. Furosemide (Lasix).
    b. Enalapril (Vasotec).
    c. Spironolactone (Aldactone).
    d. Bumetanide (Bumex).

76. A patent ductus arteriosus (PDA) results when the fetal ductus arteriosus fails to close and blood flows from the aorta back into the pulmonary circulation. In neonates this can often be closed without surgery using certain medications. What class of medications is often used to close this congenital heart defect non-surgically?

    a. Antibiotics.
    b. Adrenergic steroids.
    c. Prostaglandin synthetase inhibitors.
    d. Beta blockers.

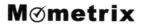

77. The most common congenital heart defect is:

    a. patent foramen ovale.
    b. atrial septal defect.
    c. ventricular septal defect (VSD).
    d. patent ductus arteriosus (PDA).

78. Which of the following congenital heart defects would lead to right ventricular hypertrophy and right heart failure if not treated?

    a. Aortic stenosis.
    b. Pulmonic stenosis.
    c. Coarctation of the aorta.
    d. Tricuspid atresia.

79. The most common cause for heart failure in children is congenital heart defects. Numerous medications can be used to improve functioning in addition to surgical procedures. Which of the following medications used in heart failure has a narrow therapeutic window requiring blood draws to monitor the blood level?

    a. Digoxin (Lanoxin).
    b. Propranolol (Inderal).
    c. Hydrochlorothiazide (HCTZ).
    d. Aspirin.

80. Rheumatic fever is a systemic inflammatory autoimmune disease that occurs after an untreated infection with bacteria. What is the causative bacterium in rheumatic fever?

    a. *Haemophilus influenza.*
    b. *Bacillus anthracis.*
    c. *Mycobacterium avium.*
    d. Group A beta-hemolytic *Streptococcus.*

81. Rheumatic fever is assessed using the Jones criteria that divide the signs and symptoms of the disease into major and minor criteria. Which of the following characteristics is considered a minor and NOT a major criterion?

    a. Polyarthritis.
    b. Fever.
    c. Carditis.
    d. Chorea.

82. Following a diagnosis of a urinary tract infection, an adolescent is counseled to maintain acidic urine to help speed healing of the infection. Which of the following liquids would NOT be a good choice?

    a. Cranberry juice.
    b. Prune juice.
    c. Carbonated sodas.
    d. Apple juice.

83. The most common genetic bone disease is osteogenesis imperfecta (OI). This is an inherited disorder that results from an abnormality in which of the following aspects of bone formation?

    a. Collagen synthesis.
    b. Calcium deposition.
    c. Phosphorus deposition.
    d. Iron deposition.

84. A 14-year-old sustained a blow to the medial forearm. He has a fracture that is incomplete and does not extend all the way through the ulna. What is this type of fracture?

a. Buckle fracture.
b. Greenstick fracture.
c. Bend fracture.
d. Open fracture.

85. Duchenne's muscular dystrophy is the most common form of muscular dystrophy and causes progressive degeneration and weakness of the skeletal muscles. At what age is Duchenne's muscular dystrophy usually first evident?

a. 6 months to 1 year.
b. 12 to 15 years.
c. 9 to 12 years.
d. 3 to 5 years.

86. Which type of seizure is characterized by a sudden loss of muscle tone and then a postictal period of confusion?

a. Tonic seizures.
b. Clonic seizures.
c. Atonic seizures.
d. Absence seizures.

87. What should women of childbearing age consume in the preconceptual period to decrease their risk of neural tube defects in their children?

a. Iron.
b. Vitamin B12.
c. Magnesium.
d. Folic acid.

88. The pituitary gland regulates many other components of the endocrine system and is composed of the anterior pituitary (adenohypophysis) and posterior pituitary (neurohypophysis). Which of the following is NOT secreted by the anterior pituitary?

a. Growth hormone.
b. Thyroid stimulating hormone.
c. Oxytocin.
d. Prolactin.

89. The islets of Langerhans in the pancreas secrete several hormones that regulate body functions. Which of the following is NOT a hormone secreted by the islets of Langerhans?

a. Aldosterone.
b. Insulin.
c. Glucagon.
d. Somatostatin.

90. Following surgery for a brain tumor, a 6-year-old female exhibits symptoms of syndrome of inappropriate antidiuretic hormone (SIADH). Which of the following is NOT a classic symptom of SIADH?

a. Fluid retention.
b. Weight loss.
c. Weakness.
d. Decreased urinary output.

91. What is the most common type of cancer in childhood?

    a. Kidney tumors.
    b. Brain tumors.
    c. Lymphomas.
    d. Leukemias.

92. During resuscitation of a 9-month-old male, what is the proper ratio of chest compressions to breaths?

    a. 1:1.
    b. 5:1.
    c. 10:2.
    d. 30:2.

93. Which of the following characteristics is NOT part of the Apgar scoring method for assessment of newborns?

    a. Heart rate.
    b. Respiratory effort.
    c. Skin color.
    d. Eye tracking.

94. A 2-year-old male is found to be in ventricular fibrillation. What is the proper initial voltage for defibrillation?

    a. 20 J/kg.
    b. 15 J/kg.
    c. 10 J/kg.
    d. 2 J/kg.

95. In the treatment of ventricular fibrillation in children what is the initial medication used if defibrillation is not effective?

    a. Amiodarone.
    b. Magnesium.
    c. Epinephrine.
    d. Lidocaine.

96. In cases of inability to obtain peripheral IV access, an interosseous line (IO) can be placed to infuse medications and fluid. Blood can also be aspirated and sent to the lab for analysis. Which of the following lab tests CANNOT be done reliably from an IO sample?

    a. White blood cell count.
    b. Type and cross.
    c. Electrolytes.
    d. Hemoglobin count.

97. For a rapid-sequence intubation of a pediatric patient, paralyzing drugs are often used. One of the more commonly used medications is succinylcholine (Anectine). Which of the following is NOT a common side effect of the use of succinylcholine?

    a. Increased intracranial pressure.
    b. Decreased heart rate.
    c. Hypokalemia.
    d. Increased eye pressure.

98. Depressed or inverted T-waves on ECG analysis can occur with many different clinical situations in pediatric patients. Which of the following is NOT a common reason for depressed or inverted T-waves?

 a. Hypokalemia.
 b. Myocarditis.
 c. Digitalis toxicity.
 d. Hyperthyroidism.

99. A child has a wide complex tachycardia and needs medication for this condition. Which one of the following medications used in the treatment of tachycardias commonly causes a brief asystolic episode that quickly resolves?

 a. Lidocaine.
 b. Amiodarone.
 c. Adenosine.
 d. Procainamide.

100. A 7-year-old has a history of intermittent blood in her stools. She and her mother are instructed on using stool Guaiac cards at home for analysis. Which of the following does NOT cause false positive results for stool Guaiac tests?

 a. Red meat.
 b. Fresh cherries.
 c. Horseradish.
 d. Vitamin C.

101. Hemolytic uremic syndrome (HUS) is a post-infectious disorder causing nephropathy, hemolytic anemia, and thrombocytopenia. It is seen following upper respiratory illnesses and following GI infections after eating meat contaminated with bacteria. What enteric bacteria have been linked to HUS?

 a. *Escherichia coli* O157:H7.
 b. *Clostridium difficile.*
 c. Rotavirus.
 d. *Vibrio cholerae.*

102. Hypertension can be seen in the pediatric population. What is the most common cause of secondary hypertension in children?

 a. Coarctation of the aorta.
 b. Renal disease.
 c. Neuroblastomas.
 d. Drug toxicity.

103. A 16-year-old female is brought into the ED with an intentional overdose of acetaminophen. In order to prevent liver toxicity what medication can be given?

 a. N-Acetylcysteine (Mucomyst).
 b. Activated charcoal.
 c. Ipecac syrup.
 d. Naloxone (Narcan).

104. Following a severe motor vehicle accident, a 10-year-old male has a hemisection of the spinal cord with associated ipsilateral weakness and loss of proprioception and contralateral loss of pain and temperature sensation. What is this spinal cord syndrome called?

   a. Anterior cord syndrome.
   b. Complete cord injury.
   c. Brown-Sequard syndrome.
   d. Posterior cord syndrome.

105. A 2-year-old male inadvertently ingests some opiates from his parent's prescription medication. Which of the following would NOT be a likely physical finding?

   a. Decreased respiratory rate.
   b. Lethargy.
   c. Decreased bowel sounds.
   d. Pupillary dilation.

106. A 10-year-old child is to have a venipuncture done at the femoral site. Which of the following anatomic structures is most medial in the inguinal area?

   a. Femoral vein.
   b. Femoral artery.
   c. Femoral nerve.
   d. Anterior superior iliac crest.

107. An early-adolescent female is described by her mother as having no interest in participating in any activities with her parents. What aspect of psychosocial development does this reflect?

   a. Identity.
   b. Peer pressure.
   c. Body Image.
   d. Independence.

108. A 16-year-old female presents to the clinic asking for oral contraceptive pills. Which of the following medical problems in the past would contraindicate the use of oral contraceptives?

   a. Migraine headaches.
   b. Depression.
   c. Deep vein thrombosis.
   d. Pneumonia.

109. A 7-year-old male has a history of supraventricular tachycardia. His ECG shows a shortened PR interval, a delta wave, and a wide QRS pattern. What is the most likely conduction disturbance?

   a. Left bundle branch block (LBBB).
   b. Wolff-Parkinson-White syndrome (WPW).
   c. Right bundle branch block (RBBB).
   d. Mobitz type II second-degree heart block.

110. Molluscum contagiosum is a papular dome-shaped skin lesion that can occur on many parts of the body and spread by autoinoculation. What is the causative organism for this skin condition?

   a. Human papillomavirus.
   b. Poxvirus.
   c. Herpes virus.
   d. Anaerobic bacteria.

111. The prevalence of type 2 diabetes in children is rising, especially among the African-American and Hispanic populations. What is the principle risk factor for type 2 diabetes?

a. Premature birth.
b. Maternal smoking.
c. Obesity.
d. Asthma.

112. A 15-year-old female has been diagnosed with hyperthyroidism due to Graves's disease. Which of the following symptoms would NOT likely be present in this patient?

a. Bradycardia.
b. Insomnia.
c. Heat intolerance.
d. Weight loss.

113. Pediatric patients are often found to have a decreased potassium level (hypokalemia). Which of the following is NOT a common reason for hypokalemia?

a. Diarrhea.
b. Laxative use.
c. Diabetic ketoacidosis.
d. Renal failure.

114. A neonate has anorexia, lethargy, vomiting, and seizures. He is thought to have an inborn error of metabolism with a high ammonia level. Which of the following is NOT an inborn error of metabolism disease?

a. Argininosuccinase deficiency
b. Ornithine transcarbamylase deficiency
c. Cystic fibrosis
d. HMG-CoA lyase deficiency

115. Patients with Turner's syndrome have 45 autosomal chromosomes and only one X sex chromosome. Which of the following is NOT a common component of Turner's syndrome?

a. Webbed neck.
b. Male sex organs.
c. Short stature.
d. Broad chest.

116. Which of the following common genetic syndromes involves dilation of the aortic root and possible development of aortic aneurysms?

a. Trisomy 21.
b. Trisomy 18.
c. Fragile X.
d. Marfan's syndrome.

117. Which lab test measures the new production of red blood cells by the body in response to any blood loss?

a. Ferritin level.
b. Mean corpuscular volume.
c. Total iron binding capacity.
d. Reticulocyte count.

118. Fresh frozen plasma (FFP) is used in the treatment of active bleeding or to reverse the effects of warfarin. Which of the following clotting factors does FFP NOT contain?

    a.   Factor IX.
    b.   Platelets.
    c.   Factor V.
    d.   Factor VII.

119. A 13-year-old male has had nasal congestion, rhinorrhea, and headaches for the past 6 months. He uses an OTC nasal spray that alleviates the symptoms but has prompt recurrence once the spray wears off. What is his likely diagnosis?

    a.   Nonallergic rhinitis with eosinophilia syndrome (NARES).
    b.   Rhinitis medicamentosa.
    c.   Vasomotor rhinitis.
    d.   Nasal polyps.

120. Many systemic diseases have skin manifestations that accompany the disorder. Erythema migrans is an annular rash with a target lesion and a clear or necrotic center. It is often accompanied by fever, headache, and myalgias. What is the systemic disease associated with erythema migrans?

    a.   Tuberculosis.
    b.   Syphilis.
    c.   Lyme disease.
    d.   HIV.

121. Infectious bacteria can be classified based by their morphology as cocci, bacilli, and spirochetes. Which of the following pediatric diseases is NOT caused by a spirochete?

    a.   Lyme disease.
    b.   Syphilis.
    c.   Yaws.
    d.   Gonorrhea.

122. Infectious protozoa are eukaryotic organisms that can cause gastrointestinal diseases, especially in developing countries, where travelers may become infected. Which of the following organisms is a protozoan?

    a.   *Giardia lamblia.*
    b.   *Salmonella typhi.*
    c.   *Escherichia coli (E. coli).*
    d.   *Vibrio cholera.*

123. Estimation of gestational age may be done in many ways. Nagele's rule is the most accurate and involves calculations using which parameter?

    a.   Mother's last menstrual period.
    b.   Fundal height.
    c.   Crown-rump length (CRL) on ultrasound.
    d.   Estimated weight on ultrasound.

124. What is the normal baseline fetal heart rate (FHR) in a term fetus?

    a.   120-160 bpm.
    b.   80-100 bpm.
    c.   100-120 bpm.
    d.   160-190 bpm.

125. Body mass index (BMI) is a valuable tool of measure healthy weight and a good predictor of future morbidity and mortality. It can be used to classify underweight, overweight, and obese status. What is the formula to calculate BMI using weight in kilograms and height in meters?

    a.   Weight x height.
    b.   Height/weight.
    c.   Weight/(height x height).
    d.   Height/(weight x weight).

126. Although vitamin supplementation is occasionally needed, an overdose of fat-soluble vitamins can lead to liver toxicity. Which of the following is a water-soluble vitamin that is NOT fat-soluble?

    a.   Vitamin A.
    b.   Vitamin E.
    c.   Vitamin C.
    d.   Vitamin K.

127. Treatment for asthma is based on guidelines related to symptom severity to determine whether medical control is adequate. If a 7-year-old female has daily daytime symptoms and symptoms more than one night per week, her asthma is in which of the following categories?

    a.   Severe persistent.
    b.   Moderate persistent.
    c.   Mild persistent.
    d.   Mild intermittent.

128. A humanistic theorist of the 20th century described a hierarchy of basic needs for all humans. His "hierarchy of needs" builds from the most basic for survival (physiologic) and ends to the most developed (self-actualization). What is the name of this philosopher?

    a.   Carl Rogers.
    b.   Lawrence Kohlberg.
    c.   John Bowlby.
    d.   Abraham Maslow.

129. In Piaget's stages of cognitive development, the "concrete operational thinking" stage involves the child thinking in terms of absolute right and wrong without the ability to reason more complex issues. What age range does this occur in?

    a.   Birth to 2 years.
    b.   2 to 7 years.
    c.   7 to 12 years.
    d.   Over 12 years.

130. A parent is noted to be very strict with harsh discipline, high expectations, low support, and low parent-child communication. What parenting style would this be considered as?

    a.   Authoritative parenting.
    b.   Permissive-neglectful parenting.
    c.   Democratic-indulgent parenting.
    d.   Authoritarian parenting.

131. Which permanent teeth eruption usually occurs first?

    a.   Central incisors.
    b.   Lateral incisors.
    c.   Cuspids (canines).
    d.   First premolars (Bicuspids).

132. A 10-year-old male has a repetitive and persistent dysfunctional pattern of aggressive behavior and violation of the law, social norms, and the rights of others. With which psychological disorder is this most consistent?

    a. Oppositional-defiant disorder.
    b. Conduct disorder.
    c. ADHD.
    d. Autism.

133. Oppositional-defiant disorder is a pattern of behavior characterized by negative and defiant behavior towards parents, teachers, and authority figures. Which of the following would NOT be an expected clinical finding consistent with this disorder?

    a. Argumentative with parents.
    b. Defiance of rules and requests.
    c. Avoids activities that require focused mental attention.
    d. Loses temper easily.

134. Learning disabilities refer to difficulties in various aspects of learning and a significantly lowered school performance than expected. Which of the following conditions is NOT commonly associated with learning disabilities?

    a. Lead poisoning.
    b. Cystic fibrosis.
    c. Fetal alcohol syndrome.
    d. Fragile- X syndrome.

135. After traumatic birth, a neonate is found to have diffuse edema of the soft tissue of the scalp, crossing suture lines. What is this finding in a neonate called?

    a. Macrocephaly.
    b. Caput succedaneum.
    c. Cephalohematoma.
    d. Microcephaly.

136. A 16-year-old male is found to have a tall stature, small penis and testes, scoliosis, and decreased testosterone levels. On genetic typing, he is found to have an extra X chromosome (47XXY). What is this syndrome called?

    a. Trisomy 21.
    b. Trisomy 18.
    c. Turner's syndrome.
    d. Klinefelter's syndrome.

137. A 6-year-old uncircumcised male has a foreskin that cannot easily be retracted over the glans penis. What is the name for this urologic condition?

    a. Cryptorchidism.
    b. Hydrocele.
    c. Varicocele.
    d. Phimosis.

138. While performing an exam on a newborn, the examiner flexes the hip and adducts the thigh and palpates a "clunk" indicating displacement of the femoral head. What is this physical exam test called?

    a. Ortolani's test.
    b. Gower's sign.
    c. Allis's sign.
    d. Barlow test.

139. The Mantoux skin test is used for tuberculosis screening and involves subcutaneous injection of PPD derivative in the skin and the reading of the result 48 to 72 hours later. What aspect of the skin is evaluated at this time?

    a. Erythema.
    b. Degree of pruritus.
    c. Induration.
    d. Bleeding.

140. An infant has microcephaly with head circumference 2 standard deviations (SD) below the mean for his age. Which of the following is NOT a common cause for microcephaly?

    a. Intrauterine TORCH infections.
    b. Hydrocephalus.
    c. Fetal alcohol syndrome.
    d. Phenylketonuria.

141. An infant has strabismus with an inwardly deviated right eye (esotropia). Which eye muscle is likely to be the weak in this case?

    a. Lateral rectus.
    b. Medial rectus.
    c. Superior oblique.
    d. Inferior oblique.

142. A 5-year-old male has an acute illness with a vesicular exanthema on tongue, gums, and palate with fever and dysphagia. He is diagnosed with hand, foot, and mouth disease. What is the causative organism for this disease?

    a. Adenovirus.
    b. Herpes simplex virus.
    c. Streptococcus.
    d. Coxsackievirus A16.

143. Due to persistent asthma, a 7-year-old female is started on long-term control medications. Which of the following medications works to stabilize mast cells?

    a. Fluticasone (Advair).
    b. Budesonide (Pulmicort).
    c. Cromolyn (Intal).
    d. Theophylline (Theodur).

144. A newborn had a collection of small white inclusion cysts filled with cheesy material on the face, but these cysts resolved spontaneously in a few weeks. What is the most likely diagnosis?

    a. Milia.
    b. Erythema toxicum neonatorum.
    c. Cutis marmorata.
    d. Nevus Flammeus.

145. An African-American 13-year-old male has several patches of hypopigmentation on his skin surface. These have developed slowly over the past several years. What is his most likely diagnosis?

    a. Albinism.
    b. Vitiligo.
    c. Pityriasis rosacea.
    d. Pityriasis alba.

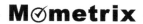

146. Which of the following common skin conditions is caused by a fungal infection?

    a. Molluscum contagiosum.
    b. Plantar warts.
    c. Tinea corporis.
    d. Shingles.

147. A 7-year-old male is treated for an anaphylactic reaction to a bee sting. What type of antibody is the prime mediator for type I hypersensitivity reactions?

    a. IgA.
    b. IgM.
    c. IgG.
    d. IgE.

148. The most common form of viral hepatitis in children is hepatitis A. Which of the following is NOT considered a characteristic of this condition?

    a. Transmission by blood contact only.
    b. Highest rate of infection in ages 5 to 14.
    c. 15- to 50-day incubation.
    d. Commonly seen in daycare centers.

149. Which of the following patients would be LEAST at risk for sepsis if presenting to the ED with a fever of 103 °F?

    a. 5-year-old with HIV.
    b. 8-year-old with Trisomy 21.
    c. 12-year-old on chemotherapy for leukemia.
    d. 2-week-old newborn.

150. A 4-year-old child is found to have a lateral bowing of the tibia that does not increase after walking. What is this condition known as?

    a. Metatarsus adductus.
    b. Metatarsus varus.
    c. Genu varum.
    d. Genu valgum.

Answer Key and Explanations

1. C: Projectile vomiting in a 6-week-old male is the classic presentation for pyloric stenosis, obstruction of the pyloric sphincter between the gastric pylorus and the small intestine, caused by hypertrophy and hyperplasia of the circular muscle of the pylorus, which obstructs the sphincter. This diagnosis can be confirmed with an ultrasound.

2. D: The 2-year-old brother, who has had the vaccine, is likely immune to varicella, so contact is safe. All of the other relatives have some form of immunosuppression from infection (HIV) or medications (chemotherapy and steroids) and should avoid contact with the patient.

3. A: Lumbar puncture is the method of choice for detecting the bacteria causing bacterial meningitis and sending a sample for culture, as meningitis infects the meninges and bacteria is present in the cerebrospinal fluid.

4. D: Caries in the posterior front teeth is a sign of sleeping with sugared drinks in the nighttime bottle (such as juice) because fluid pools in the mouth when the child falls to sleep.

5. A: Humeral head fractures usually need open reduction and internal fixation to maintain proper future functioning. Distal phalanx and toe fractures are treated with splints and fracture of the radial head with a sling.

6. C: A vaccine for Hepatitis C does not currently exist. Hepatitis A, hepatitis B and influenza vaccines are all recommended for the infant.

7. D: Anxiety and the sensation of breathlessness are signs of possible anaphylactic shock, a reaction to the packed red blood cells, so the nurse should stop the infusion immediately and notify the physician.

8. C: A decreased peak flow is the most reliable indicator that asthma may be worsening. It is therefore vital that the client's family know what the baseline is so that any deviation can be quickly addressed. Coughing and fever may trigger asthma, so peak flows should be monitored. Fatigue may result from poor oxygenation but alone it is not a reliable indicator of worsening asthma.

9. B: Respiratory alkalosis results from hyperventilation, during which extra CO_2 is excreted, causing a decrease in carbonic acid (H_2CO_3) concentration in the plasma. Symptoms include tachycardia, arrhythmias, lightheadedness, nausea, and vomiting.

10. D: In addition to IV fluids, the other primary initial treatment for sickle cell crisis resulting in vascular occlusion is pain medication because pain is often severe. Other treatments include oxygen, hydroxyurea (anti-sickling medication), blood transfusions if anemia is pronounced, and antibiotics if the crisis was triggered by an infection.

11. A: The patency of an AV shunt is assured by assessing for bruit and thrill. Continuous wave Doppler ultrasound can also assess patency. Venipuncture and blood pressure measurements should never be done on the arm with an AV shunt.

12. C: People with eating disorders, such as bulimia and anorexia, often use laxatives as well as diuretics to control weight. New patients should be checked for these items. Bulimics may purge by vomiting after eating.

13. A: An arteriogram is needed to assess the vascular supply in the arm after a gunshot wound to ensure that no injury to the ulnar and radial artery has occurred.

14. C: Accutane is a vitamin A derivative and can lead to severe birth defects if given to pregnant females. Two forms of contraception and a lengthy consent form are needed. Benzoyl peroxide and ultraviolet light treatment pose no risks to the fetus. Tetracycline has a low risk during the first trimester of pregnancy but can cause discoloration of the child's teeth if taken during the second trimester.

15. B: The Psoas sign consists of extension of the thigh while lying on the left side and causes pain with a posterior pointing appendix. Rovsing's sign also assesses for appendicitis and elicits referred pain in the right lower quadrant with palpation in the left lower quadrant. Kernig's sign and Brudzinski's sign are used to assess for meningitis.

16. A: In order to minimize contaminants, blood cultures are taken from the site (most commonly the antecubital fossa) after sterilizing it with chlorhexidine gluconate and using sterile gloves. This sample does not need to be collected from a femoral site and the culture bottles are not getting pulled from, therefore do not need to be wiped with an alcohol pad. Shaving the collection site is not required for a blood culture sample.

17. B: An unauthorized person's looking at any patient's chart is a clear HIPAA violation and must be reported to the supervisor in charge so that appropriate disciplinary action can be taken.

18. A: Only the potato is a suitable source of carbohydrate for a person with celiac disease. Celiac disease is an allergic sensitivity to gluten in wheat products. Pasta, bread, and saltine crackers are all made with flour, which contains gluten.

19. C: Circumcision has been shown to decrease the rates of transmission of HIV but does not affect rates of syphilis, HPV, or hepatitis C.

20. B: Varicella (chickenpox) is not a reportable disease, and most children are vaccinated for varicella; however, the CDC requires reporting of TB, syphilis, and rabies as these are public health concerns.

21. C: PPD tests should be read 48 to 72 hours after administration. Any sign of induration is measured. Induration of 15 mm or blistering is a positive finding for general screening, but if the person has been exposed to someone with active TB, then 10 mm induration is considered positive.

22. B: A chloride sweat test is used in the diagnosis of cystic fibrosis, which affects excretion of sodium and chloride in the sweat. A child with cystic fibrosis will have up to 5 times the normal level of sodium and chloride in his sweat.

23. D: IUD's offer no protection for HPV and only provide birth control. Abstinence, condom use, and Gardasil vaccine, recommended for girls/women ages 9 to 26, all provide protection against HPV.

24. A: Spiral fractures in children are considered due to abuse until proven otherwise. These fractures result from a twisting force that the child would not be able to perform on her own.

25. A: An undescended testis increases the risk of testicular cancer in adulthood in the affected testis as well as the contralateral testis. Hernias are unrelated to incidence of testicular cancer.

26. D: Difficult examinations should be initially attempted while the child is sitting on a parent's lap. This will allow examination while under the calming care of the parent. Restraints are psychologically traumatic and should be used as a last resort only. Sedation in the operating room is not necessary.

27. B: CF is not directly associated with deafness, so education in sign language is not indicated although repeated treatment with antibiotics (aminoglycosides) can cause sensorineural hearing deficit. Cystic fibrosis is an autosomal recessive disease and the parents should receive genetic counseling about the risk of the disease in future offspring. CF has both pulmonary and pancreatic manifestations so chest percussions and dietary modifications would be appropriate.

28. C: Use of aspirin in febrile children has been linked to the development of Reye's syndrome, a severe respiratory condition. Therefore, aspirin is not recommended for use in children. Fever in children is usually treated with acetaminophen or ibuprofen.

29. A: Jaundice is caused by an elevation of bilirubin, which is monitored to ensure treatment success. As red blood cells break down, bilirubin forms and is excreted through the liver, but the infant's liver may be immature and unable to remove bilirubin fast enough, so bilirubin levels in the blood rise. Ultraviolet light helps to break down bilirubin.

30. D: A nighttime Ph probe requires a special monitoring device be inserted through the nose and down the esophagus to assess for acid reflux into the esophagus, confirming the diagnosis.

31. B: The erythrocyte sedimentation rate is a non-specific marker for inflammation and would be elevated with rheumatoid arthritis. Monospot tests for the Epstein-Barr virus, which causes mononucleosis. WBC tests for infection, and MCV assesses the average volume of red blood cells.

32. C: The posterior superior pelvic area is the preferred choice for bone marrow biopsy site because it is a large flat bone. The skull is too thin and the radius and calcaneus too small.

33. B: An intraosseous line is inserted into the proximal anterior tibia in infants and children to 5 years old for rapid infusion of fluids and medications if another IV site is not accessible. The medial malleolus is used for older children and adults. Other possible sites include the distal femur, clavicle, humerus, and ileum.

34. C: Parvovirus B19 can cause birth defects if contracted by a pregnant mother, so the child should be counseled to avoid anyone pregnant until the disease resolves. Parvovirus B19 is contagious in the time from onset until the bright red rash occurs on the cheeks and a lacy rash on the body. Once the rash appears, the child is probably no longer contagious and can resume normal contacts and activity.

35. A: The most common cause for C. difficile colitis is recent antibiotic use that disrupts the normal colonic flora, allowing overgrowth of the offending bacteria. C. difficile produces a lethal cytotoxin (Toxin B) and an endotoxin with cytotoxic action (Toxin A), which cause fluid to accumulate in the colon and severe damage to mucous membranes.

36. B: A Monospot test for Epstein-Barr virus is used to confirm infectious mononucleosis. The test requires one drop of serum mixed with a special solution. The test can confirm mononucleosis between 2 and 9 weeks after infection. It is not accurate during the incubation period.

37. D: BCG (Bacille Calmette-Guérin) is a tuberculosis vaccine routinely administered to children in countries with high incidences of childhood tuberculous meningitis. PPD can show false positive although PPD may still be used. QuantiFERON-TB®-TB Gold test is not affected by prior BCG vaccination.

38. A: Umbilical hernias are more common in African-American children. They usually resolve with growth of the child by age 4 and do not require surgical correction.

39. B: Breast buds and sparse downy pubic hair are characteristics of Tanner stage 2. Tanner's 5 stages assess maturity of both males and females based on direct observation of breasts and genitals. Females are evaluated on breast development, onset of menses, and pubic hair distribution. Males are evaluation on penis and testes development and pubic hair distribution.

40. D: Apocrine sweat glands develop with the increase in hormones during the onset of puberty and are located primarily in the axilla and pubic area, opening into hair follicles. These sweat glands cause body odor.

41. B: Prolonged exposure to loud noises (music, power tools, firearms) can lead to high frequency hearing loss at the 4000-Hertz level, making it hard for the child to hear high-pitched voices and certain sounds, such as consonants. Digital hearing aids may be programmed to compensate for high frequency hearing loss.

42. D: Cellulitis, a bacterial skin infection, is not associated with dehydration. Burns, diabetic ketoacidosis, and hyperventilation may all contribute to dehydration in children.

43. A: The ingestion of aspirin (salicylic acid) puts the patient at risk for a metabolic acidosis due to the acidic medication. Symptoms include drowsiness, confusion, headache, decreased blood pressure, flushed skin, nausea, vomiting, diarrhea and tachypnea.

44. B: Tachycardia, not bradycardia, is a common sign of dehydration in pediatric patients. Children with dehydration typically are thirsty and have dry mucous membranes, reduced skin turgor, and depressed fontanelles (in infants).

45. C: Due to volume loss, the hematocrit will be elevated as red blood cells become more concentrated in the blood. The MCV test shows the average size of the red blood cells and helps to determine the type of anemia while RDW shows the variations in cell size, important for some types of anemia (such as pernicious anemia).

46. D: Infectious diarrhea remains the leading cause of death in developing countries. Outbreaks of diarrhea are common in areas with poor sanitation that allows food and water to become contaminated with bacteria, such as *E. coli* or *Shigella*.

47. A: Rotavirus is the most common cause for viral diarrhea in children and may be accompanied by nausea and vomiting that lead to severe dehydration. Parainfluenza, influenza, and parvovirus B19 cause mainly upper respiratory illnesses.

48. B: Giardia Lamblia is a parasite that is commonly spread via the drinking of contaminated water, especially streams that are contaminated with animal feces. A broad spectrum of gastrointestinal symptoms can occur.

49. B: Celiac disease is not infectious and not related to travel. Celiac disease (sprue) is sensitivity to gluten products and is more commonly seen in children with relatives with the disease, those with trisomy 21, or those with type 1 diabetes.

50. B: A burn area that is red with blistering is consistent with a second-degree burn. A first-degree burn would have erythema but no blistering, and a third-degree burn would be dry and leathery. Burns are not classified as fourth-degree.

51. A: IgE is the primary antibody used in the defense of parasitic infections and is involved in allergic responses. IgM increases in response to infection, and IgG provides a secondary response to infection. IgA provides immune response in mucous membranes and decreases with immunosuppression and some infections (gonorrhea).

52. A: Children less than 6 months of age have immature immune systems, so a fever in a 3-month-old child would necessitate a full work up for sepsis.

53. D: As the varicella vaccine is live, it should not be given to anyone with a potentially suppressed immune system, such as a child with HIV, as it may cause infection even in such a small dose. Hep B, DTaP (diphtheria, tetanus, and acellular pertussis), and influenza are not live vaccines and are all recommended in this patient population.

54. C: Patients with no spleen function (either from removal after trauma or autoinfarction due to sickle cell disease) should have the pneumococcal vaccine to prevent infection with encapsulated bacteria.

55. D: A patient with streptococcal pharyngitis does not have a chronic medical condition for which influenza administration is recommended. Children with chronic diseases, such as renal disease, HIV, and type 1 diabetes, should receive the influenza vaccine as influenza infection could be life threatening.

56. C: Peri-orbital cellulitis can spread to the central nervous system and lead to meningitis due to the venous drainage from this area. The infection can travel along vessels and nerve pathways into the lining of the brain. Peri-orbital cellulitis should be treated with antibiotics and the patient closely monitored.

57. A: An elevated WBC, not a decreased level, is consistent with a diagnosis of bacterial meningitis along with elevated protein, decreased glucose, and cloudiness in the cerebrospinal fluid.

58. C: Prednisolone is a corticosteroid and is used to reduce inflammation but is not a bronchodilator. Albuterol, theophylline, and levalbuterol are all bronchodilators used to treat asthma by increasing airflow.

59. A: Mucomyst is a mucolytic agent that is used to thin secretions and is especially useful in patients with cystic fibrosis. Prednisolone is used to treat inflammation, and albuterol and theophylline are bronchodilators.

60. C: *C. difficile* is a bacterial pathogen found in the GI tract and is not a common cause of acute otitis media. *Streptococcus pneumoniae*, *Haemophilus influenzae*, and *Moraxella catarrhalis* can all cause otitis media.

61. D: Epiglottiditis is the acute inflammation of the epiglottis and is usually caused by *Haemophilus influenza* infection. Children often present sitting forward (tripod position) with their heads tilted backward to try to relieve the airway obstruction. In addition to possible intubation, oxygen and steroids are the mainstays of treatment.

62. B: Cystic fibrosis is an autosomal recessive genetic disease, so both parents must pass on a recessive gene to the child. Parents of a child with CF should have genetic counseling so they are aware that they have a 1 in 4 chance of any additional children being born with CF.

63. B: Cystic fibrosis patients often need pancreatic enzymes supplementation because the pancreatic ducts may become plugged with mucous plugs. Fat-soluble vitamins A, D, E, and K assist with digestion. Constipation is common, but routine use of laxatives should be avoided.

64. D: The infant should be fed in a semi-upright position rather than Trendelenburg to direct the formula away from the cleft and to the back of the mouth to prevent aspiration. Feeding slowly, burping often, using special nipples, and stimulating sucking by rubbing the nipple against the infant's lower lip are all strategies to facilitate feeding.

65. A: The pressure of a barium enema against the intussusception is often enough to reduce it, returning the intestine to its normal position, although the intussusception can recur and may require surgical repair.

66. D: The typical life span of a red blood cell is 120 days. Red blood cells contain hemoglobin, which carries oxygen to cells and carbon dioxide back to the lungs.

67. C: Pale, not pink oral mucosa would be present with anemia. Fatigue, bruising, and conjunctival pallor all indicate anemia.

68. C: The mean corpuscular volume (MCV) measures the average size of the red blood cells. This helps to classify anemia as microcytic, normocytic, or macrocytic.

69. A: A smaller RBC size (decreased MCV) rather than larger would be found in iron-deficiency anemia. Other indicators include decreased hemoglobin, decreased RBC mass, and decreased oxygen carrying capacity, as iron is necessary for the formation of hemoglobin, which carries oxygen.

70. B: Sickle cell disease is a genetic hemolytic disease and is the most common hemoglobinopathy in African-Americans. It causes sickling of the red blood cells because of abnormal strands in the hemoglobin.

71. A: ITP represents an acquired deficiency of platelets (thrombocytes) leading to increased risk of bleeding. ITP is believed caused by an autoimmune process. Normal minimal platelet count is 140,000 for newborns and 150, 000 for older children. If the platelet count drops below 50,000, the child is at high risk for hemorrhage.

72. D: Potatoes do not provide a good source of iron in the diet. Green leafy vegetables, such as spinach, and all meats, including lean beef and chicken, are good iron sources.

73. D: A blood pressure reading of 80/40 is considered in the normal range for infants of 3 months old. Blood pressure in older children varies according to height and weight.

74. B: The P-wave represents atrial depolarization and is used to mark the starting point of a new PQRS wave, which represents right and left ventricular depolarization. The T-wave represents ventricular repolarization (a resting period).

75. B: Enalapril is an angiotensin-converting enzyme inhibitor and is not a diuretic. Furosemide, spironolactone, and bumetanide are commonly-used diuretics.

76. C: Prostaglandin synthetase inhibitors, such as indomethacin, can be used in neonates to close PDA's non-surgically. They are 80% effective if given within 10 days of birth. Some children require surgical repair.

77. C: Ventricular septal defect, the most common congenital heart defect, is an abnormal opening in the septum between the right and left ventricles. Depending on the size of the defect, some may close spontaneously and others may require surgical closure using a graft.

78. B: Pulmonic stenosis can lead to right heart failure if not treated. Pulmonic stenosis is a stricture of the pulmonary blood vessel that controls the flow of blood from the right ventricle to the lungs, resulting in right ventricular hypertrophy, as the pressure increases in the right ventricle, and decreased pulmonary blood flow. Aortic stenosis, coarctation of the aorta, and tricuspid atresia would lead to left heart failure.

79. A: Digoxin has a narrow therapeutic window and requires monitoring for the blood level to prevent toxicity in children.

80. D: Rheumatic fever is an autoimmune disease that results from a response after an untreated infection with group A beta-hemolytic *Streptococcus*. RF can result in damage to the heart valves and to the joints.

81. B: Fever, along with arthralgias and lab findings, such as elevated erythrocyte sedimentation rate and C-reactive protein, are considered minor Jones criteria. Polyarthritis, carditis, and chorea are major criteria. Rheumatic fever is diagnosed when 2 major criteria or one major and 2 minor criteria are met.

82. C: Carbonated sodas actually alkalinize the urine and are a poor choice in the treatment of a bladder infection. Cranberry juice apple juice, and prune juice are good choices to acidify urine. Citrus juices, such as lemonade and orange juice, alkalinize the urine.

83. A: OI is a genetic disorder that results from the reduction in the synthesis of collagen, causing connective tissue and bone defects, such as "brittle bones," that lead to multiple fractures.

84. B: An incomplete fracture that does not fully extend through a bone is a greenstick fracture. A buckle fracture is common in children and involves an incomplete fracture with buckling of bone on one side only. Bend fractures involve bending of the soft bone without breaking. Open fractures break through the skin.

85. D: Muscular dystrophy is usually first evident at age 3 to 5 and observed with delays in motor development and weakness in the pelvic girdle. Children may have trouble standing and may fall easily. Calf muscles may begin to enlarge.

86. C: Atonic seizures are characterized by a loss of muscle tone and often a fall and then a period of confusion from a postictal state. Tonic seizures include muscle twitching and changes in consciousness. Clonic seizures are generalized seizures often accompanied by loss of consciousness. Absence seizures cause a lack of consciousness.

87. D: Additional folic acid (0.4 mg per day) is recommended to decrease the risk of neural tube defects during pregnancy. All women of childbearing age should have counseling regarding the importance of folic acid.

88. C: Oxytocin as well as antidiuretic hormone are the two secretions of the posterior pituitary gland. The anterior pituitary gland produces growth hormone, thyroid stimulating hormone, prolactin, adrenocorticotropic hormone, follicle stimulating hormone, beta endorphin, and luteinizing hormone.

89. A: Aldosterone is secreted by the adrenal gland. Insulin, glucagon, and somatostatin are all secretions by the islets of Langerhans.

90. B: Weight gain, not weight loss is a cardinal sign of SIADH because of fluid retention and decreased urinary output caused by the hyponatremia resulting from increased secretion of antidiuretic hormone. Weakness is an additional sign of SIADH.

91. D: Leukemias remain the most common type of cancer in childhood. Brain tumors are the most common SOLID tumors in children. Lymphomas are the third most common type of tumor. The most common type of kidney tumor is Wilms tumor.

92. D: The proper ratio of chest compressions to breaths in a child of 9 months is 30:2. Compressions should be done rapidly to a count of 30 followed by 2 breaths. Brain damage can occur within 4 minutes and death within 8 minutes if the brain is deprived of oxygen.

93. D: Eye tracking is not a component as the child is not able to focus well enough to track at birth. Heart rate, color, muscle tone, reflex irritability, and respiratory effort are the components of the Apgar scoring system.

94. D: The proper initial voltage for defibrillation of a 2-year-old child is 2 J/kg. If unsuccessful, the next shock is done with 2 to 4 J/kg and then 4 J/kg.

95. C: Epinephrine is the initial drug used in the treatment of ventricular fibrillation if defibrillation is not successful. Each dose of epinephrine is usually followed by an attempt at defibrillation. If epinephrine and defibrillation are ineffective, then an antiarrhythmic, such as amiodarone or lidocaine, is used. Magnesium sulfate is indicated with torsades de pointes (a variant form of VF).

96. A: Lab analysis of a sample from an IO line is not accurate for WBC count or platelet count but can be used to type and cross match blood and for hemoglobin and electrolytes although it is less accurate than blood samples for calcium, potassium, and glucose levels.

97. C: Hypokalemia is not a common side effect of use of succinylcholine, but the drug can cause hyperkalemia, which may result in cardiac abnormalities, such as decreased heart rate. Increased intracranial pressure, increased blood pressure, and increased eye pressure are commonly seen and need to be monitored when using this medication.

98. D: Hyperthyroidism commonly causes an increase in T-wave amplitude, not a decrease. Myocarditis, hypokalemia, and digitalis toxicity are common reasons for inverted or decreased T-waves.

99. C: Adenosine commonly causes a brief asystolic episode, which can be uncomfortable for the patient. Other side effects include a metallic taste in the mouth, chest pressure, flushing, nausea, dyspnea, arm tingling, and discomfort in the neck and jaw.

100. D: Vitamin C can cause false negative stool Guaiac results. Red meat, fresh cherries, and horseradish all can cause false positive results for the Guaiac test.

101. A: *E. coli* O157:H7 from contaminated ground meat is the most common bacterial cause of HUS although other bacteria, such as *Shigella dysenteriae*, may also cause HUS.

102. B: Renal disease is the most common cause of secondary hypertension in the pediatric population. Coarctation of the aorta, neuroblastoma, and drug toxicity are less common causes of secondary hypertension. Primary hypertension is also on the rise, related to obesity, lack of exercise, and poor nutrition

103. A: N-Acetylcysteine (Mucomyst) is the medication used for acetaminophen overdoses. Toxicity occurs with dosage >140 mg/kg in one dose or >7.5g in 24 hours. The 72-hour N-acetylcysteine (NAC) protocol includes 140 mg/kg initially and 70 mg/kg every 4 hours for 17 more doses (orally or IV). Naloxone is used for opiate overdoses, and activated charcoal is used for numerous other medication overdoses.

104. C: Hemisection of the spinal cord, severing it on one side only, and its associated symptoms are referred to as Brown-Sequard syndrome. Anterior cord syndrome results in loss of motor abilities and some sensations (temperature, pain, vibration) below injury. Posterior cord syndrome retains motor functions but some sensation is lost below injury. Complete cord injury results in bilateral paralysis and lack of sensation below injury.

105. D: Pupillary constriction, not dilation, is a hallmark of opiate overdose. Decreased respiratory rate, lethargy, and decreased bowel sounds are common physical symptoms of opiate overdose.

106. A: The femoral vein is the most medial structure in the inguinal canal, so venipuncture should be attempted medially to where the femoral artery is palpated at the femoral triangle.

107. D: Decreased interest in parental activities is consistent with independence activities in which the adolescent begins to move away from the dependence of childhood to establish her own identity. This period is often characterized by rebellion and withdrawal from the family.

108. C: A history of thromboembolic disease, such as deep vein thrombosis, is a contraindication to the use of oral contraceptive pills, as this is a side effect of the drugs.

109. B: A shortened PR interval, delta wave, and wide QRS pattern with a history of SVT are suggestive of WPW. Atrial impulses are conducted via an anomalous pathway to the ventricles leading to a premature and prolonged depolarization of the ventricles. Ablation of the pathway is often needed.

110. B: Molluscum contagiosum is caused by the poxvirus and is usually treated with debridement, liquid nitrogen, or topical salicylates. This virus often spreads from contact with someone with eczema or immunocompromised. Once infected, the lesions may persist for up to 2 years even with treatment.

111. C: Childhood obesity is the primary risk factor for type 2 diabetes, and the marked recent increase in this disease corresponds with the concomitant increase in obesity. Obesity often correlates with very high carbohydrate diets and poor overall nutrition.

112. A: Tachycardia, not bradycardia is a common symptom of hyperthyroidism due to increase in circulating thyroid hormone levels. Insomnia, heat intolerance, and weight loss are common symptoms. Ophthalmic changes, including bulging of the eyeball, may also occur.

113. D: Renal failure causes hyperkalemia rather than hypokalemia. The hyperkalemia associated with renal failure often requires medications or dialysis. Diarrhea caused by infection or use of laxatives and diabetic ketoacidosis may result in hypokalemia.

114. C: Cystic fibrosis is a disorder of chloride channels in cells and is not an inborn error of metabolism disorder, argininosuccinase deficiency, ornithine transcarbamylase deficiency, and HMG-CoA lyase deficiency are inborn errors of metabolism. Hyperammonemia is common to many diseases associated with an inborn error of metabolism.

115. B: With only one X sex chromosome and no Y, all patients with Turner's syndrome are female, not male, as males die in utero. Common indications of Turner's syndrome include webbed neck, short stature, and broad chest. In addition, females often lack functioning ovaries.

116. D: Patients with Marfan syndrome have a disorder of connective tissue and can develop dilation of the aortic root. Marfan's syndrome is characterized by tall stature and longs limbs and digits. Patients may need treatment with beta-blockers or even synthetic grafting repair if an aneurysm develops.

117. D: The reticulocyte count is a measure of the production of new red blood cells by the body. Reticulocytes are immature red blood cells. When red blood cell production increases to offset blood loss, more reticulocytes are released into the circulation. An insufficient level may indicate a problem with the red blood cell producing elements of the body.

118. B: FFP contains all of the clotting factors (V, VII, and IX) except for platelets. FFP can be used in the treatment of disseminated intravascular coagulation (DIC) and thrombotic thrombocytopenic purpura (TTP), disorders that cause excessive bleeding.

119. B: Rhinitis medicamentosa is rebound rhinitis caused from the prolonged use (usually about a week) of nasal vasoconstrictors. Discontinuation of the offending OTC medication is necessary to reduce symptoms.

120. C: Lyme disease is caused by the spirochete Borrelia burgdorferi, which is inoculated by a bite from a deer tick. About 80% of people with early Lyme disease develop erythema migrans ("bulls'-eye rash") within 1 to 30 days after infection.

121. D: Gonorrhea is caused by a cocci bacterium. Lyme disease, syphilis, and yaws are all caused by spirochetes. Syphilis and yaws are caused by Treponema while Lyme disease is caused by the Borrelia burgdorferi spirochete.

122. A: *Giardia lamblia* is a protozoan that causes infectious gastroenteritis in those who drink contaminated water or touch contaminated hands to the mouth. *Salmonella typhi*, E. coli, and *Vibrio cholera* are bacteria.

123. A: Nagele's rule uses the mother's LMP and is the most accurate determination of gestational age. It is represented as estimated date of confinement (EDC) = 280 days + 7 days from LMP.

124. A: The normal term FHR is 120 to 160 beats per minute. Some variation is normal but a change that persists for more than 15 minutes is significant. Mild bradycardia is 100 to 120 bpm and severe bradycardia is <90 bpm.

125. C: BMI is calculated by weight in kilograms divided by height in meters squared. It is a useful tool in assessing weight issues.

126. C: Vitamin C is a water-soluble vitamin. Water-soluble vitamins are excreted rapidly so they do not cause toxicity although excess dosages may have some adverse effects. Vitamins A, D, E, and K are all fat-soluble and are stored in the fat for longer periods of time, so excess dosages are more likely to result in toxic reactions, such as liver toxicity.

127. B: Asthma symptoms occurring daily and more than one night during the week are classified as moderate persistent. Treatment includes inhaled steroids with long-acting inhaled beta2-agonists.

128. D: Abraham Maslow wrote about the "hierarchy of needs" concept. Carl Rogers developed the person-centered humanistic approach to psychology. Lawrence Kohlberg described stages in moral development, and John Bowlby developed a theory of attachment.

129. C: "Concrete operational thinking" stage occurs in the 7 to 12 age range when the child is able to think more logically but relies on the concrete rather than the abstract. As children become more able to understand complex issues in adolescence, they progress to the "formal operational thinking" stage.

130. D: A strict, harsh parent with high expectations but poor communication is authoritarian. Authoritarian, permissive-neglectful, and democratic indulgent parenting styles are less effective than authoritative.

131. A: The central incisors are usually the first permanent teeth to erupt around age 7 to 8, followed by the lateral incisors, the canines, the premolars (bicuspids), and finally the molars.

132. B: A pattern of aggressive behavior with violation of the law and social norms is typical of conduct disorder. DSM-5 criteria also include aggressive behavior to people or animals, destruction of property, lying or stealing, and serious rule violations.

133. C: Avoidance of tasks that require mental attention and focus is a finding more consistent with ADHD than oppositional-defiant disorder, which involves defiant behavior rather than impaired mental ability.

134. B: Cystic fibrosis is not linked to any learning disabilities. Lead poisoning, fetal alcohol syndrome, and fragile-X syndrome are all common conditions associated with learning disabilities.

135. B: Edema of the scalp is caput succedaneum and usually resolves after 2 to 4 days. A cephalohematoma will not usually cross suture lines. Macrocephaly is an enlarged head, and microcephaly is a small head.

136. D: The 47XXY genetic typing is Klinefelter's syndrome. Turner's syndrome is 45XO. Trisomy 18 occurs with 3 copies of the 18th chromosome, causing many medical disorders. Trisomy 21 occurs with an extra 21st chromosome, resulting in intellectual disability as well as physical abnormalities.

137. D: The inability to retract the foreskin past the glans penis after the age of 5 is called phimosis. As this can lead to painful swelling, a consultation with a urologist for potential circumcision is advised. Cryptorchidism is an undescended testis. Hydrocele occurs when an abnormality causes fluid to collect in the scrotum or along the spermatic cord. Varicocele is a varicosity in the vessels about the spermatic cord.

138. D: A palpable "clunk" with a flexed, adducted hip is a positive Barlow test and indicates hip dislocation or subluxation present. Ortolani's test is also used to diagnose congenital hip dislocation. Gower's sign assesses muscle weakness in the lower limbs and is used with Duchenne's muscular dystrophy. Allis's sign indicates fracture of the femur neck.

139. C: The degree of induration determines a positive PPD Mantoux test. Blistering may also indicate a positive reaction in some children.

140. B: Hydrocephalus leads to macrocephaly in most cases while intrauterine TORCH infections, fetal alcohol syndrome, and phenylketonuria affect the development of the brain and can lead to microcephaly.

141. A: If the eye deviates inwardly, the lateral rectus is weak. If the lateral rectus muscle is weak, the medial rectus is unopposed in its adduction action, resulting in esotropia.

142. D: Hand, foot and mouth disease is most commonly caused by Coxsackievirus A16. Treatment is limited to symptomatic therapy until the lesions resolve.

143. C: Cromolyn is an inhaled medication that acts by preventing mast cell from releasing their contents. It is useful in chronic asthma to reduce attacks but is not effective for the treatment of acute asthma.

144. A: Milia are small raised lesions that spontaneously resolve. They are the result of keratinous material accumulated within the pilosebaceous follicle area. Erythema toxicum neonatorum is a self-limiting erythematous, blotchy macular rash on the face and torso. Cutis marmorata is the mottling of skin, common after birth. Nevus flammeus is a port-wine stain, a type of vascular birthmark.

145. B: Acquired hypopigmented patches on the skin surface is consistent with vitiligo. As the spots lack melanin, they should be protected from the sun. Albinism is a genetic disorder that involves lack of pigmentation. Pityriasis rosacea is a scaly rash that appears in patches about the body. Pityriasis alba causes dry scaly pale patches on the skin, lasting a year or more.

146. C: Tinea corporis (ringworm) is a fungal infection of the skin causing circular lesions primarily on the arms and legs. It is treated with anti-fungal topical medications. Molluscum contagiosum, plantar warts, and shingles (herpes zoster) are all caused by viruses.

147. D: Interaction of an antigen with IgE takes place on the surface of a mast cell and leads to degranulation of these cells. The substances in these granules can then lead to the overwhelming response seen in anaphylactic conditions.

148. A: Hepatitis A is transmitted via a fecal/oral route, from raw shellfish and contaminated water. It is not normally transmitted via a bloodborne route as is Hepatitis B and C. Transmission often occurs in daycare centers from contamination from soiled diapers with the highest rate of infection from ages 5 to 14. The incubation period is about 15 to 50 days.

149. B: A child with Trisomy 21 would not normally have a decreased immune system and would not have an increased risk for sepsis. Both the child with HIV and the one receiving chemotherapy are immunocompromised, increasing risk. The 2-week child's immune system is still immature, putting the child at risk.

150. C: Genu varum refers to bowing of the legs. Genu valgum is the abnormal closeness between the knees (knock-knees). Metatarsus varus and adductus refer to forefoot conditions.

How to Overcome Test Anxiety

Just the thought of taking a test is enough to make most people a little nervous. A test is an important event that can have a long-term impact on your future, so it's important to take it seriously and it's natural to feel anxious about performing well. But just because anxiety is normal, that doesn't mean that it's helpful in test taking, or that you should simply accept it as part of your life. Anxiety can have a variety of effects. These effects can be mild, like making you feel slightly nervous, or severe, like blocking your ability to focus or remember even a simple detail.

If you experience test anxiety—whether severe or mild—it's important to know how to beat it. To discover this, first you need to understand what causes test anxiety.

Causes of Test Anxiety

While we often think of anxiety as an uncontrollable emotional state, it can actually be caused by simple, practical things. One of the most common causes of test anxiety is that a person does not feel adequately prepared for their test. This feeling can be the result of many different issues such as poor study habits or lack of organization, but the most common culprit is time management. Starting to study too late, failing to organize your study time to cover all of the material, or being distracted while you study will mean that you're not well prepared for the test. This may lead to cramming the night before, which will cause you to be physically and mentally exhausted for the test. Poor time management also contributes to feelings of stress, fear, and hopelessness as you realize you are not well prepared but don't know what to do about it.

Other times, test anxiety is not related to your preparation for the test but comes from unresolved fear. This may be a past failure on a test, or poor performance on tests in general. It may come from comparing yourself to others who seem to be performing better or from the stress of living up to expectations. Anxiety may be driven by fears of the future—how failure on this test would affect your educational and career goals. These fears are often completely irrational, but they can still negatively impact your test performance.

Elements of Test Anxiety

As mentioned earlier, test anxiety is considered to be an emotional state, but it has physical and mental components as well. Sometimes you may not even realize that you are suffering from test anxiety until you notice the physical symptoms. These can include trembling hands, rapid heartbeat, sweating, nausea, and tense muscles. Extreme anxiety may lead to fainting or vomiting. Obviously, any of these symptoms can have a negative impact on testing. It is important to recognize them as soon as they begin to occur so that you can address the problem before it damages your performance.

The mental components of test anxiety include trouble focusing and inability to remember learned information. During a test, your mind is on high alert, which can help you recall information and stay focused for an extended period of time. However, anxiety interferes with your mind's natural processes, causing you to blank out, even on the questions you know well. The strain of testing during anxiety makes it difficult to stay focused, especially on a test that may take several hours. Extreme anxiety can take a huge mental toll, making it difficult not only to recall test information but even to understand the test questions or pull your thoughts together.

Effects of Test Anxiety

Test anxiety is like a disease—if left untreated, it will get progressively worse. Anxiety leads to poor performance, and this reinforces the feelings of fear and failure, which in turn lead to poor performances on subsequent tests. It can grow from a mild nervousness to a crippling condition. If allowed to progress, test anxiety can have a big impact on your schooling, and consequently on your future.

Test anxiety can spread to other parts of your life. Anxiety on tests can become anxiety in any stressful situation, and blanking on a test can turn into panicking in a job situation. But fortunately, you don't have to let anxiety rule your testing and determine your grades. There are a number of relatively simple steps you can take to move past anxiety and function normally on a test and in the rest of life.

Physical Steps for Beating Test Anxiety

While test anxiety is a serious problem, the good news is that it can be overcome. It doesn't have to control your ability to think and remember information. While it may take time, you can begin taking steps today to beat anxiety.

Just as your first hint that you may be struggling with anxiety comes from the physical symptoms, the first step to treating it is also physical. Rest is crucial for having a clear, strong mind. If you are tired, it is much easier to give in to anxiety. But if you establish good sleep habits, your body and mind will be ready to perform optimally, without the strain of exhaustion. Additionally, sleeping well helps you to retain information better, so you're more likely to recall the answers when you see the test questions.

Getting good sleep means more than going to bed on time. It's important to allow your brain time to relax. Take study breaks from time to time so it doesn't get overworked, and don't study right before bed. Take time to rest your mind before trying to rest your body, or you may find it difficult to fall asleep.

Along with sleep, other aspects of physical health are important in preparing for a test. Good nutrition is vital for good brain function. Sugary foods and drinks may give a burst of energy but this burst is followed by a crash, both physically and emotionally. Instead, fuel your body with protein and vitamin-rich foods.

Also, drink plenty of water. Dehydration can lead to headaches and exhaustion, especially if your brain is already under stress from the rigors of the test. Particularly if your test is a long one, drink water during the breaks. And if possible, take an energy-boosting snack to eat between sections.

Along with sleep and diet, a third important part of physical health is exercise. Maintaining a steady workout schedule is helpful, but even taking 5-minute study breaks to walk can help get your blood pumping faster and clear your head. Exercise also releases endorphins, which contribute to a positive feeling and can help combat test anxiety.

When you nurture your physical health, you are also contributing to your mental health. If your body is healthy, your mind is much more likely to be healthy as well. So take time to rest, nourish your body with healthy food and water, and get moving as much as possible. Taking these physical steps will make you stronger and more able to take the mental steps necessary to overcome test anxiety.

Mental Steps for Beating Test Anxiety

Working on the mental side of test anxiety can be more challenging, but as with the physical side, there are clear steps you can take to overcome it. As mentioned earlier, test anxiety often stems from lack of preparation, so the obvious solution is to prepare for the test. Effective studying may be the most important weapon you have for beating test anxiety, but you can and should employ several other mental tools to combat fear.

First, boost your confidence by reminding yourself of past success—tests or projects that you aced. If you're putting as much effort into preparing for this test as you did for those, there's no reason you should expect to fail here. Work hard to prepare; then trust your preparation.

Second, surround yourself with encouraging people. It can be helpful to find a study group, but be sure that the people you're around will encourage a positive attitude. If you spend time with others who are anxious or cynical, this will only contribute to your own anxiety. Look for others who are motivated to study hard from a desire to succeed, not from a fear of failure.

Third, reward yourself. A test is physically and mentally tiring, even without anxiety, and it can be helpful to have something to look forward to. Plan an activity following the test, regardless of the outcome, such as going to a movie or getting ice cream.

When you are taking the test, if you find yourself beginning to feel anxious, remind yourself that you know the material. Visualize successfully completing the test. Then take a few deep, relaxing breaths and return to it. Work through the questions carefully but with confidence, knowing that you are capable of succeeding.

Developing a healthy mental approach to test taking will also aid in other areas of life. Test anxiety affects more than just the actual test—it can be damaging to your mental health and even contribute to depression. It's important to beat test anxiety before it becomes a problem for more than testing.

Study Strategy

Being prepared for the test is necessary to combat anxiety, but what does being prepared look like? You may study for hours on end and still not feel prepared. What you need is a strategy for test prep. The next few pages outline our recommended steps to help you plan out and conquer the challenge of preparation.

STEP 1: SCOPE OUT THE TEST

Learn everything you can about the format (multiple choice, essay, etc.) and what will be on the test. Gather any study materials, course outlines, or sample exams that may be available. Not only will this help you to prepare, but knowing what to expect can help to alleviate test anxiety.

STEP 2: MAP OUT THE MATERIAL

Look through the textbook or study guide and make note of how many chapters or sections it has. Then divide these over the time you have. For example, if a book has 15 chapters and you have five days to study, you need to cover three chapters each day. Even better, if you have the time, leave an extra day at the end for overall review after you have gone through the material in depth.

If time is limited, you may need to prioritize the material. Look through it and make note of which sections you think you already have a good grasp on, and which need review. While you are studying, skim quickly through the familiar sections and take more time on the challenging parts. Write out your plan so you don't get lost as you go. Having a written plan also helps you feel more in control of the study, so anxiety is less likely to arise from feeling overwhelmed at the amount to cover.

STEP 3: GATHER YOUR TOOLS

Decide what study method works best for you. Do you prefer to highlight in the book as you study and then go back over the highlighted portions? Or do you type out notes of the important information? Or is it helpful to make flashcards that you can carry with you? Assemble the pens, index cards, highlighters, post-it notes, and any other materials you may need so you won't be distracted by getting up to find things while you study.

If you're having a hard time retaining the information or organizing your notes, experiment with different methods. For example, try color-coding by subject with colored pens, highlighters, or post-it notes. If you learn better by hearing, try recording yourself reading your notes so you can listen while in the car, working out, or simply sitting at your desk. Ask a friend to quiz you from your flashcards, or try teaching someone the material to solidify it in your mind.

STEP 4: CREATE YOUR ENVIRONMENT

It's important to avoid distractions while you study. This includes both the obvious distractions like visitors and the subtle distractions like an uncomfortable chair (or a too-comfortable couch that makes you want to fall asleep). Set up the best study environment possible: good lighting and a comfortable work area. If background music helps you focus, you may want to turn it on, but otherwise keep the room quiet. If you are using a computer to take notes, be sure you don't have any other windows open, especially applications like social media, games, or anything else that could distract you. Silence your phone and turn off notifications. Be sure to keep water close by so you stay hydrated while you study (but avoid unhealthy drinks and snacks).

Also, take into account the best time of day to study. Are you freshest first thing in the morning? Try to set aside some time then to work through the material. Is your mind clearer in the afternoon or evening? Schedule your study session then. Another method is to study at the same time of day that you will take the test, so that your brain gets used to working on the material at that time and will be ready to focus at test time.

STEP 5: STUDY!

Once you have done all the study preparation, it's time to settle into the actual studying. Sit down, take a few moments to settle your mind so you can focus, and begin to follow your study plan. Don't give in to distractions or let yourself procrastinate. This is your time to prepare so you'll be ready to fearlessly approach the test. Make the most of the time and stay focused.

Of course, you don't want to burn out. If you study too long you may find that you're not retaining the information very well. Take regular study breaks. For example, taking five minutes out of every hour to walk briskly, breathing deeply and swinging your arms, can help your mind stay fresh.

As you get to the end of each chapter or section, it's a good idea to do a quick review. Remind yourself of what you learned and work on any difficult parts. When you feel that you've mastered the material, move on to the next part. At the end of your study session, briefly skim through your notes again.

But while review is helpful, cramming last minute is NOT. If at all possible, work ahead so that you won't need to fit all your study into the last day. Cramming overloads your brain with more information than it can process and retain, and your tired mind may struggle to recall even previously learned information when it is overwhelmed with last-minute study. Also, the urgent nature of cramming and the stress placed on your brain contribute to anxiety. You'll be more likely to go to the test feeling unprepared and having trouble thinking clearly.

So don't cram, and don't stay up late before the test, even just to review your notes at a leisurely pace. Your brain needs rest more than it needs to go over the information again. In fact, plan to finish your studies by noon or early afternoon the day before the test. Give your brain the rest of the day to relax or focus on other things, and get a good night's sleep. Then you will be fresh for the test and better able to recall what you've studied.

STEP 6: TAKE A PRACTICE TEST

Many courses offer sample tests, either online or in the study materials. This is an excellent resource to check whether you have mastered the material, as well as to prepare for the test format and environment.

Check the test format ahead of time: the number of questions, the type (multiple choice, free response, etc.), and the time limit. Then create a plan for working through them. For example, if you have 30 minutes to take a 60-question test, your limit is 30 seconds per question. Spend less time on the questions you know well so that you can take more time on the difficult ones.

If you have time to take several practice tests, take the first one open book, with no time limit. Work through the questions at your own pace and make sure you fully understand them. Gradually work up to taking a test under test conditions: sit at a desk with all study materials put away and set a timer. Pace yourself to make sure you finish the test with time to spare and go back to check your answers if you have time.

After each test, check your answers. On the questions you missed, be sure you understand why you missed them. Did you misread the question (tests can use tricky wording)? Did you forget the information? Or was it something you hadn't learned? Go back and study any shaky areas that the practice tests reveal.

Taking these tests not only helps with your grade, but also aids in combating test anxiety. If you're already used to the test conditions, you're less likely to worry about it, and working through tests until you're scoring well gives you a confidence boost. Go through the practice tests until you feel comfortable, and then you can go into the test knowing that you're ready for it.

Test Tips

On test day, you should be confident, knowing that you've prepared well and are ready to answer the questions. But aside from preparation, there are several test day strategies you can employ to maximize your performance.

First, as stated before, get a good night's sleep the night before the test (and for several nights before that, if possible). Go into the test with a fresh, alert mind rather than staying up late to study.

Try not to change too much about your normal routine on the day of the test. It's important to eat a nutritious breakfast, but if you normally don't eat breakfast at all, consider eating just a protein bar. If you're a coffee drinker, go ahead and have your normal coffee. Just make sure you time it so that the caffeine doesn't wear off right in the middle of your test. Avoid sugary beverages, and drink enough water to stay hydrated but not so much that you need a restroom break 10 minutes into the test. If your test isn't first thing in the morning, consider going for a walk or doing a light workout before the test to get your blood flowing.

Allow yourself enough time to get ready, and leave for the test with plenty of time to spare so you won't have the anxiety of scrambling to arrive in time. Another reason to be early is to select a good seat. It's helpful to sit away from doors and windows, which can be distracting. Find a good seat, get out your supplies, and settle your mind before the test begins.

When the test begins, start by going over the instructions carefully, even if you already know what to expect. Make sure you avoid any careless mistakes by following the directions.

Then begin working through the questions, pacing yourself as you've practiced. If you're not sure on an answer, don't spend too much time on it, and don't let it shake your confidence. Either skip it and come back later, or eliminate as many wrong answers as possible and guess among the remaining ones. Don't dwell on these questions as you continue—put them out of your mind and focus on what lies ahead.

Be sure to read all of the answer choices, even if you're sure the first one is the right answer. Sometimes you'll find a better one if you keep reading. But don't second-guess yourself if you do immediately know the answer. Your gut instinct is usually right. Don't let test anxiety rob you of the information you know.

If you have time at the end of the test (and if the test format allows), go back and review your answers. Be cautious about changing any, since your first instinct tends to be correct, but make sure you didn't misread any of the questions or accidentally mark the wrong answer choice. Look over any you skipped and make an educated guess.

At the end, leave the test feeling confident. You've done your best, so don't waste time worrying about your performance or wishing you could change anything. Instead, celebrate the successful completion of this test. And finally, use this test to learn how to deal with anxiety even better next time.

> **Review Video: Test Anxiety**
> Visit mometrix.com/academy and enter code: 100340

Important Qualification

Not all anxiety is created equal. If your test anxiety is causing major issues in your life beyond the classroom or testing center, or if you are experiencing troubling physical symptoms related to your anxiety, it may be a sign of a serious physiological or psychological condition. If this sounds like your situation, we strongly encourage you to seek professional help.

Tell Us Your Story

We at Mometrix would like to extend our heartfelt thanks to you for letting us be a part of your journey. It is an honor to serve people from all walks of life, people like you, who are committed to building the best future they can for themselves.

We know that each person's situation is unique. But we also know that, whether you are a young student or a mother of four, you care about working to make your own life and the lives of those around you better.

That's why we want to hear your story.

We want to know why you're taking this test. We want to know about the trials you've gone through to get here. And we want to know about the successes you've experienced after taking and passing your test.

In addition to your story, which can be an inspiration both to us and to others, we value your feedback. We want to know both what you loved about our book and what you think we can improve on.

The team at Mometrix would be absolutely thrilled to hear from you! So please, send us an email at tellusyourstory@mometrix.com or visit us at mometrix.com/tellusyourstory.php and let's stay in touch.

Additional Bonus Material

Due to our efforts to try to keep this book to a manageable length, we've created a link that will give you access to all of your additional bonus material:

mometrix.com/bonus948/pediatricnurse